Basic Human
Immunology

First Edition

Edited by

Daniel P. Stites, MD
Professor and Vice Chairman
Department of Laboratory Medicine
Director, Immunology Laboratory
University of California, San Francisco

Abba I. Terr, MD
Clinical Professor of Medicine, Stanford
University School of Medicine,
Stanford, California

APPLETON & LANGE
Norwalk, Connecticut/San Mateo, California

0-8385-0543-0

Notice: Our knowledge in clinical sciences is constantly changing. As new
information becomes available, changes in treatment and in the use of drugs
become necessary. The authors and the publisher of this volume have taken
care to make certain that the doses of drugs and schedules of treatment are
correct and compatible with the standards generally accepted at the time of
publication. The reader is advised to consult carefully the instruction
and information material included in the package insert of each drug or
therapeutic agent before administration. This advice is especially
important when using new or infrequently used drugs.

91 92 93 94 95 / 10 9 8 7 6 5 4 3 2 1

Prentice Hall International (UK) Limited, *London*
Prentice Hall of Australia Pty. Limited, *Sydney*
Prentice Hall Canada Inc., *Toronto*
Prentice Hall Hispanoamericana, S.A., *Mexico*
Prentice Hall of India Private Limited, *New Delhi*
Prentice Hall of Japan, Inc., *Tokyo*
Simon & Schuster Asia Pte. Ltd., *Singapore*
Editora Prentice Hall do Brasil, Ltda., *Rio de Janeiro*
Prentice Hall, *Englewood Cliffs, New Jersey*

ISBN: 0-8385-0543-0
ISSN: 1050-9399

PRINTED IN THE UNITED STATES OF AMERICA

Table of Contents

Authors

David H. Broide, MB, ChB
Assistant Professor of Medicine, University of California School of Medicine, San Diego, California

Richard A. Bronson, MD
Associate Professor, Obstetrics & Gynecology and Pathology, State University of New York, Stony Brook, New York

Steven D. Douglas, MD
Section Chief for Immunology, Professor of Pediatrics and Microbiology, Children's Hospital of Philadelphia, Philadelphia

Davendra P. Dubey, PhD
Assistant Professor, Dana Farber Cancer Institute and Harvard Medical School, Boston

Connie R. Faltynek, PhD
Scientist, Program Resources, Inc., NCI-FCRF, Frederick, Maryland; Senior Research Scientist, Sterling Research Group, Sterling Drug Inc., Malvern, Pennsylvania

Michael M. Frank, MD
Clinical Director, NIAID; Chief, Laboratory of Clinical Investigation, Bethesda, Maryland

Joel W. Goodman, PhD
Professor and Vice-Chairman, Department of Microbiology and Immunology, University of California School of Medicine, San Francisco

Joan Goverman, BA, PhD
Senior Research Fellow, Division of Biology, California Institute of Technology, Pasadena, California

Stephen P. James, MD
Senior Investigator, Mucosal Immunity Section, National Institute of Allergy and Infectious Diseases, Bethesda, Maryland

Naynesh R. Kamani, MD
Assistant Professor of Pediatrics, University of Pennsylvania School of Medicine, Philadelphia

Daniel V. Landers, MD
Assistant Professor, University of California, San Francisco General Hospital, San Francisco

Lewis L. Lanier, PhD
Associate Research Director, Immunobiology, Becton Dickinson Monoclonal Center, Inc., San Jose, California

Joost J. Oppenheim, MD
Chief, Laboratory of Molecular Immunoregulation, National Cancer Institute, Frederick, Maryland

Jane R. Parnes, MD
Associate Professor of Medicine, Stanford University, Stanford, California

Tristram G. Parslow, MD, PhD
Assistant Professor of Pathology & Microbiology and Immunology, University of California School of Medicine, San Francisco

Charles S. Pavia, PhD
Associate Professor of Medicine, Microbiology and Immunology, New York Medical College, Director of Sprirochete Research Laboratory, Valhalla, New York

Francis W. Ruscetti, PhD
Head, Lymphokine Section, National Cancer Institute, Frederick, Maryland

Benjamin D. Schwartz, MD, PhD
Professor of Medicine and Molecular Microbiology, Washington University School of Medicine; Chief, Division of Rheumatology, Jewish Hospital at Washington University Medical Center, St. Louis

Raymond G. Slavin, MD
Professor of Internal Medicine & Microbiology, Director, Division of Allergy & Immunology, St. Louis University School of Medicine, St. Louis

Daniel P. Stites, MD
Professor and Vice Chairman, Department of Laboratory Medicine, University of California School of Medicine, San Francisco

Warren Strober, MD
Head, Mucosal Immunity Section, Laboratory of Clinical Investigation, NIAID, Bethesda

David W. Talmage, MD
Distinguished Professor, University of Colorado, Denver

Abba I. Terr, MD
Clinical Professor of Medicine, Stanford University School of Medicine, Stanford, California

Robert H. Waldman, MD
Dean, College of Medicine, and Professor, Department of Internal Medicine, University of Nebraska Medical Center, Omaha

Stephen I. Wasserman, MD
Professor and Chairman, Department of Medicine, University of California School of Medicine, San Diego, California

H. James Wedner, MD
Associate Professor of Medicine, and Chief, Clinical Allergy & Immunology, Washington University School of Medicine, St. Louis

Preface

During the past 20 years, knowledge of the human immune system and its workings has exploded into an enormous data-base of scientific reports, reviews, and textbooks. Clinical application of this knowledge has made possible successful transplantation of organs and tissues, a better understanding of the immunologic nature of allergic diseases, and exploration of the role of immunologic phenomena in cancer. The emergence of Acquired Immunodeficiency Syndrome (AIDS) 10 years ago generated both interest and new knowledge in the field of immunology. A knowledge explosion in immunology occurred almost simultaneously with a technological revolution in molecular and cellular biology and genetics, permitting a level of understanding of the immune response and its consequences equal to or exceeding that of many other physiologic processes.

The sheer volume of knowledge in immunology is one of several challenges to the student. Another is the absence of any fixed anatomic structure that would help explain the function of the immune system. Most major body systems—circulatory, respiratory, digestive, genitourinary, musculoskeletal, and nervous systems—have obvious form and function relationships that help the student visualize the activities of the system. However, the immune system presents a mix of discrete organs (thymus, spleen), scattered discontinuous organs and tissues (lymph nodes, bone marrow), the hemolymphatic circulation, and unorganized cells in all body tissues. Finally, the immune response itself is an exceedingly complex interplay of cells and chemicals proceeding through interrelated and self-regulating pathways.

PURPOSE

Basic Human Immunology is a comprehensive, authoritative introductory text designed to help the student meet the challenges in understanding immunology. It will be useful to the beginner, and can serve as a thorough review for the more advanced student.

ORGANIZATION AND APPROACH

This new book makes immunology understandable by organization and selectivity of the subject matter, rather than by oversimplification. Unlike traditional texts organized by the time sequence of scientific discovery, *Basic Human Immunology* is organized to facilitate understanding of function. First, the normal immune response is described in broad detail; this is followed by a description of the cells, their function, and their secreted chemicals, including antibodies. There is a discussion of inflammation and other effector mechanisms. Finally, chapters dealing with physiological and environmental influences on immune system function and reproductive immunology–topics not usually covered in introductory texts–are included.

Illustrations are essential for teaching this difficult subject. Thus whenever possible, we have provided diagrams in which a standard set of symbols is used to identify immune and inflammatory cells, and their chemical products and receptors. A glossary of these symbols is provided at the end of the book for easy reference.

FOCUS ON HUMAN IMMUNOLOGY

Basic Human Immunology covers the structure and normal functioning of the human immune system. Though research with animals as experimental models will remain critical to the advancement of medical science, the material in this text deals exclusively with humans to avoid confusion arising from the differences in structures, functions, and terminology between animals and humans. In rare instances, animal experiments are discussed when they are needed for clarity.

Basic Human Immunology is the first section of the larger text, *Basic & Clinical Immunology, 7th edition,* which includes additional information on laboratory immunology, human immunopathology, clinical immunology, and therapy.

The editors wish to acknowledge the assistance, encouragement, and patience of the staff of Appleton & Lange during the preparation of this text. We are particularly grateful to Jack Lange, MD, Alex Kugushev, Yvonne Strong, Linda Harris, and Nancy Evans.

Daniel P. Stites, MD
Abba I. Terr, MD
San Francisco, November, 1990

History of Immunology

David W. Talmage, MD

THE ORIGIN OF IMMUNOLOGY

Immunology began as a branch of microbiology; it grew out of the study of infectious diseases and the body's responses to them. The concepts of contagion and the germ theory of disease are attributed to Girolamo Fracastoro, a colleague of Copernicus at the University of Padua, who wrote in 1546 that "Contagion is an infection that passes from one thing to another . . . The infection is precisely similar in both the carrier and the receiver of the contagion . . . The term is more correctly used when infection originates in very small imperceptible particles." Fracastoro's conclusions were remarkable because they were contrary to the philosophy of his time in that he postulated the existence of germs that were too small to be seen. He was a practical physician who gave more credence to his own observations than to traditional beliefs.

It was more than 2 centuries later that another physician, Edward Jenner, extended the concept of contagion to a study of the immunity produced in the host. This was the beginning of immunology. Jenner, a country doctor in Gloucestershire, England, noted in 1798 that a pustular disease of the hooves of horses called "the grease" was frequently carried by farm workers to the nipples of cows, where it was picked up by milkmaids. "Inflamed spots now begin to appear on the hands of the domestics employed in milking, and sometimes on the wrists . . . but what renders the Cowpox virus so extremely singular, is, that the person who has been thus affected is for ever after secure from the infection of Small Pox; neither exposure to the variolous effluvia, nor the insertion of the matter into the skin, producing this distemper."

Jenner was unclear about the nature of the infectious agent of cowpox and its relation to smallpox, but he reported 16 cases of resistance to smallpox in farm workers who had recovered from cowpox. He described how he deliberately inserted matter "taken from a sore on the hand of a dairymaid, on the 14th of May, 1796, into the arm of the boy by means of two superficial incisions, barely penetrating the cutis, each about

half an inch long." Two months later, Jenner inoculated the same 8-year-old boy with matter from a smallpox patient, a dangerous but accepted procedure called **variolation.** However, the boy developed only a small sore at the site of inoculation. His exposure to the mild disease cowpox had made him immune to the deadly disease smallpox. In this manner Jenner began the science of immunology, the study of the body's response to foreign substances.

Immunology has always been dependent upon technology, particularly lens-making and the microscopy. Eyeglasses were introduced into Europe in the 14th century, (perhaps by Marco Polo), and telescopes were used by Galileo in 1609 to discover the moons of Jupiter. However, useful microscopes were not available until the middle of the 19th century. After that, progress in microbiology was rapid. In 1850, Davaine reported that he could see anthrax bacilli in the blood of infected sheep. In 1858, Wallace and Darwin jointly submitted reports proposing evolution through natural selection, and in the same year, Pasteur demonstrated to the French wine industry that fermentation was due to a living microorganism. In 1864, Pasteur disproved the theory of spontaneous generation; in 1867, Lister introduced aseptic surgery; and in 1871, DNA was discovered by Miescher. Anthrax was first transmitted from in vitro culture to animals by Koch in 1876, thus fulfilling **Koch's postulates,** which he had said were required to prove that the bacteria caused the disease. Between 1879 and 1881, Pasteur developed the first 3 attenuated vaccines (after cowpox); these were for chicken cholera, anthrax, and rabies.

Bacteriology and histology were recognized as established scientific fields during this period. The gonococcus, the first human pathogen, was isolated in 1879 by Neisser, and 10 other pathogens were isolated in the next decade. Of particular importance to immunology was the isolation of the diphtheria bacillus by Klebs and Loeffler in 1883; this led to the production of the first defined antigen, diphtheria toxin, by Roux and Yersin in 1888. In that same year, the first antibodies, serum bac-

1

tericidins, were reported by Nuttall, and Pasteur recognized that nonliving substances as well as living organisms could induce immunity. This led to the discovery of antitoxins by von Behring and Kitasato in 1890 and later to the development of toxoids for diphtheria and tetanus.

CELLULAR VERSUS HUMORAL IMMUNITY

In 1883, Metchnikoff observed the phagocytosis of fungal spores by leukocytes and advanced the idea that immunity was primarily due to white blood cells. This provoked an intense controversy with the advocates of **humoral immunity.** The discovery of complement in 1894 by Bordet and **precipitins** in 1897 by Kraus appeared to favor the humoral side of the controversy. Ehrlich's side chain theory, proposed in 1898, was an attempt to harmonize the 2 views. According to Ehrlich, cells possessed on their surfaces a wide variety of side chains (we would call them antigen receptors) that were used to bring nutrients into the cell. When toxic substances blocked one of these side chains through an accidental affinity, the cell responded by making large numbers of that particular side chain, some of which spilled out into the blood and functioned as circulating antibodies.

In 1903, Sir Almoth Wright reported that antibodies could aid in the process of phagocytosis, thus effectively settling the controversy over cellular versus humoral community. Wright called these antibodies "opsonins." This followed the practice of labeling antibodies according to their observed action, eg, agglutinins, precipitins, hemolysins, and bactericidins.

It was gradually realized that antibodies could have deleterious as well as beneficial effects and could produce hypersensitivity. The term "anaphylaxis" was coined by Richet and Portier in 1902 to denote the frequently lethal state of shock induced by a second injection of antigen. The term "allergy" was introduced by von Pirquet in 1906 to denote the positive reaction to a scratch test with tuberculin in individuals infected with tuberculosis.

THE PERIOD OF SEROLOGY

Blood group antigens and their corresponding agglutinins were discovered by Landsteiner in 1900. This led to the ability to give blood transfusions without provoking reactions. Landsteiner was a dominant figure in immunology for 40 years, developing the concept of the antigenic determinant and demonstrating the exquisite specificity of antibodies for chemically defined haptens, a term he applied to simple chemicals that could bind to antibodies but were by themselves incapable of stimulating antibody formation. Landsteiner rejected Ehrlich's side chain theory because he was able to make antibodies against a seemingly infinite number of different substances, synthetic as well as natural.

In 1901, Bordet and Gengou introduced the complement fixation test, which became a standard diagnostic test in the hospital laboratory. The word "immunology" first appeared in the *Index Medicus* in 1910, and the *Journal of Immunology* began publication in 1916. The first 30 years of the Journal were devoted almost exclusively to a study of serologic reactions.

Landsteiner's book, *The Specificity of Serological Reactions,* was published in German in 1933 and in English in 1936. Marrack's text, *The Chemistry of Antigens and Antibodies,* was published in 1935. Antibodies were viewed as being formed directly on antigens, which functioned as templates, in a theory published by Breinl and Haurowitz in 1930. In 1939, Tiselius and Kabat showed that antibodies were gamma globulins, and in 1940, Pauling proposed the variable-folding theory of antibody formation. According to Pauling's theory, gamma globulin peptides are folded into a complementary configuration in the presence of antigen. This fit the "Unitarian" view of antibodies generally accepted at that time, which held that all antibodies were the same except for their specificity.

Immunochemistry was a natural outgrowth of this chemical approach to immunology. The quantitative precipitin test was developed by Heidelberger, Kendall, and Kabat and was used to study the structure of polysaccharide antigens.

THE REBIRTH OF CELLULAR IMMUNOLOGY

Two events of 1941–1942 heralded the rediscovery of the cell by immunologists. Coons demonstrated the presence of antigens and antibodies inside cells by the new technique of **immunofluorescence,** and Chase and Landsteiner reported that delayed hypersensitivity could be transferred by cells but not by serum. The very next year (1943), Avery, MacCleod, and McCarty reported that DNA was responsible for the transfer of hereditary traits in bacteria.

In 1945, Owen discovered blood chimeras in cattle twins, and in 1948, Fagraeus showed that antibodies were made in plasma cells. In 1949, Burnet and Fenner published their adaptive enzyme theory of antibody formation, which again established immunology as a biologic science. They also proposed the "self-marker" concept, which was the first formal explanation of self tolerance.

In 1953, Billingham, Brent, and Medawar demonstrated acquired immunologic tolerance in bone marrow chimeras in mice injected with allogeneic bone marrow at or before birth. In that same year, Watson and Crick described the double helix of DNA. The close association in the development of immunology and molecular biology is illustrated by these two discoveries. Two years later, Jerne proposed his natural selection theory of antibody formation, in which randomly diversified gamma globulin molecules were thought to replicate after binding to injected antigen. Jerne's theory explained the known facts of immunology of that time, such as immunologic memory and the logarithmic rate of rise of antibody. However, this theory was incompatible with the new concepts of cellular and molecular biology. Within 2 years, 2 new theories of antibody production were proposed, the first by Talmage and the second by Burnet. Both theories substituted randomly diversified cells for randomly diversified gamma globulin molecules and proposed that the interaction of antigen with receptors on the cell surface stimulated antibody production and the replication of the selected cell.

After more than 30 years, the cell selection theory and the name given to it by Burnet—**clonal selection**—have become part of the established dogma of immunology. This theory has been confirmed by numerous experiments and was popularized in 1975 by the development by Köhler and Milstein of the technique of producing monoclonal antibodies.

Cellular immunology reached its zenith in 1966 with the discovery by Claman, Chaperon, and Triplett of the presence and cooperation of **B cells** and **T cells.** Since that time, the study of the development, specificity, and activation of B cells and T cells has occupied the energy of a great many immunologists.

THE ADVENT OF MOLECULAR IMMUNOLOGY

By 1959, the field of protein chemistry had reached the point at which it was possible to analyze the structure of the antibody molecule in detail. In that same year, the 3 fragments of immunoglobulins, 2 Fab's and one Fc, were separated by Porter, and the heavy and light chains were separated by Edelman. The discovery of common and variable regions by Putnam and by Hilschmann and Craig came in 1965. Edelman et al reported the first complete amino acid sequence of an immunoglobulin molecule in 1969.

The 1960s and 1970s saw similar advances in the identification, separation, and structure of other molecules important to the immune system, such as complement components, interleukins, and cell receptors. These studies were greatly enhanced by the application of monoclonal antibody technology, which allowed sensitive and specific identification and isolation of many such molecules.

The elusive T cell receptor was finally isolated in 1982–1983 by Allison et al and Haskins et al. The steps required for antigen processing and presentation and the chemical reactions required for lymphocyte activation by antigen were also elucidated.

IMMUNOGENETICS & GENETIC ENGINEERING

The major histocompatibility antigens were discovered by Gorer in 1936, but it was not until 1968 that McDevitt and Tyan showed that immune response genes were linked to the genes of the major histocompatibility complex. Six years later, Doherty and Zinkernagel reported that the recognition of antigen by T cells was restricted by major histocompatibility complex molecules. During this time, the technology of recombinant DNA was developed. This led to the demonstration of immunoglobulin gene rearrangement by Tonegawa et al in 1978 and the production of transgenic mice by Gordon et al in 1980. The identification of genes for the T cell receptor by Davis et al came in 1984.

IMMUNOLOGY TIME LINE

1798   Edward Jenner
        Cowpox vaccination.

1880   Louis Pasteur
        Attenuated vaccines.

1883   Elie I. I. Metchnikoff
        Phagocytic theory.

1888   P. P. Emile Roux and A. E. J. Yersin
        Bacterial toxins.

1888   George H. F. Nuttall
        Bactericidal antibodies.

1890   Robert Koch
        Hypersensitivity.

1890   Emil A. von Behring and Shibasaburo Kitasato
        Diphtheria antitoxin.

1894   Jules J. B. V. Bordet
Complement.

1897   Rudolf Kraus
Precipitins.

1898   Paul Ehrlich
Side chain theory.

1900   Karl Landsteiner
Blood group antigens and antibodies.

1902   Charles R. Richet and Paul J. Portier
Anaphylaxis.

1903   Almoth E. Wright
Opsonins.

1905   Clemens P. von Pirquet and Bela Schick
Serum sickness.

1906   Clemens P. von Pirquet
Allergy.

1930   Friedrich Breinl and Felix Haurowitz
Template theory.

1939   Arne Wilhelm Tiselius and Elvin A. Kabat
Identity of antibodies with gamma globulins.

1941   Albert H. Coons et al
Immunofluorescence.

1942   Karl Landsteiner and Merrill W. Chase
Transfer of delayed-type hypersensitivity with cells.

1945   Ray D. Owen
Chimeras in bovine twins.

1948   Astrid E. Fagraeus
Antibodies in plasma cells.

1949   F. Macfarlane Burnet and Frank Fenner
Adaptive enzyme theory.

1953   Rupert E. Billingham, Leslie Brent, and Peter B. Medawar
Bone marrow chimeras in mice.

1955   Niels K. Jerne
Natural selection theory.

1957   David W. Talmage and F. Macfarlane Burnet
Cell selection theories.

1959   Rodney R. Porter and Gerald M. Edelman
Structure of antibodies.

1966   Henry N. Claman et al
Cooperation of T and B cells.

1968   Hugh O. McDevitt and Marvin L. Tyan
Linkage of immune response genes to major histocompatibility complex genes.

1974   Peter C. Doherty and Rolf M. Zinkernagel
T cell restriction.

1975   Cesar Milstein and Georges J. F. Kohler
Monoclonal antibodies.

1978   Susumu Tonegawa
Immunoglobulin gene rearrangement.

1980   Jon W. Gordon et al
Transgenic mice.

1983   Kathryn Haskins et al
T cell receptor isolation.

1984   Mark Davis et al
T cell receptor genes.

NOBEL PRIZE WINNERS IN IMMUNOLOGY

1901   EMIL ADOLF VON BEHRING for his work on serum therapy, especially application against diphtheria.

1905   ROBERT KOCH for his investigations and discoveries in relation to tuberculosis.

1908   PAUL EHRLICH and ELIE METCHNIKOFF for their work on immunity.

1913   CHARLES ROBERT RICHET for his work on anaphylaxis.

1919   JULES BORDET for his discoveries relating to immunity, particularly complement.

1928   CHARLES JULES HENRI NICOLLE for his work on typhus.

1930   KARL LANDSTEINER for his discovery of human blood groups.

1960 FRANK MACFARLANE BURNET and PETER BRIAN MEDAWAR for their discovery of acquired immunologic tolerance.

1972 GERALD MAURICE EDELMAN and RODNEY ROBERT PORTER for their discoveries concerning the chemical structure of antibodies.

1977 ROSALYN YALOW for the development of radioimmunoassays of peptide hormones.

1980 BARUJ BENACERRAF, JEAN DAUSSET, and GEORGE DAVIS SNELL for their discoveries concerning genetically determined structures on the cell surface that regulate immunologic reactions.

1984 NIELS K. JERNE, GEORGES F. KÖHLER, and CESAR MILSTEIN for theories concerning the specificity in development and control of the immune system and the discovery of the principle for production of monoclonal antibodies.

1987 SUSUMU TONEGAWA for his discovery of the genetic principle for generation of antibody diversity.

SUMMARY

Immunology began as a study of the response of the whole animal to infection. Over the years, it has become progressively more basic, passing through phases of emphasis on serology, cellular immunology, molecular immunology, and immunogenetics. At the same time, immunology has grown to encompass many fields such as allergy, clinical immunology, immunochemistry, immunopathology, immunopharmacology, tumor immunology, and transplantation. Thus, it has always provided an excellent mix of fundamental and applied science.

Immunology has always depended upon and stimulated the application of technology, such as the use of microscopy, electrophoresis, radiolabeling, immunofluorescence, recombinant DNA, and transgenic mice. In general, immunology has not become an inbred discipline but has maintained close associations with many other fields of medical science. From a base in microbiology, immunologists have spread out into all of the basic and clinical departments.

REFERENCES

Alexander HL: The History of allergy. In: *Immunological Diseases*. Samter M (editor). Little Brown, 1965.

Allison JP, McIntyre BW, Bloch D: Tumor specific antigen of murine T-lymphoma defined with monoclonal antibody. *J Immunol* 1982;**129**:2293.

Billingham RE, Brent L, Medawar PB: Actively acquired tolerance of foreign cells. *Nature* 1953; 172:603.

Bordet J: *Traite de L'Immunité dans les Maladies infectieuses,* 2nd ed. Masson, 1937.

Brack C, et al: A complete immunoglobulin gene is created by somatic recombination. *Cell* 1978;**15**:1.

Burnet FM: A modification of Jerne's theory of antibody production using the concept of clonal selection. *Aust J Sci* 1957;**20**:67.

Burnet FM, Fenner F: *The Production of Antibodies.* Macmillan (Melbourne), 1949.

Claman HN, Chaperon EA, Triplett RF: Thymus-marrow cell combination. Synergism in antibody production. *Proc Soc Exp Biol Med* 1966;**122**:1167.

Coons AH, et al: Immunological properties of an antibody containing a fluorescent group. *Proc Soc Exp Biol Med* 1941;47:200.

Doherty PC, Zinkernagel RM: T-cell mediated immunopathology in viral infections. *Transplant Rev* 1974;**19**:89.

Dubos R: *The Unseen World*. Rockefeller Univ Press, 1962.

Edelman GM: Dissociation of gamma globulin. *J Am Chem Soc* 1959;**81**:3155.

Ehrlich P: On immunity with special reference to cell life. *Proc R Soc London Ser B* 1900;**66**:424.

Fagraeus A: The plasma cellular reaction and its relation to the formation of antibodies in vitro. *J Immunol* 1948;**58**:1.

Foster WD: *A History of Medical Bacteriology and Immunology*. William Heineman Medical Books, 1970.

Gay FP: Immunology, a medical science developed through animal experimentation. *J Am Med Assoc* 1911;**56**:578.

Gordon JW, et al: Genetic transformation of mouse embryos by microinjection of purified DNA. *Proc Natl Acad Sci USA* 1980;**77**:7380.

Haskins K, et al: The major histocompatibility complex restricted antigen receptor on T cells. I. Isolation with a monoclonal antibody. *J Exp Med* 1983; **157**:1149.

Hedrick SM, et al: Isolation of cDNA clones encoding T cell-specific membrane-associated proteins. *Nature* 1984;**308**:149.

Jerne NK: The natural selection theory of antibody formation. *Proc Natl Acad Sci USA* 1955;**41**:849.

Köhler G, Milstein C: Continuous culture of fused cells secreting antibody of predefined specificity. *Nature* 1975;**256**:495.

Landsteiner K: *The Specificity of Serological Reactions.* Thomas, 1936; reissued by Dover, 1962.

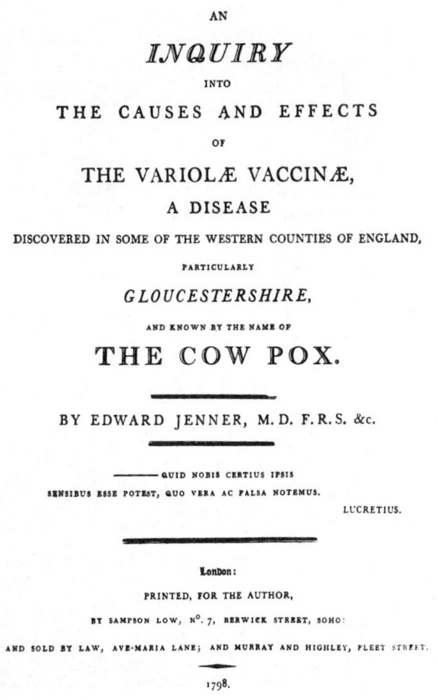

AN

INQUIRY

INTO

THE CAUSES AND EFFECTS

OF

THE VARIOLÆ VACCINÆ,

A DISEASE

DISCOVERED IN SOME OF THE WESTERN COUNTIES OF ENGLAND,

PARTICULARLY

GLOUCESTERSHIRE,

AND KNOWN BY THE NAME OF

THE COW POX.

BY EDWARD JENNER, M.D. F.R.S. &c.

——— QUID NOBIS CERTIUS IPSIS
SENSIBUS ESSE POTEST, QUO VERA AC FALSA NOTEMUS.
LUCRETIUS.

London:

PRINTED, FOR THE AUTHOR,

BY SAMPSON LOW, Nº. 7, BERWICK STREET, SOHO:

AND SOLD BY LAW, AVE-MARIA LANE; AND MURRAY AND HIGHLEY, FLEET STREET.

1798.

Figure 1-1. Face plate from first edition (1798) of Jenner's inquiry into the Causes and Effects of . . . the Cow Pox

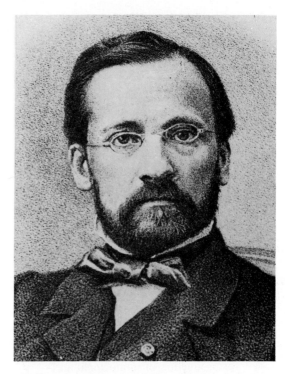

Figure 1-2. Louis Pasteur (1822–1895). (Courtesy of the Museum of the Pasteur Institute, Paris.)

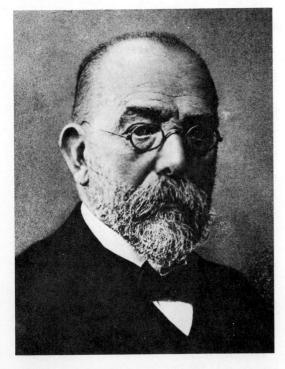

Figure 1-3. Robert Koch (1843–1910). (Courtesy of the Museum of the Pasteur Institute, Paris.)

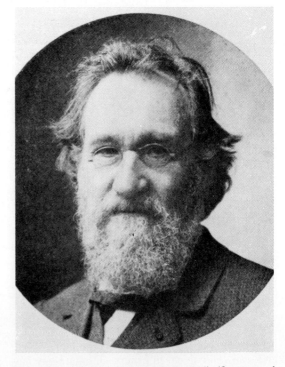

Figure 1-4. Elie Metchnikoff (1845–1916). (Courtesy of the Rare Book Library, the University of Texas Medical Branch, Galveston.)

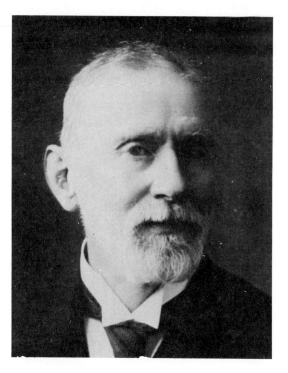

Figure 1-5. Paul Ehrlich (1854–1915). (Courtesy of the Museum of the Pasteur Institute, Paris.)

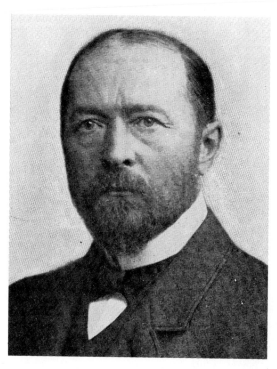

Figure 1-6. Emil von Behring (1854–1917). (Courtesy of the Museum of the Pasteur Institute, Paris.)

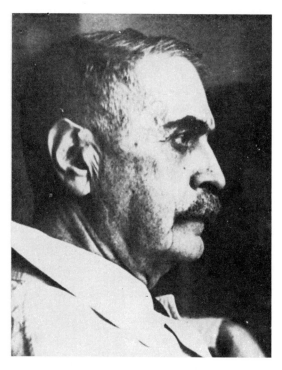

Figure 1-7. Karl Landsteiner (1868–1943). (Courtesy of the Museum of the Pasteur Institute, Paris.)

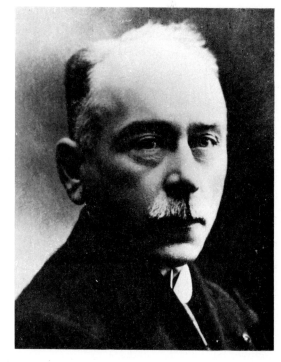

Figure 1-8. Jules Bordet (1870–1961). (Courtesy of the Museum of the Pasteur Institute, Paris.)

Landsteiner K, Chase MW: Experiments on transfer of cutaneous sensitivity to simple compounds. *Proc Soc Exp Biol Med* 1942;**49**:688.

McDevitt HO, Tyan ML: Transfer of response by spleen cells and linkage to the major histocompatibility (H-2) locus. *J Exp Med* 1968;**128**:1.

Parrish HJ: *A History of Immunization.* E & S Livingstone, 1965.

Parrish HJ: *Victory with Vaccines.* E & S Livingstone, 1968.

Pauling L: A theory of the structure and process of formation of antibodies. *J Am Chem Soc* 1940;**62**:2643.

Porter RR: The hydrolysis of rabbit gamma globulin and antibodies with crystalline papain. *Biochem J* 1959;**73**:119.

Talmage DW: Allergy and immunology. *Annu Rev Med* 1957;**8**:239.

Talmage DW: A century of progress: Beyond molecular immunology. *J Immunol* 1988;**141(Suppl)**:S5.

Structure & Development of the Immune System

2

Naynesh R. Kamani, MD, and Steven D. Douglas, MD

The cells that make up the immune system are distributed throughout the body but occur predominantly in the lymphoreticular organs, such as the lymph nodes, spleen, bone marrow, thymus, and the mucosa-associated lymphoid tissues of the gastrointestinal and respiratory tracts. In the extravascular tissues, these immune cells occupy the interstices of a network of interlocking reticular cells and fibers with a supporting framework of reticular cells. The lymphocytes are the predominant immunocytes, but monocyte-macrophages, endothelial cells, and rare eosinophils and mast cells also play roles in the immune system. All the cells of the immune system arise from pluripotent, self-renewing stem cells in the bone marrow.

Most lymphocytes are found in the spleen, lymph nodes, and Peyer's patches of the ileum. In mammals, the aggregate of lymphocytes constitutes about 1% of total body weight; the human body contains about 10^{12} lymphocytes. Approximately 10^9 lymphocytes are produced daily. Lymphocytes in the tissues are in dynamic equilibrium with those in the circulating blood and continuously recirculate through the vascular and lymphatic channels from one lymphoid organ to another.

Macrophages are found in connective tissues, lungs, liver, nervous system, serous cavities, bones and joints, and lymphoid organs. The lymphoid tissues of the body may be divided into primary or central lymphoid organs, ie, the thymus and bone marrow, and secondary or peripheral organs, eg, the lymph nodes, spleen, and Peyer's patches.

ORGANIZATION OF THE IMMUNE SYSTEM

LYMPHOID ORGANS

Thymus

The **thymus** is derived embryologically from the third and fourth branchial pouches and differenti-

ates as ventral outpocketings from these pouches during the sixth week of embryonic life. During vertebrate embryogenesis, the thymus is the first organ to begin the production of lymphocytes. It is central to the development and function of the immune system; however, it is generally protected from exposure to antigen, partly by means of a barrier created by an epithelial membrane that surrounds thymic cortical blood vessels. The thymus does not directly participate in immune reactions but, rather, provides the microenvironment necessary for the maturation of T cells.

The thymus consists of 2 lobes, each of which is divided by septae into several lobules. Each lobule contains a cortex and medulla (Fig 2–1). It is believed that a humoral factor is produced by thymic epithelium that attracts stem cells to the thymus. Whether these cells are already committed to the T lymphoid lineage is unknown. Incoming cells migrate from the cortex to the medulla and in the process differentiate, acquire newer functions and surface antigens, and then emigrate from the thymus to peripheral tissues.

The most rapidly dividing cells in the thymus are large, blastlike lymphoid cells found in the subcapsular cortex. These cells contain terminal deoxynucleotidyl transferase (TdT) and express the early thymocyte T10 antigen. Approximately three-quarters of the lymphocytes within the thymus are located in the deeper cortex. These express the T6 or CD1 marker as well as both the helper-inducer CD4 and suppressor-cytotoxic CD8 markers. The medullary thymocytes are corticosteroid-resistant mature cells that express high levels of class I **major histocompatibility complex** (MHC) antigens and either the CD4 or the CD8 antigens. They constitute about 20% of the thymic lymphocytes. The medulla also contains thymic (Hassall's) corpuscles, composed of layers of epithelial cells, some macrophages, and cell debris. The function of thymic corpuscles is not known, but these structures may be the sites where lymphocyte cells die inside the thymus. The thymus has the highest rate of cell production of any tissue of the body, but the vast majority of cells produced in the thymus die there. This remark-

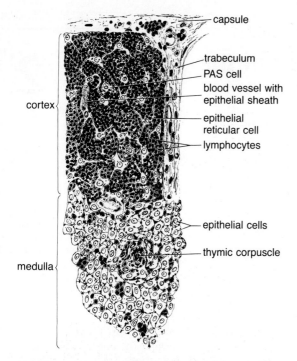

cortex

medulla

capsule

trabeculum
PAS cell
blood vessel with
epithelial sheath
epithelial
reticular cell
lymphocytes

epithelial cells

thymic corpuscle

Figure 2–1. Histologic organization of the thymus. The cortex is heavily infiltrated with lymphocytes. As a result, the epithelial cells become stellate and remain attached to one another by desmosomes. The medulla is closer to a pure epithelium, although it too is commonly infiltrated by lymphocytes. A large thymic corpuscle consisting of concentrically arranged epithelial cells is seen. The capsule and trabeculae are rich in connective tissue fibers (mainly collagen) and contain blood vessels and variable numbers of plasma cells, granulocytes, and lymphocytes. (Reproduced, with permission, from Weiss L: *The Cells and Tissues of the Immune System: Structure, Functions, Interactions.* Copyright © 1972. Reprinted by permission of Prentice-Hall, Inc., Englewood Cliffs, NJ.)

able degree of cell wastage most probably results from abortive rearrangements of genetic material that occur during the generation of T cell receptor diversity (see Chapter 6).

Lymphoid cells in the thymus are surrounded by epithelial cells and other supporting cells, including interdigitating reticular cells and macrophages. The cortical and medullary thymic epithelial cells differ in their embryologic derivation and hence also in their morphologic features. A number of thymic hormones, including thymulin, thymosin $\alpha 1$, thymosin $\beta 4$, and thymopoietin, are produced by thymic epithelial cells. These hormones are necessary for differentiation of stem cell precursors in the thymus into mature cells.

The thymus reaches its maximum size (as a percentage of body weight) in most vertebrates either at birth or shortly thereafter. The human thymus grows until puberty and then begins a gradual process of involution. It decreases from 0.27% to 0.02% of total body weight between the ages of 5 and 15 years.

Neonatal removal of the thymus has profound effects on the immune system in many species of animals. In certain strains of mice, removal of the thymus leads to "wasting disease" (runting), with marked lymphoid atrophy and death. In other strains of mice, severe lymphopenia occurs, with depletion of cells from the paracortical areas of lymph nodes and periarteriolar regions of the spleen. Since cellular immunocompetence occurs early in human fetal development, there are few significant sequelae to neonatal thymectomy in humans. Long-term follow-up studies of individuals who received thymic radiation in early infancy have revealed decreases in the numbers of T and B lymphocytes and reduction in in vitro proliferative responses of lymphocytes to mitogens.

Impaired thymic development may be associated with immunologic deficiency disorders. The classic example of this is the DiGeorge syndrome, which results from an embryologic maldevelopment of the pharyngeal pouches, leading to various degrees of thymic hypoplasia and cellular immunodeficiency, congenital cardiac defects, an abnormal facies, and hypoparathyroidism. Abnormalities of the thymus, including both lymphoid hyperplasia and the development of thymomas, frequently occur in patients with certain autoimmune diseases, particularly systemic lupus erythematosus and myasthenia gravis.

Bursa of Fabricius & Mammalian "Bursa Equivalents"

The bursa of Fabricius, which is present in birds, is a lymphoepithelial organ located near the cloaca. The bursa is lined with pseudostratified epithelium and contains lymphoid follicles divided into cortex and medulla. In chickens, removal of the bursa of Fabricius leads to marked deficiency in immunoglobulins, impairment in development of germinal centers, and absence of plasma cells. The "bursa-dependent" lymphoid system is independent of the thymus. The mammalian equivalent of the bursa of Fabricius has not yet been definitively identified, although the mammalian gut-associated lymphoid tissues, including the appendix and Peyer's patches, histologically most closely resemble avian bursal tissues. Nevertheless, the primary site for B cell differentiation in mammals is most probably the fetal liver and, following birth, the bone marrow (Fig 2–2).

Pluripotent hematolymphoid stem cells, which have as yet not been morphologically or immunophenotypically identified with certainty in hu-

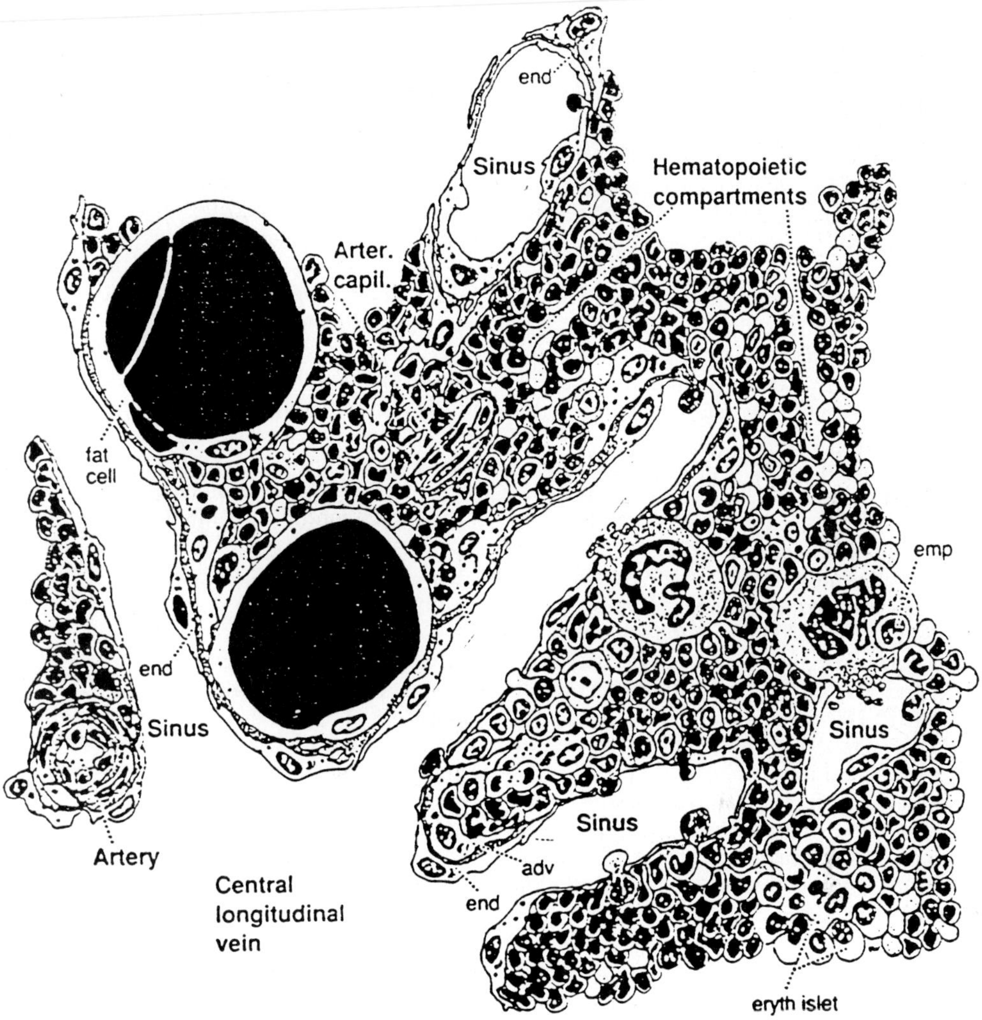

Figure 2-2. Histologic organization of the bone marrow. Hematopoietic cells lie between sinuses that drain into the central longitudinal vein. The wall of the sinus and the vein is trilaminar consisting of endothelium (end), a basement membrane, and adventitial cell (adv). With fatty change, the adventitial cells become voluminous fat cells and encroach on the hematopoietic space, whereas with active hematopoiesis, these cells become flat with the sinus wall reduced to a single endothelial cell layer. Megakaryocytes (meg) characteristically lie against the outside of the sinus wall, discharging platelets into the lumen through an aperture. Occasionally, other cell types enter megakaryocyte cytoplasm by a phenomenon known as emperipolesis (emp).

mans, are found in the fetal liver and adult bone marrow. These common progenitors give rise to lymphoid stem cells that eventually differentiate into mature lymphocytes and to hematopoietic progenitors that divide and differentiate into phagocytic cells (neutrophils and monocytes), erythrocytes, platelets, and eosinophils. Growth factors (called "cytokines"; see Chapter 7) that induce differentiation and maturation of hematopoietic cells in the bone marrow have been isolated and cloned. One of these, interleukin-4

(IL-4), previously known as B cell growth factor 1 (BCGF-1), is produced by T cells and serves as a proliferation factor not only for B cells but also for a number of other hematolymphoid progenitors, including T cells and megakaryocytic, myelomonocytic, and erythrocytic precursors.

Pre-B cells arise from lymphoid stem cells in the bone marrow and are the earliest identifiable cells of the B cell lineage. These are large lymphoid cells that express cytoplasmic μ chains but no light chains or surface immunoglobulin and are identified in fetal liver and adult bone marrow. During early B cell differentiation independent of antigen, stem cells and pre-B cells differentiate into immature and then mature B cells that express surface immunoglobulin and acquire Fc receptors for IgG. Following antigenic stimulation, B cells differentiate into immunoglobulin-secreting plasma cells or return to small, resting memory cells.

Lymph Nodes

The lymph nodes are encapsulated, bean-shaped or round structures usually located at the junction of major lymphatic tracts. In the resting state they range from 1 to 25 mm in diameter, and during states of infection or malignancy they enlarge significantly. Afferent lymphatics enter the nodes at the subcapsular sinus, from which there is centripetal flow toward the major efferent lymphatic duct, located in the hilus. Lymphocytes leave the circulation and enter the node via the **high endothelial venules (HEV)** in the paracortex, migrate toward the medulla, and eventually return to the circulation via efferent lymphatic channels that ultimately drain into the thoracic or right lymphatic duct (Fig 2–3). Lymph nodes serve as a filter for particulate foreign matter and tissue debris and participate as the central organs in lymphocyte circulation.

The histologic appearance of a lymph node depends on the state of activity of the node. The resting lymph node, which has not received recent antigenic stimulation, is morphologically divided into cortex, paracortical areas, and medulla. The margin between the cortex and paracortex may be obscure and may contain many resting lymphocytes. Within the cortex, there are a few aggregates of predominantly B lymphocytes called **primary follicles.** The paracortical areas contain postcapillary venules lined by cuboid epithelium, through which passes the blood supply to the node (Fig 2–4). The paracortex consists mostly of T lymphocytes that are situated in close proximity to interdigitating antigen-presenting cells (see the section on mononuclear phagocytes). In the resting node, the medulla is composed mostly of connective tissue surrounding the hilum. The antigen-stimulated lymph node shows an increased turnover of lymphocytes. Following antigenic stimulation, the paracortical area is hypertrophied, contains large lymphocytes and blastlike cells, and is easily distinguished from the cortex. The cortex contains germinal centers composed of metabolically active and mitotic cells, and the medulla contains numerous plasma cells, which actively secrete antibody.

Spleen

The spleen is a secondary lymphoid organ and performs a number of nonimmunologic functions, including filtration of blood and conversion of hemoglobin to bilirubin. Like the lymph nodes, it has a collagenous tissue capsule with trabeculae that penetrate the splenic parenchyma. The white and the red pulp constitute the 2 major types of splenic tissue. They are supported by a dense, close-meshed reticular network. The lymphoid

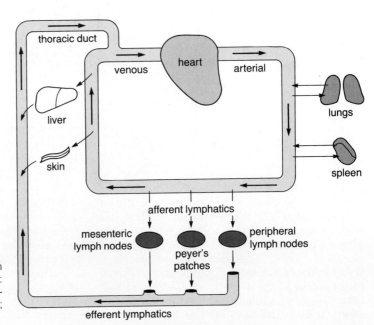

Figure 2-3. Lymphatic recirculation (Adapted from Duijvestijn A, Hamann A: Mechanisms and regulation of lymphocyte migration. *Immunol Today* 1989; **10**:23.)

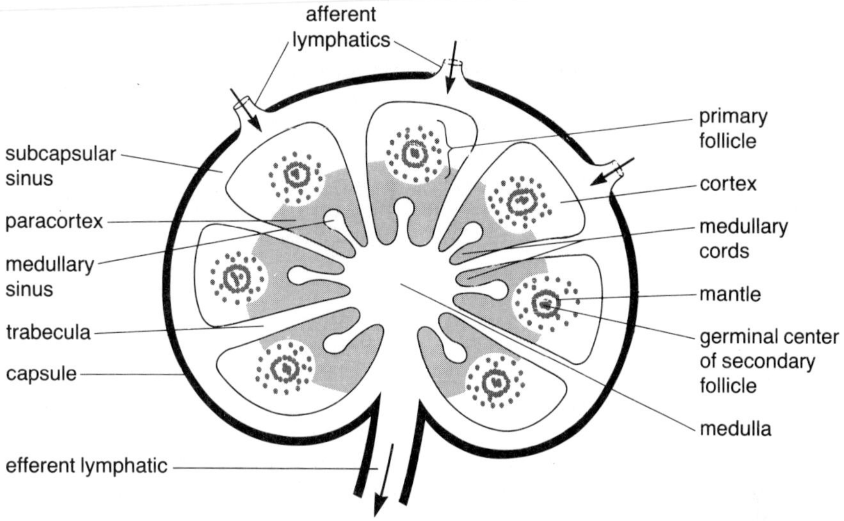

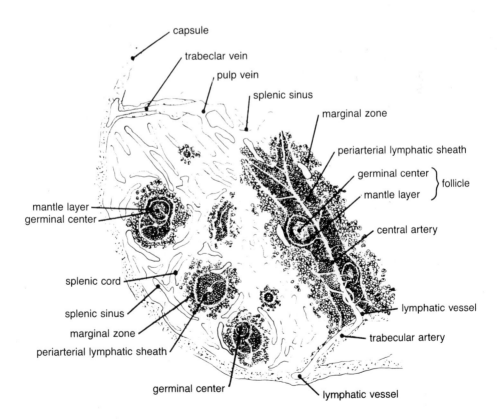

Figure 2-4. Schematic diagram of an immunologically active lymph node.

Figure 2-5. Histologic organization of the spleen. (Reproduced, with permission, from Weiss L: *The Cells and Tissues of the Immune System: Structure, Function, Interactions.* Copyright © 1972. Reprinted by permission of Prentice-Hall, Inc., Englewood, Cliffs, NJ.)

white pulp has central lymphoid follicles consisting mostly of B cells surrounded by thymus-dependent T lymphocytic regions (Fig 2–5). The erythroid red pulp serves as a filter for damaged or aged red cells and as a reserve site for extramedullary hematopoiesis (Fig 2–6). Unlike lymph nodes, lymphocytes enter and leave the spleen predominantly via the bloodstream.

Mucosa-Associated Lymphoid Tissue

The diffusely distributed, nonencapsulated lymphoid tissues of mucosal surfaces of the gastrointestinal, respiratory, and urogenital tracts are collectively referred to as the **mucosa-associated lymphoid tissues (MALT)**. Of all these tissues, the **gut-associated lymphoid tissue (GALT)** and the **bronchus-associated lymphoid tissue (BALT)** are the best-characterized. The lymphoid aggregates within these tissues are strategically located so that they are directly exposed to the external environment.

A. GALT: GALT is made up of Peyer's patches and isolated lymphoid follicles that are found predominantly in the colonic submucosa. Lymphoid cells are also scattered widely through the lamina propria, among the absorptive intestinal epithelial cells, and in small numbers in the lumen of the intestine. Peyer's patches consist of lymphoid aggregates with a central B cell–dependent follicle and surrounding T cell–dependent regions and macrophages that serve as antigen-

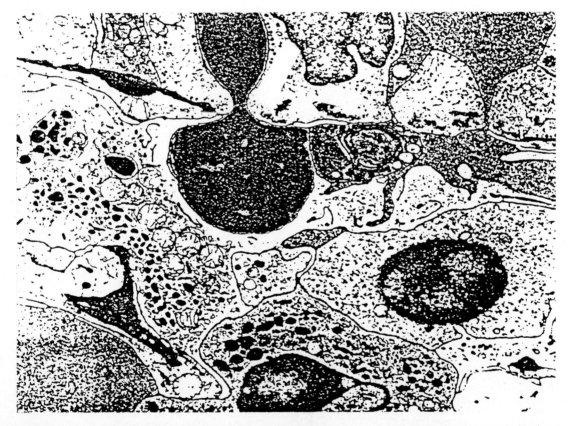

Figure 2–6. Human spleen in thalassemia. The wall of a splenic sinus crosses this field, its endothelial cells (End) cut in cross section. The base of these endothelial cells is rich in intermediate filaments and microfilaments that tend to run longitudinally. In this section, most filaments are cut in cross section and impart a stippled effect. In places the filaments are folded on one another and appear as relatively dense plaques (pl). Sinus and endothelial cells lie upon a fenestrated basement membrane (Bas Mb), represented here as short linear segments. Portions of reticular fibers (RF) branch into the perisinusal cord. Several erythrocytes (Ery), disparate in size and content, lie in interendothelial slits of the sinus. In addition, an erythroblast (Eb) is in passage through the wall, quite markedly pinched by the basal portions of the separated endothelial cells. The portion of its nuclear pole in the cord is surrounded by a macrophage (Mp), which also reaches to the cordal portion of a vesiculated, lamellated erythrocyte (Ery2) in the contiguous interendothelial slit. These slits impose a test on erythrocytes and other cells during passage through the human spleen.

presenting cells. The B cells are heterogeneous and may express any of the immunoglobulin isotypes. The T cells are predominantly regulatory and cytotoxic. These patches have efferent lymphatics that drain into mesenteric lymph nodes, but they have no afferent lymphatics. They are covered by a specialized lymphoepithelium consisting of microfold of M cells, which can be distinguished from surrounding epithelium by electron microscopy. They have short, wide, and irregular microvilli containing conspicuous axial filaments; an apical cytoplasm that has very few lysosomelike structures; and a basally situated nucleus (Fig 2–7). Luminal antigens can enter the Peyer's patches via the M cells after these cells selectively pinocytose and phagocytose particles. It is not known whether the antigens that eventually reach MALT are processed within the M cells or whether the M cells merely act as passive conduits for these antigens.

B. BALT: BALT is structurally and probably functionally quite similar to Peyer's patches and other lymphoid tissues that constitute the GALT of the intestines. It consists of large collections of lymphocytes organized into lymphoid aggregates and follicles. These are found primarily along the main bronchi in all lobes of the lungs and are situated prominently at the bifurcations of bronchi and bronchioles. The epithelium convering BALT follicles is devoid of goblet cells and cilia. In some species, BALT follicles seem to protrude into the lumen of the larger bronchi and trachea. The follicles invariably lie between branches from the pulmonary artery and the bronchial epithelium. BALT contains an elaborate network of capillaries, arterioles and venules, and efferent lymphatics; this suggests that BALT may play a role in sampling antigen not only from the lumen but also from the systemic circulation.

The M cells overlying the BALT follicles are

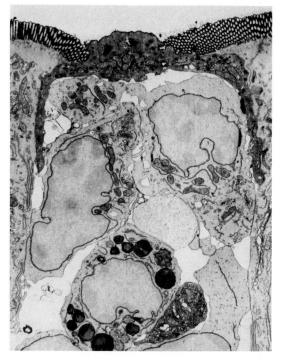

Figure 2–7. (**A**) Schematic diagram summarizing the transport of exogenous horseradish peroxidase observed by Owen and Jones. They hypothesize that the M cell transports intact macromolecules from the lumen to allow efficient "sampling" of luminal antigens by lymphocytes. L, Lymphocytes; C, columnar absorptive cells. (Reproduced with permission, from Owen RL: Sequential uptake of horseradish peroxidase by lymphoid follicle epithelium of Peyer's patches in the normal unobstructed mouse intestine: An ultrastructural study. *Gastroenterology* 1977;**72:**440.) (**B**) Electron micrograph showing the attenuated apical cytoplasm of an M cell over a cluster of intraepithelial lymphocyte (L). The protein tracer horseradish peroxidase (HRP) was introduced into the lumen 1 hour before fixation. The dense reaction product reveals the presence of HRP on the microvillous border of two adjacent absorptive cells and within small vesicles in the M cell cytoplasm. (Reproduced, with permission, from Owen RL, Nemanic P: Page 367, in: *Scanning Electron Microscopy.* Vol. II. SEM, Inc., 1978.)

structurally similar to intestinal M cells covering GALT. BALT consists mostly of collections of lymphocytes organized into follicles with infrequent germinal centers. The majority of lymphocytes in BALT are B cells.

Tonsils

By virtue of their strategic location, the palatine and nasopharyngeal **tonsils** are directly exposed to both airborne and alimentary antigens. Their architecture is similar to that of the lymph nodes. The deep crypts in tonsillar epithelium facilitate the trapping of antigens and foreign particles and greatly augment the area of contact between lymphoid tissue and airborne environmental antigens. Antigen is transported from the crypts to well-organized lymphoid follicles via the reticular epithelium. B cells predominate in these follicles, accounting for 40–50% of all lymphocytes. As in lymph nodes, the germinal centers within the follicles are antigen-dependent B cell areas, where memory clones expand and differentiate into plasma cells.

IMMUNOLOGIC CELLS

1. LYMPHOID CELLS

Morphology

The **lymphocyte** is a cell defined by certain morphologic features. Visualized by light microscopy, lymphocytes are ovoid cells 8–12 μm in diameter. They contain densely packed nuclear chromatin and a small rim of cytoplasm that stains pale blue with Romanovsky stains. The cytoplasm contains a number of azurophilic granules and a few vacuoles. In the area where most of the cytoplasmic organelles are present, the cytoplasmic rim is thickened. Phase contrast microscopy of living lymphocytes reveals a characteristic slow ameboid movement with a "hand-mirror" contour. Histochemical studies have demonstrated nucleolar and cytoplasmic ribonucleoprotein. The cytoplasm contains some glycogen. The lymphocyte contains a number of lysosomal hydrolases and mitochondrial enzymes. T and B cells are indistinguishable by conventional light microscopy.

Ultrastructure

Electron-microscopic examination of the resting circulating lymphocyte (Fig 2–8) reveals a dense heterochromatic nucleus, which contains some less electron-dense areas referred to as **euchromatin.** The nucleolus contains agranular, fibrillar, and granular zones. The nucleus is surrounded by the **nuclear membrane complex.** The cytoplasm of the resting lymphocyte contains or-

ganelle systems characteristic of eukaryotic cells (Golgi zone, mitochondria, ribosomes, and lysosomes). Many of these organelle systems, however, are poorly developed. There are many free ribosomes, a few ribosome clusters, and strands of granular endoplasmic reticulum. A small Golgi zone is present, which contains vacuoles, vesicles, and a few lysosomes. Microtubules are often present, and there are frequent mitochondria. The cytoplasm usually contains several lysosomes. The plasma membrane of the lymphocyte is a typical unit membrane, which may show small projections and, under some circumstances, longer pseudopodia or uropods. When platinum-carbon replicas of the plasma membranes of these cells are visualized by the freeze-fracture technique, they are shown to contain intramembrane particles in all membrane systems examined. Plasma membrane specialization may be related either to cell attachment to surfaces or to cell-cell interaction. By transmission electron microscopy, the cells of the plasma cell series are distinguishable from lymphocytes by the extensive development and dilation of granular endoplasmic reticulum and a well-developed Golgi zone in plasma cells (Fig 2–9). Monocular phagocytes (monocyte-macrophages) possess larger Golgi zones and more lysosomes than lymphocytes do.

The **blast cell,** in contrast to the small lymphocyte, has a nucleus characterized by loosely packed euchromatin, a large nucleolus, and a large cytoplasmic volume containing numerous polyribosomes and an extensively developed Golgi zone. It is easily identified by light microscopy and measures 15–30 μm in diameter. Blast cells are present in lymph nodes in vivo following antigenic stimulation or in cultures of lymphocytes stimulated in vitro with phytomitogens.

B & T Lymphocytes

The general features of these cell types are considered in order to provide a basic and more detailed understanding of their interactions in immune responses, their function, and their alterations in immunologic deficiency and autoimmune diseases.

A. Surface Markers: Numerous **monoclonal antibodies** have been developed that define leukocyte differentiation and cell surface molecules. As of 1989, the International Workshop on Human Leukocyte Differentiation Antigens has agreed on many clusters of differentiation (CD; see Chapter 5) groups or subgroups of distinct antigens on leukocyte cell surfaces that are recognized by the various available monoclonal antibodies. There is an important distinction between a plasma membrane **determinant,** which is a macromolecule present on the cell membrane, detected by labeled antibody methods and identifying particular cell

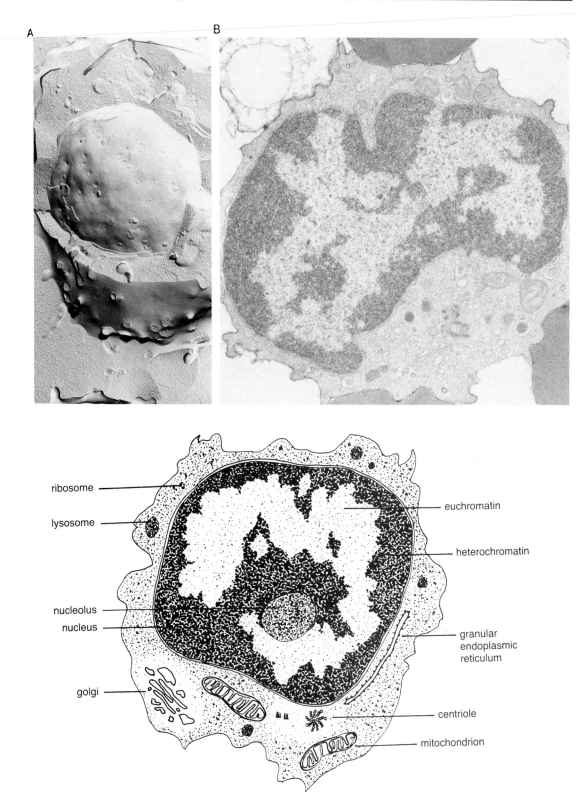

Figure 2–8. **Top:** (**A**) Freeze-fracture electron micrograph of normal human circulating lymphocyte. (Original magnification × 25,000.) (**B**) Transmission electron micrograph of normal circulating human lymphocyte. (Original magnification × 33,000.) **Bottom:** Diagrammatic representation of the micrograph shown at top right.

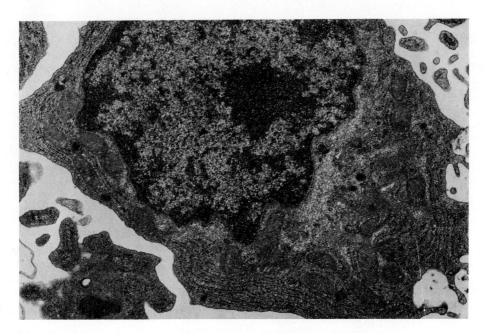

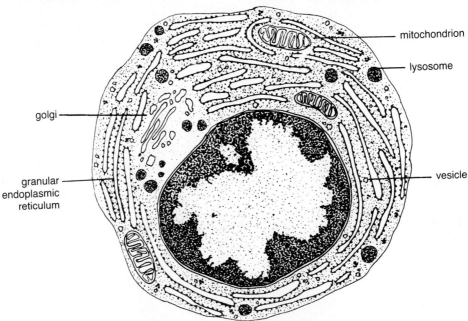

Figure 2–9. ***Top:*** Electron micrograph of bone marrow plasma cell from patient with multiple myeloma. (Original magnification × 19,000.) ***Bottom:*** Diagrammatic representation of cell shown at top.

types or subpopulations, and a **receptor,** which is a functional macromolecule characteristic of a specific cell type but with a known binding affinity for a specific ligand.

A property of most membrane determinants and receptors that is related to membrane fluidity is their ability to undergo redistribution and "cap-

ping." When a membrane component combines with its complementary molecule, it first undergoes a metabolically independent reorganization into patches over the entire cell surface ("patching") It may then undergo a metabolically dependent process by which the marker is topographically redistributed from dispersed patches to localization at one pole of the cell (capping). This capping event is usually followed by internalization of the components via membrane vesicles.

B. B Lymphocytes: The B lymphocyte in humans and most mammalian species is characterized by the presence of readily detectable surface immunoglobulin (Fig 2–10). The major immunoglobulin class on circulating B lymphocytes is IgM, which is present in monomeric form. IgD, IgG, IgA, and IgE may also be present on B lymphocyte membranes. In addition, most of the B lymphocytes have a receptor for antigen-antibody complexes, or aggregated immunoglobulin. This receptor is specific for a site on the Fc portion of the immunoglobulin molecule and is known as the **Fc receptor.** A receptor for the complement component C3d and for Epstein-Barr virus has been demonstrated on B cells (CD21 or B2). This complement receptor is distinct from the Fc receptor. A number of other B cell lineage–restricted differentiation antigens have been characterized. These include CD19 (B4) and CD20 (B1). B cells also possess other cell surface antigens not restricted to cells of the B lineage. These include CD10 (CALLA), CD9 (BA-2), and CD23, which appears to serve as the Fc receptor for IgE. B cells also express class II MHC antigens and the transferrin receptor.

C. T Lymphocytes: T lymphocytes form rosettes with sheep erythrocytes via the sheep erythrocyte receptor (CD2 or T11), and this marker is used to identify human T cells. A series of monoclonal antibodies to T cell membrane markers are used for the delineation of functional subsets of T cells. Anti-CD5 (anti-T1) is a monoclonal antibody reactive with 100% of peripheral T cells but only 10% of thymocytes. The CD5 thymocytes are the only thymocytes capable of reactivity in mixed lymphocyte culture. Anti-CD3 has essentially identical reactivity. Anti-CD4 reacts with 75% of thymocytes and 60% of peripheral T cells; it appears to identify a helper or inducer subset of peripheral blood T cells, which also are the only peripheral T cells that show a proliferative response to soluble antigens. This CD4+ subset is roughly equivalent to the $Th_1^+(Th_2^-)$ subset defined by heteroantisera. Anti-CD8 (anti-T5 and anti-T8) reacts with about 80% of thymocytes and 20–30% of peripheral T cells; anti-75 identifies a subset with both suppressor and cytotoxic capacity, similar to the Th_2^+ subset. Anti-CD1 (anti-T6), anti-T9, and anti-T10 react almost exclusively with thymocytes and not with peripheral T cells. The earliest thymocytes bear T9 and T10 markers or T10 alone; the T10 antigen is apparently lost when the cells leave the thymus for the peripheral compartment. The CD8+ subset in humans is analogous to the murine Lyt-2,3 subset, which mediates both cytotoxic and suppressor functions, and the human CD4 subset is analogous to the murine Lyt-1 subset, which has helper functions.

CD4 cells of the inducer type predominate in the thymic medulla, blood, and T cell traffic areas, including tonsillar paracortex and intestinal lamina propria. Cells of the suppressor-cytotoxic type, CD8, constitute the major T cell population in normal human bone marrow and gut epithelium. In lymph node microenvironments, there is close anatomic proximity between CD4 cells and cells expressing large amounts of Ia antigens, interdigitating cells, and macrophages (Table 2–1).

Natural Killer (NK) Cells

Functional studies have identified lymphocyte populations that serve as **natural killer (NK) cells** and antibody-dependent killer cells in the surveillance of certain tumors and virus-infected cells. The NK cell is defined as an effector cell that has the capacity for spontaneous cytotoxicity toward

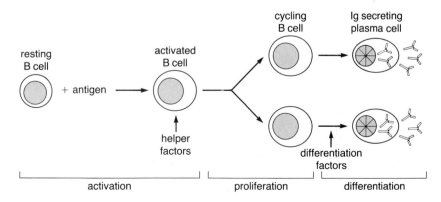

Figure 2–10. Model of B cell activation, proliferation, and differentiation.

Table 2-1. Lymphocyte distribution in various tissues in humans.[1]

Tissue	Approximate %		
	T cells		B cells
	CD4+	CD8+	
Peripheral blood	35–60	20–30	15–30
Lymph nodes and Tonsils			
Paracortex & interfollicular areas	60	20–40	Rare
Germinal centers	5–30	Rare	70–95
Lymphoid follicles (mantle zone)	Few	Few	>95
Spleen			
Periarteriolar sheath	70–90	10–30	Rare
Marginal zone–white pulp	40–55	5–20	40
Red pulp	20–40	60–80	Few
Thymus			
Cortex	>90	>90	Rare
Medulla	60–80	20–40	5–10

[1]Adapted from Hsu, S, Cossman, J, Jaffee, ES: Lymphocyte subsets in normal lymphoid tissues. *Am J Clin Pathol* 1983;**80**:21.

various target cells and is not MHC restricted. The precursor cells of these effector cells are unknown, but they lack major functional, genotypic, and phenotypic features of T cells, B cells, and monocyte-macrophages. NK cells, many of which appear as **large granular lymphocytes (LGL)**, have unique morphologic features and typically possess round or indented nuclei with abundant pale cytoplasm containing azurophilic granules (Fig 2–11). LGL contain membrane-bound granules that stain for acid hydrolases, including acid phosphatase, α-naphthyl acetate esterase, and β-glucuronidase. These granules may be related to the cytolytic capacity of the LGL. LGL lack surface immunoglobulins, are nonadherent and nonphagocytic, frequently form rosettes with sheep erythrocytes, and express IgG Fc receptors (CD16). Thus, LGL exhibit morphologic and membrane characteristics intermediate between those of lymphocytes and monocytes.

Large Granular Lymphocytes (LGL)

LGL characteristically bear the cell surface antigens CD16, CD3, and Leu 7 (HNK-1). Blood LGL with NK activity have been subdivided into a majority population of CD16+ CD3− and a minority population of CD16− CD3+. Approximately 10% of peripheral blood lymphocytes are CD16+ CD3−. Following exposure to interleukin-2 (IL-2), these cells can efficiently kill targets that are otherwise NK insensitive (ie, solid tumor cells). The CD16+ CD3+ cell type is a non-MHC-restricted cytotoxic lymphocyte. These cells may recognize their targets through the CD3-Ti receptor. A distinguishing feature of the CD16− CD3+ cells is the expression of NKH-I (Leu 19), an anti-

gen not present on the majority of T cells. These CD3+ Leu 19+ cells make up 5% or less of peripheral blood lymphocytes.

Since LGL form rosettes with sheep erythrocytes and a subset does express CD3-Ti receptors, there is debate about whether NK cells are T cells or represent a distinct (third) lineage of lymphoid cells. The study of genotypic alteration, unique to human T cells (rearrangement of α, β, and γ genes) has helped to resolve this controversy. Human CD16+ CD3− cells neither rearrange α or β genes nor produce functional mRNA for these genes. The non-MHC-restricted cytotoxic cells do, however, rearrange Ti genes and produce functional Ti mRNA. Thus, this LGL subpopulation may be from the T cell lineage.

Lymphokine-Activated Killer (LAK) Cells

Lymphokine-activated killer (LAK) cells are generated when fresh lymphoid cells from the blood or spleen are incubated in IL-2. They differ from NK cells in that they have cytotoxic activity against a broader range of target cells, including freshly isolated autologous and allogeneic tumor cells and cell lines. Characterization of LAK cells shows that they are mostly negative for CD3 and positive for the CD16 and NKH 1 markers. These phenotypic characteristics and other experimental data on the augmentation of NK activity by IL-2 suggest that most of the LAK activity can be attributed to NK cells activated by IL-2. However, LAK cell activity can also be generated from thymocytes. LAK cells have shown promise against a number of metastatic cancers in clinical studies. Recently, another population of lymphocytes that are cytotoxic to specific human tumors has been

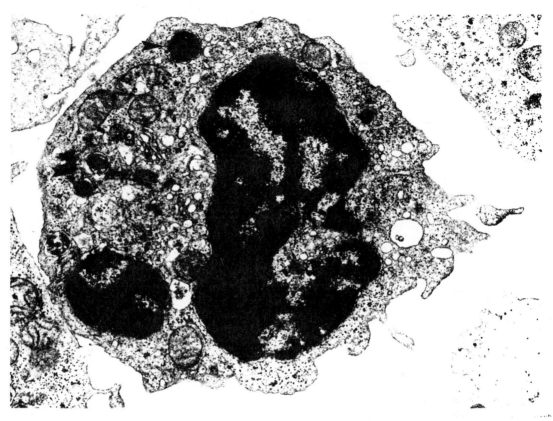

Figure 2-11. Morphology of the human NK cell. The nucleus is indented and rich in chromatin. The cytoplasm is abundant, and characteristic osmiophilic granules (spearheads) numerous mitochondria, centrioles (arrow), and the Golgi apparatus (g) are visible. (Original magnification × 17,000.) (Reproduced, with permission, from Carpen O, Virtanen I, Saksela E: *J Immunol* 1982;**126**:2692.)

identified within these solid tumors. These cells are known as **tumor-infiltrating lymphocytes (TIL).**

Dendritic Cells

Human **dendritic cells** have been identified in the peripheral blood and various peripheral lymphoid organs; they have similar cytologic features to rodent dendritic cells. They are bone marrow derived but belong to a distinct hematopoietic cell lineage, and they constitute less than 1% of peripheral blood mononuclear cells. They are potent stimulators of mixed-leukocyte reactions and are capable of presenting antigen for primary immune responses. They differ from other immunocytes in that they are Ia positive but lack Fc and sheep erythrocyte receptors, surface immunoglobulin, and other lymphocyte and monocyte markers. They have an irregular nucleus, small nucleoli, and pale blue-gray cytoplasm. They bear many mitochondria but few lysosomes and ribosomes and have scanty rough endoplasmic reticulum. Their surfaces lack ruffles and microvilli.

Functional Properties

The functions of various subpopulations of lymphocytes are discussed in Chapters 3, 5, and 6. Several reagents stimulate lymphocytes in vitro; these include plant lectins, bacterial products, polymeric substances, and enzymes. Morphologic transformation occurs following stimulation, with the formation of blast cells or, in some instances, plasma cells. Lymphocyte transformation may also be assessed biochemically by the measurement of RNA, DNA, or protein synthesis. The detailed functional aspects of B and T lymphocytes, their interaction, and their alteration in disease are discussed in subsequent chapters.

Table 2-2. Cells belonging to the mononuclear phagocytic system.[1]

Bone marrow	Tissues	Body Cavities
Monoblasts	Macrophages occurring in:	Pleural macrophages
Promonocytes	Connective tissue (histiocytes)	Peritoneal macrophages
Monocytes	Skin (histiocytes; Langerhans cells?)	
	Liver (Kupffer cells)	**Inflammation**
Blood	Spleen (red pulp macrophages)	Exudate macrophages
Monocytes	Lymph nodes (free and fixed-macrophages; interdigitating cells?)	Epithelioid cells
	Thymus	Multinucleated giant cells
	Bone marrow (resident macrophages)	
	Bone (osteoclasts)	
	Synovia (type A cell)	
	Lung (alveolar and tissue macrophages)	
	MALT	
	Gastrointestinal tract	
	Genitourinary tract	
	Endocrine organs	
	Central nervous system (macrophages, [reactive] microglia, CSF macrophages)	

[1]Reproduced, with permission, from Van Furth R: Development and distribution of mononuclear phagocytes in the normal steady state and inflammation. In: *Inflammation: Basic Principles and Clinical Correlates.* Gallin JI, Goldstein IM, Snyderman, R (editors). Raven Press, 1988.

2. MONONUCLEAR PHAGOCYTES (MONOCYTE-MACROPHAGES)

The mononuclear phagocytes include circulating pheripheral blood monocytes, promonocytes, precursor cells in the bone marrow, and tissue macrophages. Tissue macrophages are present in several tissues, organs, and serous cavities. The organization of the mononuclear phagocyte system is shown in Table 2–2. The precursor cell in the mononuclear phagocyte lineage is the **monoblast,** which is present in the bone marrow and is morphologically similar to the myeloblast. The monoblast gives rise to the **promonocyte,** a bone marrow cell that is phagocytic and adherent and contains nonspecific esterase (Fig 2–12). Circulating monocytes are heterogeneous in size, receptor expression, and phagocytic function. There is a wide spectrum of morphologic features in the various types of mononuclear phagocytes. Their surface membranes are characterized by prominent microvilli and ruffles (Fig 2–13).

Functions of Macrophages

The major functional properties of monocyte-macrophages are ingestion of particles smaller than 0.1 μm by pinocytosis and engulfment of particles larger than 0.1 μm by phagocytosis. During engulfment, the particle first adheres to the plasma membrane of the cell and is then ingested. The monocyte-macrophage is capable of both nonimmunologic and immunologic phagocytosis. It has a plasma membrane receptor that recognizes 2 of the 4 subclasses of human IgG (IgG1 and IgG3); this binding site on the IgG molecule has been localized to the C_H3 domain of the im-

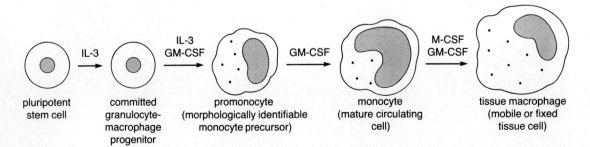

pluripotent stem cell   **IL-3**   committed granulocyte-macrophage progenitor   **IL-3 GM-CSF**   promonocyte (morphologically identifiable monocyte precursor)   **GM-CSF**   monocyte (mature circulating cell)   **M-CSF GM-CSF**   tissue macrophage (mobile or fixed tissue cell)

Figure 2-12. Cells of mononuclear phagocyte lineage.

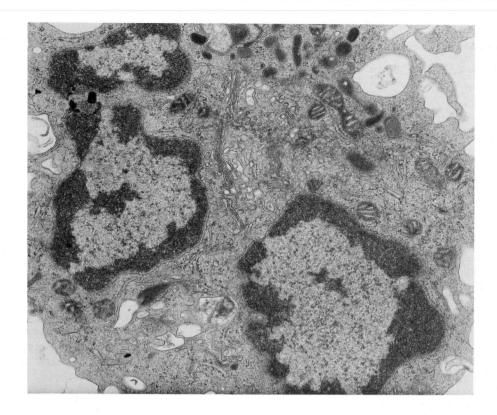

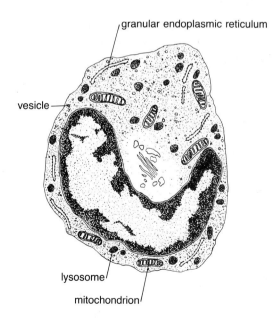

granular endoplasmic reticulum

vesicle

lysosome

mitochondrion

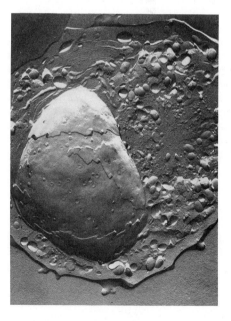

Figure 2–13. **Top:** Electron micrograph of normal human blood monocyte. (Original magnification × 34,500.) **Bottom left:** Diagrammatic representation of the monocyte. **Bottom right:** Freeze-fracture micrograph of normal human blood monocyte. (Original magnification × 10,000.)

munoglobulin molecule. Three types of human receptors for the Fc region of IgG (FcγR) have been identified. These are referred to as HuFcγRI, HuFcγRII, and HuFcγRIII. HuFcγRI is found predominantly on monocytes and macrophages, is a heavily glycosylated protein with molecular weight of 72,000, and plays a role in antibody-dependent cellular cytotoxicity reactions. HuFcγRII (CDw32) is an MW 40,000 protein found on monocytes, platelets, eosinophils, neutrophils, and B cells; its most important role may be in initiating the oxidative burst. HuFcγRIII (CD16) is expressed on tissue macrophages but not on monocytes and is also expressed on neutrophils, NK cells, and eosinophils. Its abundant presence on tissue macrophages in the liver and spleen suggests that it plays a vital role in clearance of autologous erythrocytes and other immune complexes.

Monocyte Receptors

Monocyte-macrophages also have an independent receptor system, which recognizes the activated third component of complement. Three major types of surface receptors for C3 have been identified on immunocytes. Of these, CR1 and CR3 are expressed on monocytes. CR1 is a single-chain molecule that demonstrates polymorphism, with a molecular weight (MW) ranging from 160,000 to 250,000 depending on the allotype. CR3, which is specific for C3bi, is a heterodimer with an MW 165,000 α chain and an MW 95,000 β chain. A monoclonal antibody, anti-CD11 (anti-Mac-1), recognizes this determinant on more than 95% of fresh human monocytes and macrophages. Mac-1(CR3) is a member of an interrelated family of different cell surface adhesion molecules, including LFA-1 and p150,95, that share identical 95 K β chains. CR2 is the Epstein-Barr virus receptor found on B lymphocytes.

The monoclonal MO2 antibody (anti-CDw14) appears to be specific for peripheral blood monocytes. There are a number of other monoclonal antibodies that react with monocytes and other nonmonocyte blood elements. CD4 molecules and their corresponding mRNA have been demonstrated on monocytes, macrophages, and monocytelike cell lines. This CD4 receptor on monocytes serves as the principal site of entry for the human immunodeficiency virus (HIV) into mononuclear phagocytes.

Mononuclear phagocytes play an important role as antigen-presenting cells; they bear Ia antigens, the class II MHC antigens. The macrophage receptors for the Fc portion of IgG and C3b are the principal modes of antigen binding and recognition of appropriately opsonized antigen. Cells of the monocyte-macrophage series are active in killing bacteria, fungi, and tumor cells.

3. CELL TYPES INVOLVED IN THE INFLAMMATORY PHASE OF THE IMMUNE RESPONSE

Leukocytes consisting of neutrophils, eosinophils, basophils, and mast cells all participate in inflammatory reactions. For a description of their structure and functions, refer to Chapter 12.

HEMATOLYMPHOPOIESIS

Lymphocyte Recirculation & High Endothelial Venules (HEV)

The distribution of lymphocytes in various body tissues is determined by a number of factors, including lymphocyte class, stage of differentiation, and antigenic specificity. Thus, T cells predominate in the peripheral lymph nodes, whereas B cells migrate to MALT. Studies with animals show that antigen-specific T and B cells predominate in tissues that have been challenged with antigen. After their generation and maturation in the thymus and bone marrow, lymphocytes migrate to the secondary lymphoid organs, ie, the lymph nodes, MALT, and spleen. After traversing these tissues, lymphocytes that constitute the recirculating pool reenter the circulation via the efferent lymphatics and major lymphatic channels and repeatedly travel through the secondary lymphoid tissues via the blood and lymphatics (Fig 2–3). Approximately 10^9 lymphocytes are produced per day in the primary lymphoid organs. The average lymphocyte completes a cycle of recirculation in about 1–2 days. A small fraction of lymphocytes travel through nonlymphoid tissues such as the skin and gut (intestinal lamina propria). The mechanisms that govern their migration through these tissues parallel those relevant for traffic through secondary lymphoid organs. Labeling experiments have shown that thymic lymphocytes can be seen in peripheral lymph node high endothelial venules (HEV) within 30 minutes of being labeled in the thymus. Lymphocytes take more than 6 hours to travel from an afferent lymphatic vessel to the efferent lymphatic vessel draining the lymph node.

Approximately 1% of total body lymphocytes are present in the blood. During lymphocyte trafficking and recirculation, migrating lymphocytes leave the blood at HEV, which are specialized segments of the postcapillary venules. These HEV are characterized by distinctive, cuboidal, plump endothelial cells (Fig 2–14). In the white pulp of the spleen, lymphocytes leave the circulation via capillaries in the marginal zone of the periarteriolar lymphoid sheath. Since there are no HEV in the spleen, it is unknown how this occurs. The selective nature of the interaction between

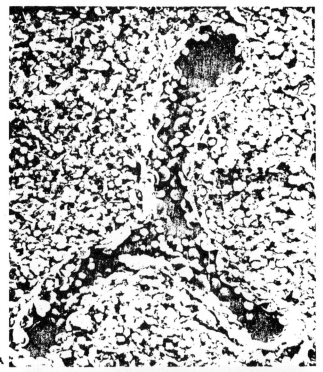

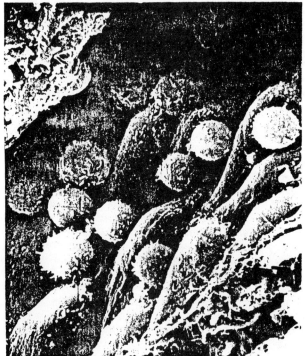

Figure 2-14. Scanning electron micrographs illustrating high endothelial venules (HEV) in mouse lymph nodes. **A:** Inverted Y-shaped HEV. The high endothelial cells bulge into the lumen. Individual small round lymphocytes can be seen attached to the endothelium, some apparently migrating between endothelial cells on their way into the lymph node parenchyma. **B:** Higher power showing numerous lymphocytes tightly bound to the high endothelial cells. Nonadherent blood elements were washed out by perfusion of the vasculature with medium prior to fixation by perfusion with glutaraldehyde in phosphate-buffered saline. (Reproduced, with permission, from Butcher EC et al: *The Pathology of the Endothelial Cell,* pp 409–424. Nossel H, Vogel H [editors]. Academic Press, 1982.)

lymphocytes and HEV and lymphocyte extravasation is mediated by organ-specific receptors, whereby lymphocytes have the capacity to distinguish between HEV in lymph nodes, mucosal tissues, and possibly other lymphoid organs.

Homing Receptors

A number of "homing" receptors have now been identified on lymphocyte surface membranes. At least 3 distinct types of homing receptors exist: one that mediates the binding of lymphocytes to peripheral lymph node HEV, one for Peyer's patch HEV, and one that mediates lymphocyte adhesion to endothelium in inflamed synovia. These receptors constitute a closely related family of MW 90,000 glycoprotein molecules. Their basic structure consists of a constant backbone region and a variable region that confers tissue specificity. This HEV-recognizing property of lymphocytes is developmentally acquired and appears to be based on lymphocyte class. Thus, "virgin" or non-antigen-exposed surface IgA-bearing B cells preferentially bind to HEV of and localize better to the mucosal lymphoid tissues such as Peyer's patches, whereas virgin regulatory T cells bind better to peripheral lymph node HEV.

The lymphocyte function-associated antigen LFA-1 is a non-tissue-specific surface molecule on lymphocytes that may play an accessory role in lymphocyte interaction with HEV. The intercellular adhesion molecule ICAM-1 has recently been identified as a ligand for LFA-1 on HEV cells, but its definitive role in HEV endothelial cell-lymphocyte interaction is unknown. Molecules on HEV endothelial cell surfaces that serve as recognition and binding sites for lymphocyte homing receptors have been identified by using monoclonal antibodies. These tissue-specific glycoproteins are referred to as "vascular addressins."

Upon exposure to antigen and following lymphocyte activation, there is a rapid increase in the blood supply to the stimulated lymphoid organ. Concurrently, a transient arrest of lymphocyte egress from these tissues occurs, allowing lymphocytes to accumulate, proliferate, and differentiate within these sites.

Common Mucosal Immune System

Support for the concept of a common mucosal immune system comes from studies showing that lymphocytes can selectively migrate between various mucosal surfaces in the body that produce secretory immunoglobulins at sites of antigen exposure. These sites include the intestines, lungs, breasts, and the female genital tract. The lymphoid tissues in these sites are all structurally similar and have plasma cells that produce secretory IgA.

For example, gut lymphoid tissue-derived cells can home to several different types of mucosal tissues but not to peripheral lymph nodes. During the late stages of gestation and lactation, gut-derived IgA-bearing plasma cells are diverted to breast connective tissue, where they secrete IgA antibodies specific for antigens to which these B cells were exposed in the gut. This results in the transfer of passive immunity to the intestinal tract of the suckling newborn (see Chapter 15).

PHYLOGENY OF IMMUNITY

The immune response originated in organisms with a nucleus (eukaryotic organisms), probably in response to a need to distinguish self from nonself. Unicellular organisms (protozoa) have undergone evolutionary changes that allow them to differentiate food or invading microorganisms from autologous cell components. Multicellular organisms (metazoa) have also evolved highly complex and functionally integrated cells and tissues that exhibit various degrees of immunologic competence. Such cell-specific or tissue-specific antigens arise from a restricted phenotypic expression of the genome (see Chapter 4). In such organisms, specialized cells or immunocytes have developed that protect the entire body from microbial invaders, from incursions of foreign tissue, and from diseases that may be caused by altered or neoplastic cells. This phemonemon is known as **immune surveillance**

From an evolutionary standpoint, cellular immunity and, particularly, phagocytosis preceded the development of antibody production in animals. Invertebrates characteristically demonstrate primitive forms of graft rejection and phagocytosis, but in no invertebrate species have molecules been identified that have a functional or physicochemical structure analogous to that of vertebrate immunoglobulins. On the other hand, all vertebrate species synthesize antibody, reject grafts, and exhibit **immunologic memory.** Thus, there is a relatively sharp delineation between the complexity of immunity in invertebrates and vertebrates; no clearly transitional forms have so far been identified.

The fully developed immune response is characterized by **specificity** and **anamnesis.** These essential criteria should be borne in mind when distinguishing true immunity from primitive or paraimmunologic phenomena in the phylogenetic analysis that follows.

IMMUNITY IN INVERTEBRATES

Unicellular invertebrate species have survived largely as a result of their remarkable reproductive capacity rather than the development of specific immune responses to environmental challenges. Perhaps the most primitive self-recognition mechanism is the ability of certain protozoa to reject transplantation of foreign nuclei. However, this phenomenon is really quasi-immunologic and probably depends on enzymatic rather than specific antigenic differences among various species.

All invertebrate species exhibit some form of self-versus-nonself recognition. However, true cellular immunity, with specific graft rejection and anamnesis, has been conclusively demonstrated only in certain earthworms (annelids) and corals (coelenterates) (Table 2–3). Although invertebrates with coelomic cavities possess a variety of humoral substances such as bacteriolysins, hemolysins, and opsonins, none of these have been specifically induced by immunization, nor do these rather ill-defined substances have any known physicochemical similarities with vertebrate antibodies. A fascinating array of primitive or quasi-immunologic phenomena, including self-recognition, phagocytosis, encapsulation, allograft and xenograft rejection, humoral defenses, and leukocyte differentiation, have been identified in invertebrates.

IMMUNITY IN VERTEBRATES

The most advanced invertebrates, the protochordates, are probably the ancestors of the true chordates, from which all higher vertebrates are descended. However, at the level of the most primitive extant vertebrate class, the agnathae, an entirely new component in the immune system is apparent, ie, **antibody.** Specific antibody synthesis is a property of all vertebrates. Cellular immunity, present in a primitive form in invertebrates, is highly developed and immunologically specific in all vertebrates. Graft rejection is accelerated after primary sensitization, and a true second-set rejection phenomenon occurs. However, some difference in the expression of immunologic functions is evident between warm-blooded and cold-blooded animals.

The hallmark of vertebrate immunity is the presence of a truly 2-component immune system; this is best demonstrated in birds, in which 2 independent central lymphoid organs exist: the thymus, which controls cellular immunity, and the bursa, which determines antibody-producing capacity. The immunologic repertoire of the various vertebrate classes is shown in Table 2–4.

Several generalizations regarding the phylogenetic emergence of immunity are possible. First, primitive and quasi-immunologic phenomena are present in the simplest forms of extant animal species. Second, T cell immunity precedes antibody immunity in evolution. Third, a truly bifunctional immune system with dual central lymphoid organs in a highly differentiated form is the most recent immunologic evolutionary development.

THE IMMUNOGLOBULIN GENE SUPERFAMILY

The immunoglobulin gene superfamily consists of a series of genes that share an evolutionary homology but do not necessarily share function, genetic linkage, or coordinate regulation. The members of this superfamily are defined by the presence of one or more structural regions homologous to the basic structural unit of the immunoglobulin molecule. This unit (the immunoglobulin homology unit) is characterized by a primary sequence of 70–110 amino acids with an essentially invariant disulfide bridge and several relatively conserved residues. The unique ability of the immunoglobulin homology unit to accommodate diversity has made possible the evolution of the complex phenotypic traits of the immunoglobulin gene superfamily. Comparisons of these sequences reveal that the similarity score between proteins that make up this superfamily is greater than 2–3 standard deviations above what would be expected between 2 random sequences.

The molecules that mediate the specific recognition of antigen, ie, the immunoglobulin molecule, the T cell receptor, and the class I and II MHC molecules, are the most significant products of this gene superfamily. However, a wide variety of gene products ranging from the above-named molecules to receptors of cartilage formation and nervous system-associated molecules are represented in this superfamily. These include (1) non-antigen-presenting β_2-microglobulin, (2) T cell-associated molecules, (3) molecules expressed on both T cells and neural cells, (4) nervous system-associated molecules, (5) immunoglobulin-binding molecules, and (6) growth factor/kinase receptors (Table 2–5).

The diversity inherent in the genes of the immunoglobulin homology unit appears to have driven the evolution of this superfamily of gene products. New functional structures have arisen during evolutionary development through the duplication of nucleotides, exons, genes, and entire families of genes. It is most likely that this superfamily arose from structures that first evolved to mediate cellular interactions and that the immune system in vertebrates developed from this group of structures.

Table 2–3. Evolution of immunity in invertebrates.[1]

Phylum or Subphylum	Graft Rejection	Immunologic Specificity of Graft Rejection	Immunologic Memory	Phago-cytosis	Encapsula-tion	Nonspecific Humoral Factors	Phagocytic Ameboid Coelomocytes	Leukocyte Differentia-tion	Inducible Specific Antibodies
Protozoa	Yes. Enzyme incompatibility.	No	No	Yes; whole organism	No	No	No	No	No
Porifera (sponges)	Yes. Aggregation inhibition; species-specific glycoprotein.	Yes	Yes	No	Yes	No	No	No	No
Coelenterata (corals, jellyfish, sea anemones)	Yes; with graft necrosis.	Yes	Yes, short term	No	Hyperplastic growth around graft.	No	No	No	No
Annelida (earthworms)	Yes	Yes. First and second set graft rejection.	Short term, either positive or negative.	Yes	Yes	Yes. Nonspecific hemagglutinins, ciliate lysins, bacteriocidins.	Yes. Chemotaxis to bacteria.	Probable phytohemagglutinin response in coelomocyte.	No
Mollusca	Yes	?	?	Yes	Yes	Yes. Hemagglutinins act as opsonins.	Yes	No	No
Arthropoda	Yes	?	?	Yes	Yes	Yes	Yes	No	No
Echinodermata	Yes. Prolonged 4–6 months.	Yes. Specific second set graft rejection.	Short term only.	Yes	Yes	Yes. Hemolysins.	Yes	Yes. Cellular infiltrate in graft injection.	No
Protochordata (tunicates)	Yes. Genetically determined alloimmunity.	Probable. Tolerance possible.	Yes	Yes	Yes	Yes	Yes. Macrophage, lymphocyte, and eosinophil.	Yes. Lymphocytes present which form E rosettes and respond to phytohemagglutinin.	No

[1]Modified from Hildemann WH, Reddy AL: Fed Proc 1973;**322**:2188.

Table 2-4. Immunologic features exhibited by various vertebrate classes.

Class	Lymphocytes	Plasma Cells	Thymus	Spleen	Lymph Nodes	Bursa	Antibodies	Allograft Rejection
Agnatha (jawless fish)	+	−	PRIM[1]	PRIM	−	−	+	+
Chondrichthyes (cartilaginous fish) Primitive	+	−	+	+	−	−	+	+
Advanced	+	+	+	+	−	−	+	+
Osteichthyes (bony fish)	+	+	+	+	−	−	+	+
Amphibia	+	+	+	+	+	−	+	+
Reptilia	+	+	+	+	+(?)[2]	−	+	+
Aves	+	+	+	+	+(?)	+	+	+
Mammalia	+	+	+	+	+	−	+	+

[1]PRIM = primitive.
[2]? = some question regarding the presence of lymphoid structures under consideration, although such structures or their functional counterparts may have been described.

ONTOGENY

In the fetus, hematopoiesis—predominantly erythropoiesis—begins in the blood islands of the yolk sac in the second week of gestation. By about the sixth week of embryonic life, foci of hematopoiesis can be seen in the liver. During the second month, the bone marrow assumes an increasing role in this process and becomes the predominant site for hematopoiesis by the second half of gestation. The fetal spleen transiently serves as a hematopoietic organ between the third and fifth months of gestation. After birth, the bone marrow is normally the only hematopoietic organ, although both the liver and the spleen can serve as sites for extramedullary hematopoiesis if the bone marrow fails for any reason.

BLOOD CELLS

All circulating peripheral blood cells, including the lymphocytes, are derived from the pluripotent stem cells. These stem cells have the ability to self-replicate and eventually differentiate into mature blood cells. It is estimated that one of every 10,000 nucleated marrow cells in adult mouse bone marrow is a stem cell. As few as 30 pluripotent stem cells in the mouse can hematopoietically reconstitute lethally irradiated mice. These cells are lymphoid-appearing cells intermediate in size between bone marrow lymphocytes and large myeloid cells. Similar cells probably also exist in humans.

T Cells

Entry into the human thymus of blood-borne stem cells derived from sites of fetal hematopoiesis and their subsequent differentiation into lymphoid cells starts around the seventh week of gestation. Contact with the thymic epithelium, the presence of which is demonstrable by the seventh week of gestation, appears to be necessary for the maturation and differentiation of T cells in the thymus. The exact role of the thymic peptide hormones in the induction of these changes is unclear.

Important insights into murine thymocyte ontogeny have been obtained from studies of developmentally regulated expression of lymphocyte cell surface molecules involved in antigen recognition, including the T cell receptor (TCR). The first stage of T cell development from a molecular standpoint involves the rearrangement of TCR gene segments and the cell surface expression of the TCR. After surface TCR expression, cellular selection can occur. Cells that express self-reactive TCRs are eliminated, whereas those expressing TCRs that can recognize foreign antigens in the context of self-MHC molecules are positively selected. Following cell selection, thymocytes progressively acquire effector functions.

The order of appearance of critical ontogenetic events in humans is believed to be very similar to that in mice. The majority of TCR gene rearrangements occur at the stage of the earliest CD4⁻ CD8⁻ CD3⁻ fetal thymocytes. The T cell γδ re-

Table 2-5. Members of the immunoglobulin gene superfamily.

Molecules of immune recognition	T cell–associated molecules
Immunoglobulin molecule	CD7, CD28
T cell receptor	CD2, CD3, CD4, CD8
MHC class I and II molecules	
β2-Microglobulin-associated molecules	Immunoglobulin-binding molecules
Qa and Tla	Mouse Fc receptor
CD1	Polyimmunoglobulin receptor (p-IgR)
T cell nervous system–associated molecules	Nervous system molecules
THY-1 antigen	Neural cell adhesion molecule (N-CAM)
Rat Ox-2 cell surface antigen	Rat myelin-associated glycoprotein (MAG)
	Peripheral myelin glycoprotein (Po)
Growth factor receptors	
Platelet-derived growth factor (PDGFR)	
Receptor for macrophage colony-stimulating factor (CSF-1R)	
Other molecules	
Carcinoembryonic antigen (CEA)	
1B-glycoprotein (1B)	
Link glycoprotein (cartilage)	

ceptor (TCR$_{\gamma\delta}$) is the first CD3-associated receptor to appear during ontogeny. This is closely followed by the expression of TCR$\alpha\beta$. In humans, thymocytes from 9.5-week-old fetuses can be shown to express the TCR$_{\gamma\delta}$, and by 10 weeks, expression of TCR$_{\alpha\beta}$ is demonstrable, followed by a progressive decrease in the number of thymocytes expressing TCR$_{\gamma\delta}$. T cells acquire maturational surface markers during corticomedullary differentiation by about 14 weeks of gestation. Although fetal thymocytes can be shown to possess several functional capabilities, detectable T cell functions appear in peripheral blood lymphocytes around birth. Responsiveness to phytohemagglutinin can be shown as early as 10–12 weeks; responses to allogeneic cells and cell-mediated lympholysis occur by 12 and 16 weeks, respectively.

Studies of neonatal immune function shows that the magnitude of the responses of neonatal lymphocytes is generally comparable to that of adult lymphocytes. When deficiencies of function are demonstrable, they are secondary both to lower levels of precursors of effector T cells and to deficiencies of accessory or antigen-presenting cells.

B Cells

B lymphocytes arise from a common lymphoid stem cell derived from the pluripotent stem cells, although some studies have suggested a closer relationship of B cell precursors to myeloid precursors than to T cell progenitors. In early fetal life, the liver is the major repository of B cell progenitors. During mammalian embryogenesis, the bone marrow becomes the primary hematopoietic organ and, with it, becomes the significant source of B cell precursors.

Pre-B cells are the earliest identifiable B cell lineage progenitors. They are large, rapidly dividing cells that contain cytoplasmic μ chains but no light chains or surface immunoglobulin. They can be detected in human fetal liver by the seventh or eighth week of gestation. With proliferation, smaller pre-B cells arise; these express first cytoplasmic light chains and then surface immunoglobulin. B cells can be detected in fetal liver by about the ninth week of gestation. At this stage, they have surface complement receptors and IgM. Between the tenth and twelfth weeks, lymphocytes expressing other classes of immunoglobulin appear. By the fifteenth, the proportions of mature surface immunoglobulin-bearing B cells in the blood, spleen, and lymph nodes and the distribution of B cells expressing different immunoglobulin classes are comparable to those found in adults. If the emerging clones of B cells that express only surface IgM are exposed to antigen, they become tolerant to that antigen, a phenomenon referred to as clonal anergy. This mechanism is important in the development of B cell tolerance to high concentrations of self-antigens.

During B cell ontogeny, all B cell clones arise from surface IgM (sIgM)-expressing progenitors. Immature sIgA- or sIgG-bearing B cells also coexpress sIgM and sIgD, whereas coexpression of both sIgA and sIgG is extremely rare. IgM synthesis can be detected as early as the tenth to twelfth weeks of gestation. IgG synthesis is demonstrable somewhat later, and synthesis of serum IgA and secretory IgA cannot be detected until about the thirtieth week of gestation. At birth, the neonatal serum contains almost no IgA, small amounts of IgM, and adult levels of IgG, most of which is passively transferred maternal IgG. The rapidity with which serum immunoglobulin levels rise from neonatal levels to normal adult levels varies according to the isotype. Functionally, the neonatal immune response is qualitatively and quantitatively different from that of the adult. The neonatal IgM response is prolonged and prominent, whereas the IgG and IgA responses are relatively deficient. This defect appears to be related to lack of T cell help rather than to a lack of B cell precursors. Neonates also appear to have a relative inability of mounting an IgG2 subclass response; this may correspond to their inability to respond to carbohydrate antigens.

Monocyte-Macrophages

The mononuclear phagocyte cell lineage arises from a committed progenitor that itself is derived from the pluripotent stem cell. Differentiation of the progenitor into monocytes is probably a random event, but the differentiation and subsequent maturation of this progenitor into mature monocytes is facilitated by a number of **colony-stimulating factors (CSF)** including granulocyte-macrophage CSF (GM-CSF), interleukin-3 (Il-3), and macrophage CSF (M-CSF). Following commitment, the first identifiable cell of this lineage in the bone marrow is the promonocyte, which constitutes approximately 3–5% of the bone marrow. Although monoblasts can be seen in bone marrow during leukemic states, they cannot routinely be differentiated from myeloblasts in normal bone marrow. Each promonocyte divides in the bone marrow, giving rise to 2 daughter monocytes, which subsequently enter the peripheral circulation, circulate for about 3 days, and then migrate to different tissues. Tissue macrophages are derived from precursors in the bone marrow. Once in the tissues, local proliferation may contribute to the tissue macrophage pool although this pool is regularly replenished from the blood monocyte pool.

Embryonic macrophages can be found in the hematopoietic tissues of the yolk sac around the third to fourth week of gestation. When hematopoiesis moves to the liver, more than half of the free intravascular hematopoietic cells in the human fetal liver are of the mononuclear phagocyte lineage. Between the eighth and twenty-second weeks of gestation, high levels of colony forming units for granulocytes and monocytes (CFU-GM) can be identified in fetal liver and peripheral blood. These CFU-GM are different from those derived from adult bone marrow in that they are more actively proliferating and give rise more consistently to pure macrophage colonies in vitro. Mature monocytes do not appear in the fetal circulation until about the fifth month of fetal life. Beyond 30 weeks, monocytes constitute about 3–7% of all hematopoietic cells. The exact kinetics of monocyte production and tissue distribution during fetal life are unknown. There is a relative monocytosis during the perinatal period, with peripheral blood monocyte counts returning to normal levels by about 1 month of age. Histologic studies of the lungs of stillborn infants and neonates have suggested that very few alveolar macrophages are present in fetal lungs prior to birth but there is a significant influx of macrophages into the lungs soon after birth.

MALT

MALT cannot be identified in animal or human tissues at birth. Mononuclear cell aggregates which may be the forerunners of MALT have been identified in the intestines and less so in the lungs of the human fetus as early as 14 weeks of gestation. This assumption is supported by studies demonstrating the development of BALT follicles in fetal lungs transplanted from 18-day-old mouse fetuses into syngeneic animals. In humans, lymphoid aggregates representative of MALT are absent at birth but appear at the end of the first week of life and subsequently increase in number with age during childhood and adolescence.

Complement

Synthesis of some of the components of **complement** starts in the human fetal liver during the first trimester of gestation. Specifically, synthesis of C3 and C1 inhibitor protein have been documented as early as the 29th day of gestation, C4 and C2 by the 8th week and C5 by the 9th week of gestation. Throughout fetal life, the liver and other tissues continue to produce complement components at varying rates. Transplacental passage of complement proteins does not occur. The levels of immunochemically and hemolytically detectable complement components in newborn sera range between 60 and 90% of adult levels. They rise steadily in the first few years of life to reach normal adult levels.

SUMMARY

The immune system is composed of cells within the lymphoreticular organs, which include the primary lymphoid organs (the bone marrow and thymus) and the secondary organs such as the spleen, lymph nodes, and the MALT. Thymus-derived (T) lymphocytes and bone marrow-derived (B) lymphocytes are the predominant immunocytes. The structural architecture of lymphoid organs is generally characterized by discrete T and B cell areas interspersed with endothelial, stromal, and reticuloendothelial cells. The peripheral lymphoid tissues, ie, the tonsils, lymph nodes, and MALT, are situated in strategic areas where they are intimately and continuously exposed to antigens.

T lymphocyte precursors arise in the bone marrow, migrate to the thymus, and undergo maturation and differentiation within the thymic microenvironment. A number of differentiational and functional cell surface markers are acquired during this process. These immunocompetent T lymphocytes then emigrate from the thymus and populate the T cell areas of peripheral lymphoid organs. Postnatally, maturation of B lymphocytes occurs exclusively in the bone marrow. These short-lived B lymphocytes then travel to B cell areas of peripheral lymphoid tissues, where they can differentiate into long-lived B cells upon antigenic stimulation.

All lymphocytes continuously recirculate throughout the lymphoid tissues of the body. They leave the blood circulation via the HEV in the peripheral lymphoid tissues and eventually return to the venous circulation after traversing afferent lymphatics, lymph nodes, and the efferent lymphatics, which ultimately empty into the thoracic duct. There is preferential migration of B lymphocytes to MALT, whereas T cells migrate to peripheral lymph nodes. This selective migration is mediated via lymphocyte-endothelial interaction involving receptors on lymphocyte cell surfaces and ligands on specialized vascular endothelium.

Teleologically, the immune response arose to meet a need for organisms to distinguish self components from foreign or nonself components. Primitive forms of graft rejection and phagocytosis are present in invertebrates, but truly immunologic responses, with specificity and anamnesis, are present only in vertebrates. Ontogenetic studies of the human immune system show that although hematopoiesis begins in the fetal yolk sac in the second week of gestation, the earliest T and B cell functional characteristics cannot be demonstrated until the seventh or eighth week of gestation. The neonatal immune response is immature in comparison with the fully developed response in the immunocompetent adult.

REFERENCES

LYMPHOID ORGANS

Bienenstock J: The mucosal immunologic network. *Ann Allergy* 1984;**53**:535.

Hsu S, Cossman J, Jaffe, ES: Lymphocyte subsets in normal lymphoid tissues. *Am J Clin Pathol* 1983;**80**:21.

Janossy G et al: Cellular differentiation of lymphoid subpopulations and their microenvironments in the human thymus. *Curr Top Pathol* 1986;**75**:89.

Weiss L: The blood cells and hematopoietic tissues. Page 423 in: *Cell and Tissue Biology. A Textbook of Histology,* 6th ed. Weiss L (editor). Urban & Schwarzenberg, 1988.

Immunologic Cells

Douglas SD, Hassan NF: Morphology of monocytes and macrophages. Chapter 93 in: *Hematology,* 4th ed. Williams WJ (editor). McGraw-Hill, 1989.

Douglas SD, Hassan, NF, Blaese, RM: The mononuclear phagocyte system. Page 81 in: *Immunologic Disorders in Infants and Children,* 3rd ed. Stiehm ER (editor). Saunders, 1988.

Douglas SD, Kay NE: Morphology of plasma cells. Chapter 101 in: *Hematology,* 4th ed. Williams WJ (editor). McGraw-Hill, 1989.

Herberman RB et al: Lymphokine-activated killer cell activity. Characteristics of effector cells and their progenitors in blood and spleen. *Immunol Today* 1987;**8**:178.

Hersey P, Bolhuis R: "Nonspecific" MHC-unrestricted killer cells and their receptors. *Immunol Today* 1987;**8**:233.

Kay NE, Douglas SD: Antigenic phenotype and morphology of human blood lymphocytes. Chapter 100 in: *Hematology,* 4th ed. Williams WJ (editor). McGraw-Hill, 1989.

Sprangrude GJ, Heimfeld S, Weissman IL: Purification and characterization of mouse hematopoietic stem cells. *Science* 1988;**241**:58.

Steinman RM, Nussenzweig MC: Dendritic cells: Features and functions. *Immunol Rev* 1980;**53**: 127.

Trinchieri, G: Biology of natural killer cells. *Adv Immunol* 1989;**47**:187.

Voorhis WC et al: Human dendritic cells. Enrichment and characterization from peripheral blood. *J Exp Med* 1982;**155**:1172.

Zola H: The surface antigens of human B lymphocytes. *Immunol Today* 1987;**8**:308.

Hematolymphopoiesis

Butcher EC: The regulation of lymphocyte traffic. *Curr Top Microbiol Immunol* 1986;**128**:85.

Duijvestijn A, Hamman A: Mechanisms and regulation of lymphocyte migration. *Immunol Today* 1989;**10**:23.

Yednock TA, Rosen SD: Lymphocyte homing. *Adv Immunol* 1989;**44**:313.

Phylogeny

Cohen N: Phylogeny of lymphocyte structure and function. *Am Zool* 1975;**15**:119.

Goetz D (editor): *Evolution and Function of the Major Histocompatibility System.* Springer-Verlag, 1977.

Hildemann WH, Clark EA, Raison RL: *Comprehensive Immunogenetics.* Elsevier, 1981.

Hood L, Prahl J: The immune system: A model for differentiation in higher organisms. *Adv Immunol* 1971;**14**:291.

Ontogeny

Hunkapiller T, Hood L: Diversity of the immunoglobulin gene superfamily. *Adv Immunol* 1989; **44**:1.

Kincade, PW: Experimental models for understanding B lymphocyte formation. *Adv Immunol* 1987; **41**:181.

Lawton AR, Cooper MD: Ontogeny of immunity.

Chapter 1 in: *Immunologic Disorders in Infants and Children,* 3rd ed. Stiehm ER (editor). Saunders, 1988.

Stutman O: Ontogeny of T cells. *Clin Immunol Allergy* 1985;**5**:191.

Vogler LB, Lawton AR: Ontogeny of B cells and humoral immune functions. *Clin Immunol Allergy* 1985;**5**:235.

Williams AF: A year in the life of the immunoglobulin superfamily. *Immunol Today* 1987;**8**:298.

The Immune Response

Joel W. Goodman, PhD

The **immune response** is made up of a complex sequence of events; it is triggered by the introduction of a stimulus (immunogen or antigen) and usually culminates in the elimination of the provoking agent. Indeed, the primary function of the immune response is to discriminate between self and nonself and thereby to eliminate the latter, be it a pathogenic microorganism, a tissue allograft, or an innocuous environmental substance such as proteins in pollens, grasses, or food.

The immune response depends primarily on 3 major cell types: macrophages, thymus-derived lymphocytes (T cells), and bone marrow–derived lymphocytes (B cells). These interact with one another, either directly or via interleukins. In addition, the immune system is integrally connected with the complement, kinin, clotting, and fibrinolytic systems, all of which are involved in inflammation.

The interplay of these elements, which are still imperfectly understood despite the rapid pace of progress in immunology during recent years, can be bewildering to the uninitiated. The purpose of this chapter is to clarify a very complex subject by considering the essential elements of the immune response in a stepwise, simplified fashion, from the initial encounter with an immunogen to the final products of the response, which function to eliminate the antigenic stimulus.

INNATE & ADAPTIVE IMMUNITY

All living things are continually under environmental assault. There are 2 levels of defense against invasion by external agents: **innate immunity** and **adaptive immunity** (also known as acquired immunity) (Table 3–1). The principal differences between the two relate to specificity and immunologic memory, which are properties of acquired immunity only.

Innate Immunity

Innate immunity, sometimes called natural immunity, is present from birth and includes numerous nonspecific elements.

Body surfaces, especially skin, form the first line of defense against penetration by microorganisms. When penetration does occur, the invading organisms initially encounter other elements of the innate immune system. The enzyme lysozyme is widely distributed in secretions and can damage the cell walls of many bacteria. Similarly, the alternative complement pathway (see Chapter 14) is directly activated by a variety of bacteria; this may result in clearance of the bacteria via lysis or via facilitation of phagocytosis by macrophages (see Chapter 11), which possess receptors for certain components of the complement system, and by **polymorphonuclear neutrophils (PMN),** for which activated complement components are chemotactic. The serum concentration of certain proteins, called **acute-phase proteins,** increases during infection. One of these is **C-reactive protein (CRP),** so called because it binds to the C protein of pneumococci. This interaction activates the alternative complement pathway, which can then aid in eliminating the bacteria as described above.

Innate immunity against viruses, as opposed to bacteria, is implemented by natural killer NK cells and by **interferons.** NK cells are lymphocytes that are capable of binding to and killing virus-infected and tumor cells by a mechanism not yet understood (see Chapter 5). They are distinguishable from cytotoxic T lymphocytes (see below) on the basis of surface antigens and their failure to exhibit immunologic memory. NK cells are activated by interferons, which are also components of the innate immune system. Alpha and beta interferons (see Chapter 7) are produced by certain leukocytes and by virus-infected cells. Aside from their action on NK cells, interferons elevate the resistance of normal cells to viral infection and thus constitute a vital early defense mechanism against many viruses.

Adaptive Immunity

If the defenses provided by the innate immune system fail to fully prevent infection (or completely halt dissemination of nonliving immunogens), the adaptive immune response comes into

Table 3-1. Comparison of innate and adaptive immunity.

Property	Innate Immunity	Adaptive Immunity
Physical barriers	Skin and mucous membranes	None
Soluble factors	Enzymes (eg lysozyme and complement) Acute-phase proteins (eg CRP) Alpha and beta interferons	Antibodies Lymphokines
Cells	Macrophages, PMN, eosinophils, NK cells	T and B lymphocytes
Self-nonself discrimination	Yes	Yes
Specificity	No	Yes
Memory	No	Yes

play. Adaptive immunity is a more recent evolutionary development (see Chapter 2) than innate immunity and is distinguished by a remarkable specificity for the offending immunogen (see Chapter 8) and by its memory (ie, intensified responses upon subsequent encounters with the same or closely related immunogens). In this adaptive immune response, the foreign agent or immunogen triggers a chain of events that lead to the activation of lymphocytes and the production of antibodies and effector lymphocytes which are highly specific for the immunogen.

The principal players in adaptive immunity are **antigen-presenting cells (APC)**, thymus-derived lymphocytes (T cells), and bone marrow–derived lymphocytes (B cells). T cells produce soluble molecules with many effects, and B cells eventually result in antibody formation. The roles of these important lymphocytes are described here, but a more detailed account of their properties is given in Chapters 2 and 5.

The Adaptive Immune Response

The adaptive immune response is triggered by the presence of a foreign agent that escapes early elimination by the innate immune system. A "grand scheme," necessarily somewhat oversimplified, of the major events in the adaptive immune response is shown in Figure 3–1. These events are considered in turn.

IMMUNOGENS & ANTIGENS

This subject is covered thoroughly in Chapter 8. Briefly, an **immunogen** is a molecule that can induce an immune response in a particular host. The term "antigen," which is frequently used interchangeably with immunogen, actually refers to the ability of a molecule to react with the products of adaptive immunity, particularly antibodies, not necessarily to its ability to induce their formation. Thus, although all immunogens are also antigens, the converse is not true.

In general, the more complex the foreign agent, the more distinct are the immunogens it contains. Thus, a single foreign molecule is a single immunogen, but foreign cells such as bacteria are composed of many immunogens, each of which may elicit a unique immune response. The foreign agent in Figure 3–1 is a virus, which usually contains several immunogenic proteins. Most immunogens are composed largely or exclusively of protein (lipoproteins, glycoproteins, nucleoproteins). Pure carbohydrates may be immunogenic, but they fall into a special class of immunogens called **T cell-independent antigens** (see Chapter 8).

The fate of an immunogen that penetrates the physical barriers of the innate immune system depends partially on its route of entry. In general, an immunogen may take 3 routes. If the immunogen enters the bloodstream, it is carried to the spleen, which becomes the principal site of the immune response. If the immunogen remains localized in the skin, a local inflammatory response ensues and it travels through afferent lymphatic channels to regional lymph nodes draining the affected area, which then serve as the major site of the immune response. Finally, the immunogen may enter the mucosal immune system in the respiratory or gastrointestinal tract (see Chapter 15), both of which have lymphoid tissue (tonsils and Peyer's patches) for mounting an immune response. Antibodies produced there are deposited locally, but immune lymphocytes from those organs may be transported via the thoracic duct to other lymphoid organs, thereby spreading the response systemically. There is always some trafficking of lymphocytes via the blood and lymphatics, so although a response may be initiated locally, it eventually spreads throughout the body (see Chapter 2).

Antigen Processing & Presentation

Responses to most immunogens, with the possible exception of T cell-independent antigens (see Chapter 8), require processing of the immunogen by APC. The reason for this is that T cells, which are the principal orchestrators and regulators of the immune response, ordinarily recognize immunogens only together with major histocompatibility complex (MHC) antigens (see Chapter 4) on the surfaces of other cells. Thus, the first steps in the immune response following entry of the im-

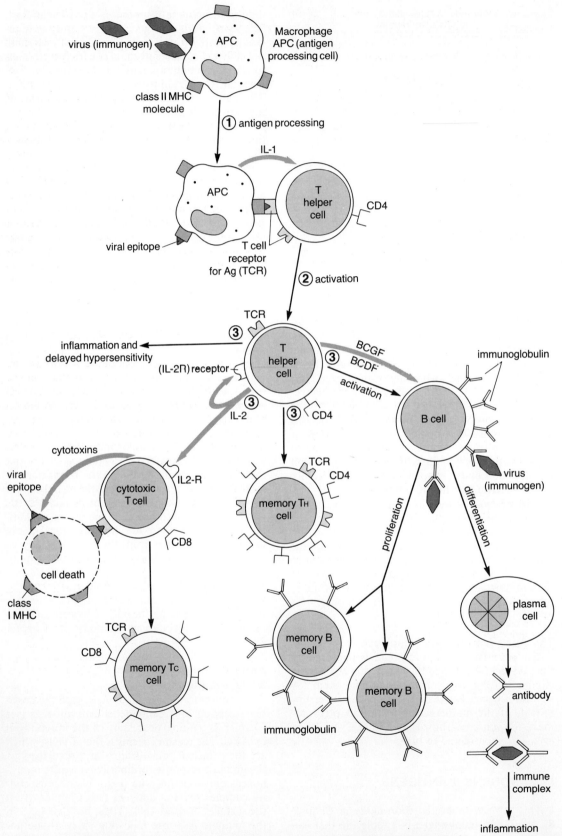

Figure 3-1. Grand scheme of adaptive immune system (see text for explanation)

munogen involve capture and processing of the immunogen by APC and presentation of a processed form of the immunogen in association with class II MHC molecules to a subset of T cells called **helper T (T**H**) cells** (Table 3–2).

Although all somatic cells express class I MHC proteins, relatively few cell types express class II proteins. Those that do include macrophages, dendritic cells in lymphoid tissue, Langerhans cells in the skin, Kupffer's cells in the liver, and microglial cells in central nervous system tissue, all of which are very similar and may have a common precursor. B cells, the precursors of antibody-secreting cells (plasma cells), also express class II MHC molecules. The common denominator among these diverse cells is the expression of class II antigens and hence their role as APC (Table 3–2).

These cells phagocytose or pinocytose the immunogen, which is then modified in endocytic vacuoles in the cytoplasm. The precise steps of antigen processing have not been definitively established and may range from denaturation and unfolding to proteolysis. If an agent undergoes proteolysis, fragments of the original immunogen (epitopes; see Chapter 8) become noncovalently associated with class II molecules and the complex is transported to the cell surface, where it is then accessible to the T cell (Fig 3–2). Only a limited number of the peptide fragments from a protein antigen are capable of associating with class II molecules to form an immunogenic complex. Such peptides are termed **immunogenic epitopes** (see Chapter 8). It is believed that all immunogenic epitopes become bound to a single binding site on the class II molecule.

Although it is unexpected, B cells, the precursors of antibody-secreting cells, can also present antigen to T cells. B cells not only express class II proteins but also have a very efficient capture mechanism for specific antigens through their immunoglobulin antigen receptors (see Chapter 5).

B cells alone are relatively poor activators of resting or virgin T cells when presenting antigens, possibly because such T cells require auxiliary activating factors, such as interleukins, that B cells fail to provide. However, B cells require only about one-thousandth as much immunogen as do macrophages for activating memory T cells. Because B cells specific for a particular immunogen are rare in an unimmunized individual and virgin T cells do not respond well to antigen presented by B cells, it is believed that macrophages probably play the predominant role as APCs in the initial, or primary, immune response, whereas B cells may dominate in the memory, or secondary, response (see below).

ACTIVATION OF HELPER T CELLS

TH cells are the principal orchestrators of the immune response because they are needed for the activation of the major effector cells in the response, ie, cytotoxic T (TC) cells and antibody-producing B cells. The activation of TH cells occurs early in the immune pathway (Fig 3–1) and requires at least 2 signals. One signal is provided by the binding of the T cell antigen receptor to the class II MHC-antigen complex on the APC. The second signal derives from interleukin-1 (IL-1), a soluble protein produced by the APC. Macro-

Table 3–2. Cells of the acquired immune system.

Cell Type	Antigen-Specific	Immunologic Functions	Distribution	Selected Markers
Antigen-presenting cells				
Macrophages	No		Wide	Class II MHC molecules
Dendritic cells	No		Lymphoid tissues	Class II MHC molecules
Langerhans cells	No		Skin	Class II MHC molecules
Kupffer's cells	No	Process and present	Liver	Class II MHC molecules
Microglial cells	No	antigen to T cells	Central nervous system	Class II MHC molecules
B lymphocytes	Yes		Wide	Class II MHC molecules and surface immunoglobulin
T lymphocytes				
TH cells	Yes	Perform positive regulation	Wide	CD4
TC cells	Yes	Kill cells bearing foreign antigens	Wide	CD8
TS cells	Yes	Perform negative regulation	Wide	CD8
B lymphocytes	Yes	Produce antibody	Wide	Surface immunoglobulin

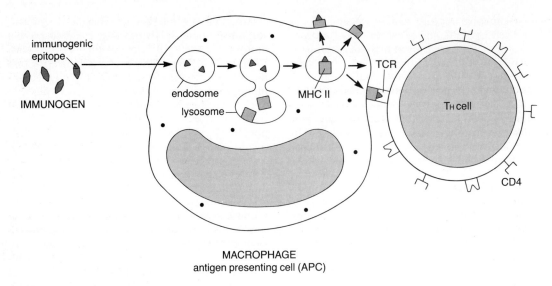

Figure 3-2. Uptake and processing of immunogen by APC. Fragmentation of the immunogen takes place in an acidic compartment (produced by fusion of endosome with lysosome), and the immunogenic epitope becomes associated with class II MHC molecules. This complex is transported to the cell surface, where it is accessible to TH cells specific for that particular epitope-class II combination. An immunogen usually has more than one epitope, each of which may be processed and presented in this manner. The initial contact between processed antigen and class II MHC is depicted as occurring in the endosome, but that is uncertain.

phages produce much more IL-1 than B cells do, which may account for their ability to activate virgin T cells.

Together, the 2 signals induce the expression of receptors for another lymphokine, IL-2, as well as the production of a battery of cell growth and differentiation factors (cytokines) that are important for triggering B cells and activating macrophages (Fig 3–3). IL-2 induces the growth of cells expressing IL-2 receptors, including the very same TH cells that produce it (autocatalytic effect) and TC cells that do not ordinarily produce it. Thus, the main function of IL-2 is to amplify the response initiated by contact of TH cells with APCs.

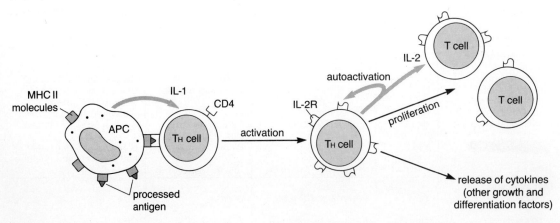

Figure 3-3. TH cell activation. The APC presents an epitope in the context of class II molecules in the TH cell. This interaction constitutes one of the 2 essential activating signals for the TH cell. The other is provided by IL-1 produced by the APC. The activated TH cell expresses IL-2 receptors and produces IL-2, which triggers growth of the TH cell and production of other lymphokines important in the activation of other cell types.

ACTIVATION OF CYTOTOXIC T CELLS

The activated TH cell is the key to further steps along the immune pathway, notably the triggering of TC cells, whose major function is the killing of cells that express foreign or nonself antigens, and B cells, which differentiate into antibody-producing plasma cells. The TC cell can be distinguished from the TH cell by the presence of CD8 rather than CD4 (Table 3–2) and by its recognition of foreign antigen in the context of class I rather than class II MHC molecules. CD4 and CD8 proteins on T cells have been shown to bind to class II and class I molecules, respectively, on APC, and thereby these CD molecules participate in T cell recognition of antigen-MHC complexes.

TC cells, like TH cells, also require 2 activating signals. One is provided by interaction of the T cell antigen receptors with a complex of a foreign epitope and class I MHC on the target cell; these cells may be virus-infected or tumor cells or foreign tissue grafts. The second signal is furnished by IL-2 produced by the activated TH cell. The activated TC cell then releases cytotoxins that kill the target cell (Fig 3–4).

ACTIVATION OF B CELLS

Antibody production requires both the activation of B lymphocytes and their differentiation into antibody-producing plasma cells. The sequence of events in this process can be visualized as follows. While the TH cell is being activated as described above, relevant B cells have also been engaging immunogen through their antigen receptors, which are membrane-bound forms of the antibodies they will later secrete (see Chapters 5 and 9). Antigen binding is followed by endocytosis of the antigen-receptor complex, which appears to

furnish an activating signal; however, this is insufficient for full activation of B cells, which require additional signals from TH cells. These additional signals are lymphokines (BCGF and BCDF; see below) that are released by activated TH cells and have a short radius of activity. Thus, the relevant T and B cells must be in close proximity to participate in an immune response.

Because B cells can also function as APC, they process endocytosed antigen and transport immunogenic epitopes complexed with class II molecules to their surface. These complexes then activate T cells or induce the formation of memory T cells. Effector T cells can then deliver the appropriate lymphokines at close range, which affects other T and B cells and probably nonlymphoid cells as well (Fig 3–5).

B Cell-Stimulating Lymphokines

At least 2 lymphokines produced by TH cells are needed for growth and differentiation of B cells. The first lymphokine is descriptively called **B cell growth factor** (BCGF), which, in concert with antigen, stimulates proliferation of B cells. The second lymphokine, termed **B cell differentiation factor** (BCDF), induces activated B cells to differentiate into antibody-secreting plasma cells. Thus, the complete process of B cell activation and differentiation requires at least 3 signals, one provided by the immunogen and at least 2 furnished by TH cells. Other TH products may also be involved; the process has not yet been fully delineated.

A fraction of activated B cells proliferate but do not differentiate into plasma cells, possibly because they receive insufficient BCDF. Such B cells form a pool of **memory cells,** which can respond to subsequent encounters with the relevant immunogen. TH cells are also long-lived, providing memory in the T cell compartment of the immune system.

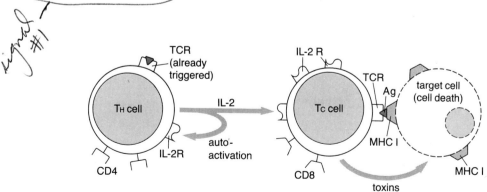

Figure 3-4. Activation of TC cell by antigen. A complex of MHC class I and processed antigenic epitope together with IL-2 produced by TH cells triggers activation in TC. The TC activated by the 2 signals secretes toxins that kill the target cell.

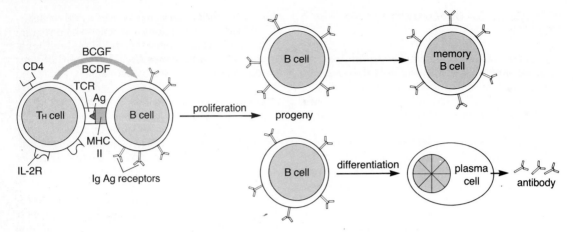

Figure 3–5. B cell–activation pathway. Signals from antigen and TH cells induce growth and differentiation of B cells. Some B cells progress to the plasma cell stage and secrete antibody, while others form a pool of memory B cells.

KINETICS OF THE IMMUNE RESPONSE

An individual's first encounter with a particular immunogen is called a **priming event** and leads to a relatively weak, short-lived antibody response designated the **primary immune response** (Fig 3–6). The response is divisible into several phases.

The **lag** or **latent phase** is the time between the contact with the immunogen and the detection of antibodies in the circulation, which averages about 1 week in humans. During this period, activation of T and B lymphocytes is taking place. The **exponential phase** marks a rapid increase in the quantity of antibodies in the circulation. Antibodies are secreted by plasma cells, the terminal phase of the pathway depicted in Figure 3–1. After an interval during which the antibody level remains relatively constant because synthesis and degradation are occurring at approximately equal rates (**steady-state phase**), the antibody level gradually declines (**declining phase**) as synthesis of new antibody wanes. The regulatory mechanisms involved in turning off the antibody response are considered below.

Subsequent encounters with the same immunogen lead to responses that are qualitatively similar to the primary response but manifest marked

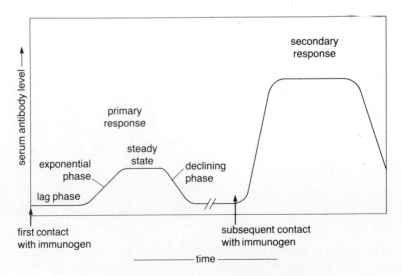

Figure 3–6. Primary and secondary immune responses.

but is slope of phase lift? decline phase lift? YES, less than in 1°

quantitative differences (Fig 3–6). In the **secondary** or **anamnestic response,** the lag period is shortened, and antibody levels rise more rapidly to a much higher steady-state level (steeper slope), remaining detectable in serum for much longer periods. Memory T and B cells generated during the primary response are responsible for the more rapid kinetics and greater intensity and duration of secondary responses; this explains why booster injections of vaccines are so efficacious.

CLONAL SELECTION

The properties of the immune response are fully consistent with the theory of clonal selection proposed by Sir Macfarlane Burnet and for which he was awarded the Nobel Prize in medicine in 1960. The clonal selection theory postulates that virgin lymphocytes express antigen receptors before ever encountering antigen. Thus, the immune cell population is composed of a very large number of individual clones of lymphocytes, each with its own antigen receptor, permitting it to recognize and respond to only a very small part of the total universe of antigenic epitopes. The whole library of lymphocyte clones, however, is sufficiently diverse to deal with any potential immunogen. Antigen, then, serves as a selective agent in the immune response, recruiting only clones that recognize its epitopes, which are then selectively expanded without affecting the rest of the lymphoid population. Thus, primary and secondary responses are strictly specific for the provoking immunogen, and the kinetic differences between them are explicable in terms of the antigen-specific clones expanded during the primary response.

The clonal selection theory further proposes that immature lymphocytes which contact antigen are somehow eliminated predominantly in the embryonic thymus, whereas mature lymphocytes are responsive to their antigens. This aspect of the theory can account for self-nonself discrimination, because clones reactive with self antigens (autoreactive lymphocytes) would contact antigen early in development and be aborted. The basic tenets of clonal selection have been extensively confirmed experimentally and are now firmly established.

MECHANISMS OF ANTIGEN ELIMINATION

The ultimate function of the immune system is to seek and destroy alien substances in the body. This is accomplished in several different ways.

One, described above, is the direct killing of target cells expressing foreign antigens by activated Tc cells via elaboration of cytotoxins. Antibodies perform the task in a variety of ways, the most important of which are discussed below.

Toxin Neutralization

Antibodies specific for bacterial toxins or the venom of insects or snakes bind these antigenic toxins, thus causing inactivation and promoting elimination of the antigen-antibody complexes via the reticuloendothelial system. Because of their effectiveness, antibodies against toxins and venom are used to passively protect nonimmune individuals who have been exposed and are consequently at risk.

Virus Neutralization

Antibodies specific for epitopes on the surface of a virus may block the attachment of the virus to target cells, particularly if the antibodies bind at or close to the site of attachment on the virus. This mechanism is probably less important in defense against viral infection than the killing of virus-infected target cells by Tc cells.

Opsonization of Bacteria

Antibodies can coat bacteria, thereby promoting their clearance by macrophages, which have receptors for certain classes of antibodies (see Chapter 9). Binding to macrophages via these receptors facilitates phagocytosis of the coated antigen. The antibody in this situation is called an **opsonin.**

Activation of Complement

Certain classes of antibodies can activate the complement cascade when they are complexed with antigen (see Chapter 9). If the epitope is on the surface of a cell, such as a bacterium, activated complement can lyse the cell through its enzymatic activity (see Chapter 14). Some of the components of complement also have opsonic activity. They bind to the antigen-antibody complex and subsequently to receptors on macrophages, further facilitating phagocytosis of the coated antigen. Other components of activated complement are chemotactic for phagocytic neutrophils. Still other components cause the release of histamine by mast cells or basophils. The responses mediated by the complement system are complex and are involved in the induction of inflammation, which is itself a very important defense mechanism (see Chapters 11 and 12). Other enzyme systems that interact with the immune system in inflammation include the kinin system, the clotting system, and the fibrinolytic system (see Chapter 11).

receptors on NK cell (all Robbers)?
NK cell
NK & FcR

Antibody-Dependent Cellular Cytotoxicity (ADCC)

The major class of antibodies, IgG (see Chapter 9) binds to a subclass of NK cells that expresses receptors for it. NK cells armed with antibody bind to the target cell, be it a bacterium or a tumor cell, and kill it with cytotoxins. This NK cell can be distinguished from the Tc cell by the fact that it does not express the CD8 marker and requires antibody for its activity.

INFLAMMATION & DELAYED HYPERSENSITIVITY

Another inflammatory response, **delayed-type hypersensitivity (DTH),** is mediated by a subset of TH cells. These T cells, following activation by APC, release lymphokines that attract and activate macrophages, setting up an inflammatory reaction. The response is called "delayed" because inflammatory responses mediated by antibody become apparent within minutes or hours, whereas DTH takes 24–48 hours to appear. The two are also distinguished by the nature of the cellular infiltrate: antibody complement-mediated inflammation features predominantly PMN, whereas DTH features mononuclear cells.

It is noteworthy that inflammatory responses have a "Jekyll-and-Hyde" characteristic. In addition to their value for the elimination of infectious agents, inflammatory responses may be mounted against normally innocuous environmental substances and thereby cause disease. Allergic reactions to poison oak and poison ivy are typical DTH reactions, whereas inflammatory responses to grasses, pollens, drugs, and antibiotics are more commonly triggered by antibodies.

REGULATION OF THE IMMUNE RESPONSE

We have now traced the adaptive immune response from its initiation by entry of the immunogen to the induction of effector functions of cellular and antibody immunity. After the elimination of the offending immunogen, the response is damped, thereby preventing uncontrolled activation of lymphocytes and unregulated production of antibody.

One regulatory mechanism is reflected by the declining phase of the antibody response (Fig 3–6). Negative regulatory mechanisms constrain the response, but positive regulation that heightens the response exists as well. The TH cell is the cardinal positive regulatory element in the immune response. Imbalances in the exquisitely tuned immune regulatory system may occur by virtue of genetic defects, infectious or neoplastic disease, or hormonal imbalance and may lead to immune deficiencies or to a loss of self-nonself discrimination and autoimmunity. For example, acquired immunodeficiency syndrome (AIDS) results from depletion of the TH cell population by infection with human immunodeficiency virus (HIV), which cripples an individual's ability to mount immune responses, leading to susceptibility to normally innocuous microorganisms (opportunistic infection) and possibly to certain cancers, the most common of which is Kaposi's sarcoma. On the other hand, myasthenia gravis is an autoimmune disease caused by inappropriate production of antibodies reactive with the acetylcholine receptor, which blocks transmission of nerve impulses.

Major Regulatory Influences on the Immune Response

Many factors influence the intensity of the immune response. The dose and immunogenic potency of the antigen, its route of entry, and the presence or absence of adjuvants when vaccines are administered (see Chapter 8) all play a role in the magnitude and duration of the response. However, once the response is under way, there are 3 tightly interwoven major mechanisms that limit its growth and longevity (Fig 3–7).

A. Antibody: The production of antibody results in **feedback inhibition** of further production of the same antibody. This feedback inhibition may operate in several ways. The antibody could simply remove residual antigen, thus limiting the immunogenic stimulus. Levels of circulating antigen decline sharply following the appearance of antibodies in the circulation, as would be expected. However, antibodies may also limit the response through their role in **idiotypic regulatory circuits,** as described below.

B. Idiotype-Specific Regulation: Idiotypes are antigenic epitopes located in the antigen-binding regions of antibody molecules (see Chapter 9). An individual is believed to have on the order of 10^7 B cell clones, each genetically programmed to make its antibody possessing a unique profile of idiotypic epitopes (**idiotopes**). Upon immunogenic stimulation, the number of clones capable of recognizing epitopes on the antigen is expanded, as described above, and so the level of their particular idiotopes is elevated. This perturbation in the steady-state level of these idiotopes serves as an immunogenic stimulus, inducing anti-idiotype antibody responses. Therefore, despite being self antigens, idiotypes are apparently immunogenic when their level is increased, although the basis for this apparent contradiction of self tolerance is not clearly understood. It may be due to the min-

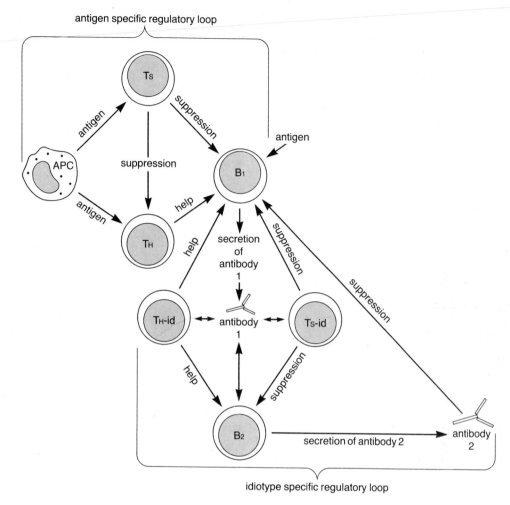

antigen specific regulatory loop

idiotype specific regulatory loop

Figure 3-7. Regulatory circuits in the adaptive immune response involving suppressor Ts cells and idiotypes. The original antigen activates TH and Ts cells, which exert opposing influences on specific B cells (B₁). B₁ cells secrete antibody-1, which stimulates anti-idiotypic responses by TH (TH-id), Ts (Ts-id), and B₂ cells. Antibody-2 expresses idiotypes that may stimulate anti-id responses, and so on along the network.

ute quantity of any particular idiotype in the virgin lymphocyte population, which could escape notice as a "self-marker" during lymphocyte development.

Anti-idiotype antibodies have been shown to appear in the circulation of animals during the declining phase of a number of carefully studied immune responses; this suggests that they may be instrumental in turning off the response (Fig 3-7). It is also conceivable that reaction of anti-idiotype antibody with B cell (or T cell) antigen receptors serves as an immunogenic signal for the lymphocyte in much the same way that ordinary immunogens do. However, the appearance of anti-idiotype antibody in the course of a normal immune response has not been found to trigger a resurgence of antibody to the original immunogen.

If antibodies against exogenous immunogens have sets of idiotopes, anti-idiotype antibodies should have their own idiotopes and consequently induce anti-anti-idiotype responses, sometimes referred to as antibody-3 (anti-idiotype being antibody-2; Fig 3-7). These theoretic considerations led Nobel laureate Niels Jerne to propose that the lymphoid system is a closed interacting network of cells that communicate via idiotype–anti-idiotype recognition. In other words, every lymphocyte expresses idiotypes that will be recognized by the antigen receptors of other lymphocytes. Jerne further proposed that every possible epitope is represented in the total population of more than 10^7 idiotopes. He called idiotopes "internal images" of epitopes because they are structural parts of the antibody molecules themselves but resemble the epitopes of molecules outside the immune system (ie, on bacteria and viruses).

Some features of Jerne's idiotype network theory have been confirmed experimentally. As already mentioned, anti-idiotype antibodies arise normally during the course of immune responses, and in some instances it has been demonstrated that at least a fraction of the anti-idiotype antibody resembles the epitope that induced the original antibody response. It has been difficult to detect the successive waves of anti-idiotypes beyond antibody-3, possibly because the immunogenic signals diminish with increasing time from the original stimulus. Even though it has not been possible to verify the network in all details, it is believed to play an important role in immune regulation.

C. Suppressor T Cells: Another type of T cell we have not previously considered is able to suppress the activity of TH cells and may also act directly on B cells. These suppressor T cells (Ts cells) express CD8, which distinguishes them from CD4 TH cells. Cytotoxic T cells also express CD8, but Ts cells do not appear to exert cytotoxic activity; they seem to be a distinct subset of T cells. Ts cells may be specific for the epitopes of exogenous antigens or for idiotype markers on the antigen receptors of B cells (antibodies) or T cells (Fig 3–7).

The mechanism of action of Ts cells is less clear than their existence, but they have been reported to secrete factors that can suppress the activities of TH and B cells. Thus, Ts cells and idiotypic regulation interface with each other in the complex control of the immune response, as depicted simplistically in Figure 3–7.

It can readily be visualized that such complex, delicately balanced, interacting regulatory networks may malfunction at any of a number of points. As mentioned above, a number of diseases have been associated, with varying degrees of certainty, with defects in these regulatory networks. Such diseases are treated in depth later in this volume and collectively represent one of the most intensive areas of biomedical research.

SUMMARY

There are 2 levels of protection against infection. Innate or natural immunity is present from birth, lacks specificity and memory, and consists of physical barriers such as skin and mucous membranes, certain enzymes, and phagocytic cells. Acquired or adaptive immunity is specific for the invading antigen, exhibits memory, and is based on the responses of T and B lymphocytes.

In the adaptive immune response, antigen is initially taken up and processed by APC, which express fragments of it called immunogenic epitopes complexed with class II MHC molecules to TH cells; these recognize features of both the epitope and the class II molecule.

Activated TH cells regulate the activities of other lymphocytes in a positive fashion through the secretion of soluble factors called lymphokines. One of these, IL-2, is an activating signal for Tc cells, which recognize antigens in the context of class I MHC molecules on target cells.

TH cells also furnish growth and differentiation signals to B cells, which then differentiate into antibody-secreting plasma cells.

The basis for memory in the immune response is the generation of antigen-specific TH and B cells following initial exposure to an antigen in the primary response. These memory cells are prepared to make amplified responses upon subsequent encounters with the same antigen in secondary, or anamnestic, responses.

Tc cells and antibodies use a variety of mechanisms to eliminate foreign antigens, some of which are integrally linked to inflammation.

The regulation of immune responses is accomplished through complex interacting networks involving antibody feedback, Ts cells, and idiotype-anti-idiotype interactions.

REFERENCES

Asherson GL, Colizzi V, Zembala M: An overview of T-suppressor cell circuits. *Annu Rev Immunol* 1986;**4**:37.

Goodman JW, Sercarz EE: The complexity of structures involved in T cell activation. *Annu Rev Immunol* 1983;**1**:465.

Kishimoto T, Hirano T: Molecular regulation of B lymphocyte response. *Annu Rev Immunol* 1988; **6**:485.

Singer A, Hodes RJ: Mechanisms of T-cell B-cell interaction. *Annu Rev Immunol* 1983;**1**:211.

von Boehmer H: The developmental biology of T lymphocytes. *Annu Rev Immunol* 1988;**6**:309.

The Human Major Histocompatibility Human Leukocyte Antigen (HLA) Complex

4

Benjamin D. Schwartz, MD, PhD

IMMUNE SYSTEM MECHANISMS

The immune system has evolved to protect the individual from a hostile environment containing innumerable viruses, bacteria, fungi, worms, and other parasites. To do so effectively, the immune system must distinguish between antigens against which an immune response would be beneficial and those against which it would be harmful. In other words, the immune system must discriminate "nonself" from "self." This crucial discrimination is achieved via the molecules of the major histocompatibility complex (MHC).

It now appears that every antigen, both nonself and self, is recognized by T cells only in conjunction with MHC molecules. Thus, CD4 (generally helper) T cells recognize antigens in conjunction with class II MHC molecules, whereas CD8 (generally cytotoxic) T cells recognize antigens in the context of class I MHC molecules (see below).

During embryogenesis, a process of T cell "education" occurs in the thymus, whereby T cells recognizing self antigens in the context of MHC molecules are eliminated and T cells potentially recognizing foreign antigens in the context of the individual's own MHC molecules are selected for survival. Breakdown in the elimination of self-recognition can result in autoimmune disease, whereas failure to recognize foreign antigens can lead to immunodeficiency with overwhelming infections and possibly uncontrolled spread of tumors.

The MHC Molecules

The MHC molecules are part of the immunoglobulin "supergene" family and appear to have evolved from the same primordial gene as immunoglobulin and T cell receptor molecules. Most probably as a result of repeated duplication and mutations of this primordial MHC gene during evolution, the genes encoding the MHC molecules are found clustered into a relatively small chromosomal region. It is this cluster of genes that constitutes the MHC.

The Human MHC

The human MHC was discovered in the mid-1950s, when leukoagglutinating antibodies were first found in the sera of both multiply transfused patients and 20–30% of multiparous women. Each antiserum gave a positive reaction with the cells of some but not all individuals, and different antisera reacted with the cells of different but overlapping populations of individuals. This pattern suggested that these antisera were detecting alloantigens (ie, antigens present on the cells of some individuals of a given species) that were the products of at least one polymorphic genetic locus.

Human Leukocyte Antigens (HLA Antigens)

The importance of matching these antigens for success in organ transplantation was soon realized and provided an important impetus for studying the genes that determine **human leukocyte antigens (HLA antigens).** Over the past 2 decades, the role played by the HLA complex in the regulation of human immune responses has become widely appreciated. By 1973, certain HLA antigens were found to be associated with specific diseases in a high proportion of cases. Together, these findings provided a second impetus for the study of the HLA complex.

The initial delineation of the HLA system resulted from cytotoxicity testing for identification of specific HLA antigens in this system, combined with the use of computers to codify reaction patterns of literally thousands of anti-HLA alloantisera. Recently, recombinant DNA methods have helped to delineate HLA genes and the amino acid sequence of many HLA molecules. Very recently, the elucidation of the crystal structure of an HLA molecule has provided insight into how HLA molecules function in an immune response. An international workshop now meets every 2–3 years to update the description of the organization and nomenclature of the HLA complex.

EVOLUTIONARY ORIGINS OF THE HLA COMPLEX

The origins of the MHC can be traced to the advanced invertebrates. It has been proposed that in these lower organisms, a recognition system arose that allowed individuals to distinguish self from nonself, especially in regard to other individuals of the species. Presumably, this recognition system prevented fusion of members of the species, which, in turn, promoted genetic diversity and dissemination of the species over a wider habitat.

Evidence for such a recognition system can be observed, for example, in tunicates. If a colony of sea squirts, which is an example of advanced invertebrates, is divided in half, each half will grow independently. If brought back into contact, the 2 colonies fuse and grow again as a single colony. In contrast, if 2 unrelated colonies of sea squirts are brought into contact, they almost never fuse. Rather, the cells at the contact point die, and a barrier of necrotic material results that keeps the 2 colonies separate. Furthermore, if this experiment is repeated with many different unrelated colonies, the vast majority of such fusions fail, suggesting that this recognition system is highly polymorphic.

This ability to distinguish self from nonself—and subsequent graft rejection of nonself—becomes increasingly evident as the phylogenetic ladder is ascended (see Chapter 2). These processes are reminiscent of syngeneic (self) and allogeneic (foreign) recognition phenomena seen in mammals and suggest the premium that nature has placed on self-recognition. It is likely that this primitive recognition system has evolved into the modern immune system, with the MHC functioning as a central element.

STRUCTURE, TISSUE DISTRIBUTION, & FUNCTION OF HLA MOLECULES

HLA molecules and the genes that encode them fall into 3 categories: classes I, II, and III. Class I and class II HLA molecules are cell surface glycoproteins and are members of the immunoglobulin supergene family, as shown by amino acid homologies. (This family includes a wide variety of cell surface molecules including immunoglobulins, T cell receptors, CD4, and CD8.)

The class I and class II molecules are distinguishable on the basis of their structure, tissue distribution, and function (Table 4–1). The class I molecules, also termed the classic histocompatibility molecules, include the HLA-A, -B, and -C molecules. Class II molecules include HLA-DR, -DQ, and -DP molecules.

The class III molecules include the second and fourth (C2 and C4) components of the classic complement pathway and properdin factor B of the alternative pathway. The class III HLA molecules are soluble and do not act as transplantation antigens, nor do they present antigen to T cells. The location of complement genes within the HLA complex remains unexplained (see Chapter 14).

1. CLASS I HLA MOLECULES

Structure of Class I HLA Molecules

The HLA-A, -B, and -C molecules each consist of a 2-chain structure. The heavy or α chain (MW 44,000) is a polymorphic glycoprotein determined by genes in the HLA complex on chromosome 6 and is noncovalently linked to a nonpolymorphic MW 12,000 protein, β_2-microglobulin, determined by a gene on chromosome 15. A schematic picture of a class I molecule is shown in Figure 4–1.

The entire molecule is anchored in the cell membrane by the MW 44,000 α chain. The α chain contains 338 amino acid residues and can be divided into 3 regions. Starting at the N-terminal end of the molecule, these regions are an extracellular hydrophilic region (residues 1–281), a transmembrane hydrophobic region (residues 282–

Table 4–1. Comparison of class I and II HLA.

Properties	Class I	Class II
Antigens included	HLA-A, -B, -C	HLA-D, -DR, -DQ, -DP
Tissue distribution	Ubiquitous on virtually every cell	Restricted to immunocompetent cells, particularly B cells, and macrophages
Functions	Present processed antigenic fragment to CD8 T cells. Restrict cell mediated cytolysis of virus-infected cells.	Present processed antigenic fragment to CD4 T cells. Necessary for effective interaction among immunocompetent cells.

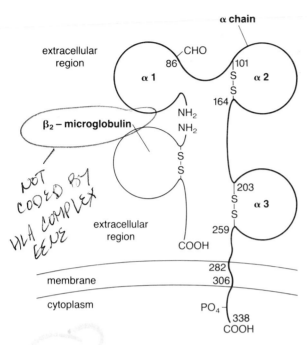

α chain

extracellular region

CHO

86

α 1

101

S–S

α 2

164

NH₂

β₂ – microglobulin

NH₂

S–S

NOT CODED BY HLA COMPLEX GENE

203

S–S

α 3

extracellular region

259

COOH

282

306

membrane

cytoplasm

PO₄

338

COOH

Figure 4-1. Schematic representation of a class I HLA molecule. The molecule consists of an MW 44,000 polymorphic transmembrane glycoprotein termed the α chain, which bears the antigenic determinant, in noncovalent association with an MW 12,000 nonpolymorphic protein termed β_2 microglobulin. The α chain has three extracellular domains termed α_1, α_2, and α_3. Abbreviations: NH₂, amino terminus; COOH, carboxy terminus; CHO, carbohydrate side chain; -SS-, disulfide bond; PO₄, phosphate. Numbers indicate amino acid residues where certain features are found (see text).

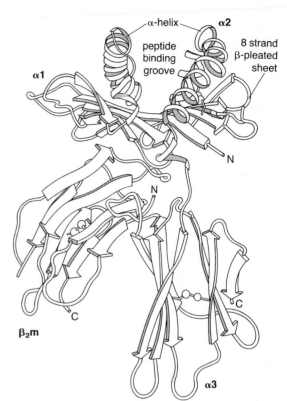

α-helix α2

peptide binding groove

8 strand β-pleated sheet

α1

N

N

β₂m

C

C

α3

Figure 4-2. The diagrammatic crystalline structure of a class I HLA molecule (side view). The extracellular part of the molecule is depicted in side view with the portion distal to the cell membrane on top and the portion proximal to the membrane at the bottom. The transmembrane and intracytoplasmic domains are not shown. The β_2 microglobulin (β_2m) and α_3 domain support an interactive structure formed by the α_1 and α_2 domains. This interactive structure consists of a β-pleated sheet platform supporting two α helixes, which form a cleft that binds antigenic peptide fragments. β strands are shown as broad arrows; α helices are shown as ribbonlike structures. N indicates the amino terminus; C indicates the carboxy end.

306), and an intracellular hydrophilic region (residues 307–338). The extracellular region is divided into 3 domains termed α1, α2, and α3, which are composed of amino acid residues 1–90, 91–180, and 181–271, respectively. Comparison of the amino acid sequences of several HLA antigens has shown that the vast majority of the HLA antigenic determinants reside in the α1 or α2 domain.

Structure-Function Relationships of Class I HLA Molecules

The structure-function relationships of the class I molecule were advanced with the elucidation of the crystalline structure of the HLA-A2 molecule. A side view of the molecule is shown in Figure 4-2. β_2-Microglobulin and the α3 domain have a β-pleated sheet* structure similar to that of an immunoglobulin domain and form the lower part of the molecule. The α1 and α2 domains each consist of 4 β strands and an α helix, and they form the upper portion of the molecule. The 8 β strands of

these 2 domains form a β-pleated sheet that acts as a platform supporting the 2 α helices. These α helices create a groove or cleft that serves as the antigen-binding site to accept a peptide fragment appropriately processed from a larger antigen. Most of the polymorphism of class I molecules is

*A β-pleated sheet is a structure in which sections of a polypeptide chain or different polypeptide chains are aligned side by side and held together by hydrogen bonds to form a relatively flat surface or "sheet." The pleating maximizes the number of hydrogen bonds possible between the polypeptide chains.

localized to these α helices and to the portion of the β-pleated sheet platform that forms the floor of this cleft. Thus, the antigen-binding site varies from one class I molecule to another, and a given class I molecule can bind only a limited number of peptide fragments.

It should be emphasized that although the antigen-binding site of a class I molecule displays some selectivity in the peptide fragments it binds, this site is quite different from an immunoglobulin antigen-binding site that displays exquisite specificity. The 2 α helices, together with the bound antigenic fragment, make up a ligand recognized by the T cell receptor on a class I restricted CD8 T cell. A top view of the class I molecule, as it would appear to the T cell receptor of a CD8 T lymphocyte, is shown in Figure 4–3.

Function of Class I HLA Molecules

Class I HLA molecules are present on all nucleated cells, which is appropriate for their physiologic role. For an antigen to be recognized by a CD8 (generally cytotoxic) T lymphocyte, the antigen must be recognized in combination with a class I molecule. This phenomenon is termed **HLA restriction.** When, for example, a virus infects a cell, certain of the viral antigens are metabolized to peptide fragments that are then bound by the class I molecule and presented to CD8 cytotoxic (killer) T cells. The antigen receptor of a given T lymphocyte will recognize a particular viral peptide only in the context of a particular class I HLA molecule. These receptors do not recognize the *particular* viral peptide bound by a *different*

class I molecule, a *different* viral peptide bound by the *particular* class I molecule, or the class I molecule *by itself*. Once recognition occurs, the cytotoxic T lymphocyte kills the target cell bearing the viral antigen. In the nonphysiologic condition of transplantation, it is the foreign class I molecules (with as yet unidentified bound peptides) that are recognized by the host CD8 T lymphocytes during graft rejection.

2. CLASS II HLA MOLECULES

The class II HLA-DR, -DP, and -DQ molecules are also 2-chain structures. Unlike the class I molecules, however, both chains are encoded by genes within the HLA complex.

Structure of Class II HLA Molecules

Each class II molecule is a heterodimer consisting of 2 glycoprotein chains, an α chain (MW 34,000) and a β chain (MW 29,000), in noncovalent association. Because the structures of all class II molecules are similar, the detailed structure of a class II HLA-DR molecule is described as the prototype.

The α chain and β chain are composed of 229 and 237 amino acids, respectively (Fig 4–4). Like the class I heavy chain, the α and β chains each consist of 3 regions: an extracellular hydrophilic region, a transmembrane hydrophobic region, and an intracellular hydrophilic region. The last 2 of these anchor the chains in the cell membrane.

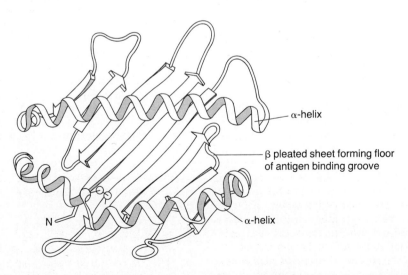

Figure 4–3. The diagrammatic crystalline structure of a class I HLA molecule (top view). The molecule is shown as the T cell receptor would see it. The antigen-binding site formed by the α helices (ribbonlike structures) and β-pleated strands (broad arrows) is shown. N indicates the amino terminus.

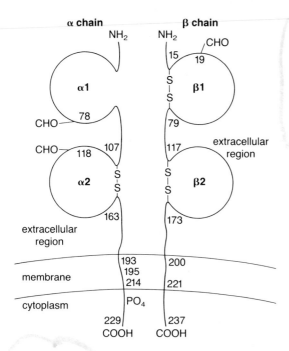

Figure 4-4. Schematic representation of an HLA-DR molecule. The molecule consists of an MW 34,000 glycoprotein (the α chain) in a noncovalent association with an MW 29,000 glycoprotein (the β chain). (Abbreviations and numbers are as in Fig 4–1.)

The extracellular hydrophilic region of the α chain contains 2 domains (residues 1–84 and 85–178), termed α1 and α2, respectively. The extracellular hydrophilic region of the β chain also contains 2 domains (residues 1–91 and 92–192), termed β1 and β2, respectively. The α2 and β2 domains both show significant homology to domains of immunoglobulin constant regions.

The structural features of the DQ and DP molecules are similar to those of DR. The DQ α and β chains have 234 and 229 amino acids, respectively, whereas the DP α and β chains each have 229 amino acids.

Although the crystalline structure of the class II molecules is not yet known, similarities between the structures of class I and class II molecules have allowed hypothetical models of class II structure to be generated by computer. It is thought that the class II α2 and β2 domains constitute the portion of the molecule proximal to the cell membrane that supports the portion distal to the cell membrane formed by the α1 and β1 domains. This latter portion is an interactive structure composed of 8 β strands and 2 α helices and is very similar to that created by the α1 and α2 domains of the class I molecule. The 2 α helices and a portion of the β-pleated sheet of the class II molecule also form a cleft or groove.

The polymorphism of the class II molecules is located in this cleft, resulting in different antigen-binding sites for each class II molecule. Thus, a given class II molecule can bind only a limited number of antigenic peptide fragments. This binding site of the class II molecule therefore shows some selectivity for antigens, but it lacks the fine specificity of an immunoglobulin antigen-binding site.

A top view of the class II α1 and β1 domains, as it would appear to a T cell receptor on a CD4 T lymphocyte, is shown in Figure 4–5. A processed antigenic peptide fragment can be accepted by the antigen-binding groove created by the 2 α helices and the platform. The α helices and antigenic peptide fragment then make up the ligand recognized by the receptor on CD4 T lymphocytes. Constraints on the recognition of the class II antigenic peptide complex by CD4 T lymphocytes are similar to those on the recognition of the class I antigenic peptide complex by CD8 T lymphocytes.

Function of Class II HLA Molecules

Class II HLA molecules have a limited cellular distribution. They are found chiefly on immunocompetent cells, B lymphocytes, antigen-presenting cells (macrophages and dendritic cells), and, in humans, activated T cells. In addition, cells that do not normally express class II molecules (such as resting T cells, endothelial cells, and thyroid cells) can be induced to express them. This abnormal expression has been postulated as an important element of one theory to account for HLA-disease associations (see below).

The function of class II molecules is to present processed antigenic peptide fragments to CD4 T lymphocytes during the initiation of immune responses. Just as CD8 T lymphocytes recognize peptide fragments only in the context of a class I molecule (see above), CD4 (generally helper) T lymphocytes recognize peptide fragments only in the context of class II molecules (Fig 4-6). In the nonphysiologic condition of bone marrow transplantation, class II molecules that have bound unidentified antigenic peptides on the host cells elicit a response from the engrafted donor T cells, resulting in a graft-versus-host reaction.

NOMENCLATURE & GENETIC ORGANIZATION OF THE HLA SYSTEM

Nomenclature & Genetic Loci

The nomenclature of the HLA system is devised by the HLA Nomenclature Committee of the World Health Organization. The entire histocompatibility complex is termed the HLA complex. It occupies a segment of approximately 3500 kilo-

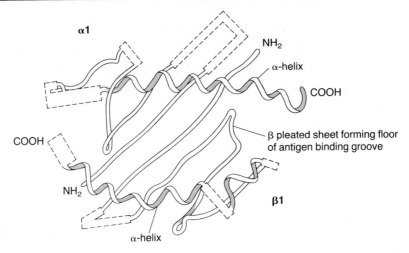

Figure 4–5. The crystalline structure of a class II HLA molecule (top view). The molecule is shown as it might appear to a T cell receptor. The antigen-binding site formed by the α chain α_1 domain and β chain β_1 domain consists of the β-pleated sheet platform (thin strands) supporting two α helices (ribbonlike structures) and is very similar to that of the class I molecule. NH_2 indicates the amino terminus; COOH indicates the carboxy end.

bases (kb) on the short arm of chromosome 6. Figure 4–7 schematically depicts the current map of the HLA complex, showing the genetic regions containing the various HLA loci. A **locus** is the position of a given gene on the chromosomes. The positions of the regions with respect to one another and to the centromere, as well as the approximate distances between regions, are shown in kilobases.

The HLA-A, -B, and -C gentic loci determine the class I molecules, which bear the class I antigens, and the HLA-DR, -DQ, and -DP genetic subregions, each of which contains several additional loci, determine the class II molecules, which bear the class II antigens (see above for an explanation of classes I and II).

Several other genetic regions are part of the HLA complex. The complement or HLA class III

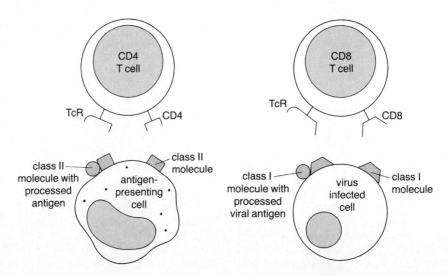

Figure 4–6. CD4 T cells (left) recognize processed antigen in the context of class II molecules through the T cell receptor and recognize an epitope on the nonpolymorphic region of the class II molecule through CD4. In contrast, CD8 T cells (right) recognize processed antigen in the context of class I molecules through their T cell receptor and an epitope on the nonpolymorphic region of the class I molecule through CD8.

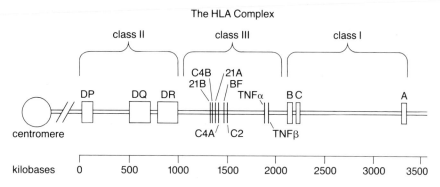

The HLA Complex

Figure 4–7. The HLA complex. The HLA complex is found on the short arm of chromosome 6. Locations of various MHC classes are indicated by brackets. The locations of these genes have been determined by molecular biologic techniques. Distances are given in kilobases. 21A and 21B are 21-hydroxylase A and B, respectively. BF is properidin factor, and BG is the alternative complement pathway. C2, C4A, and C4B are complement components. TNFα and TNFβ are tumor necrosis factor α and β, respectively. The DP, DQ, and DR subregions each contain multiple loci.

region has been mapped between the HLA-B and -DR regions and contains genes for the second and fourth components (C2 and C4) of the classic complement pathway and properdin factor B (BF) of the alternative pathway. The genes determining 21-hydroxylase A and B of the steroid biosynthetic pathway are also found here. The genes for tumor necrosis factors α and β (lymphocytotoxin) have recently been mapped between the complement and HLA-B regions.

The HLA system is extremely polymorphic, having multiple alternative forms or alleles of the gene at each known locus (Table 4–2). For example, there are at least 24 distinct alleles at the

Table 4–2. Complete listing of recognized HLA specificities.

A	B		C	D	DR	DQ	DP
A1	B5	B51(5)	Cw1	Dw1	DR1	DQw1	DPw1
A2	B7	Bw52(5)	Cw2	Dw2	DR2	DQw2	DPw2
A3	B8	Bw53	Cw3	Dw3	DR3	DQw3	DPw3
A9	B12	Bw54(w22)	Cw4	Dw4	DR4	DQw4	DPw4
A10	B13	Bw55(w22)	Cw5	Dw5	DR5	DQw5(w1)	DPw5
A11	B14	Bw56(w22)	Cw6	Dw6	DRw6	DQw6(w1)	DPw6
Aw19	B15	Bw57(17)	Cw7	Dw7	DR7	DQw7(w3)	
A23(9)	B16	Bw58(17)	Cw8	Dw8	DRw8	DQw8(w3)	
A24(9)	B17	Bw59	Cw9(w3)	Dw9	DR9	DQw9(w3)	
A25(10)	B18	Bw60(40)	Cw10(w3)	Dw10	DRw10		
A26(10)	B21	Bw61(40)	Cw11	Dw11(w7)	DRw11(5)		
A28	Bw22	Bw62(15)		Dw12	DRw12(5)		
A29(w19)	B27	Bw63(15)		Dw13	DRw13(w6)		
A30(w19)	B35	Bw64(14)		Dw14	DRw14(w6)		
A31(w19)	B37	Bw65(14)		Dw15	DRw15(2)		
A32(w19)	B38(16)	Bw67		Dw16	DRw16(2)		
Aw33(w19)	B39(16)	Bw71(w70)		Dw17(w7)	DRw17(3)		
Aw34(10)	B40	Bw70		Dw18(w6)	DRw18(3)		
Aw36	Bw41	Bw72(w70)		Dw19(w6)			
Aw43	Bw42	Bw73		Dw20	DRw52		
Aw66(10)	B44(12)	Bw75(15)		Dw21	DRw53		
Aw68(28)	B45(12)	Bw76(15)		Dw22			
Aw69(28)	Bw46	Bw77(15)		Dw23			
Aw74(w19)	Bw47			Dw24			
	Bw48	Bw4		Dw25			
	B49(21)	Bw6		Dw26			
	Bw50-(21)						

[1]See text for explanation. Numbers in parentheses indicate parent HLA antigen from which these antigens split (see text and Table 4–4).

HLA-A locus and at least 50 distinct alleles at the HLA-B locus. Each allele determines the structure of a glycoprotein chain. The products of the HLA-A, -B, -C, -DR, -DQ, and -DP alleles are all cell surface molecules that carry their own antigenic determinants, which are detectable by various in vitro histocompatibility tests (see Chapter 21).

The 7 groups of antigens officially recognized by the HLA Nomenclature Committee are HLA-A, -B, -C, -D, -DR, -DQ, and -DP. These are designated by the locus (for class I) or subregion (for class II) determining the antigenic specificity and a number; thus, HLA-A1 is the number 1 specificity determined by a gene at the HLA-A locus, and HLA-DR3 is the number 3 specificity determined by the HLA-DR subregion. Antigens that have not yet been officially recognized are designated by a "w" (for "workshop") placed before the number, eg, HLA-DRw1. Official recognition results in the elimination of the "w," eg, HLA-DR1. The entire listing of officially and tentatively recognized HLA-A, -B, -C, -D, -DR, -DQ, and -DP antigens is presented in Table 4–2.

HLA Public & Private Antigens

HLA antigens found on a single molecule (and no other) are termed **HLA private antigens.** In contrast, **HLA public antigens** are determinants common to several HLA molecules each of which additionally bears a distinct HLA private antigen. HLA-Bw4 and -Bw6 are the best-known examples of HLA public antigens, and one or the other is found on every molecule determined by HLA-B alleles. The distribution of the HLA-Bw4 and -BW6 public antigens on HLA-B molecules bearing HLA-B private antigens is shown in Table 4–3.

Several HLA antigens initially thought to be single private antigens were later found to be a group of 2 or 3 closely related antigens, each of narrower specificity. These latter antigens are termed "splits" of the original broad-specificity

Table 4-4. Splits of HLA antigens.

Original Broad Specificities	Splits
A9	A23, A24
A10	A25, A26, Aw34, Aw66
Aw19	A29, A30, A31, A32, Aw33, Aw74
A28	Aw68, Aw69
B5	B51, Bw52
B12	B44, B45
B14	Bw64, Bw65
B15	Bw62, Bw63, Bw75, Bw76, Bw77
B16	B38, B39
B17	Bw57, Bw58
B21	B49, Bw50
B21	B49, Bw50
Bw22	Bw54, Bw55, Bw56
B40	Bw60, Bw61
Bw70	Bw71, Bw72
Cw3	Cw9, Cw10
DR2	DRw15, DRw16
DR3	DRw17, DRw18
DR5	DRw11, DRw12
DRw6	DRw13, DRw14
DQw1	DQw5, DQw6
DQw3	DQw7, DQw8, DQw9
Dw6	Dw18, Dw19
Dw7	Dw11, Dw17

antigens. Biochemical analysis has indicated that splits are, in fact, closely related structural variants. In Table 4–2, HLA antigens that are splits are followed in parentheses by their original broad antigen. Thus, for example, the terms HLA-A25(10) and -A26(10) indicate that HLA-A25 and -A26 are splits of HLA-A10. Conversely, HLA-A10 can be considered a public antigen on the HLA molecules bearing the private HLA-A25 and -A26 antigens. Table 4–4 lists the currently recognized splits of the broad-specificity antigens.

Conversely, HLA private antigens can be organized into groups based on apparent serologic cross-reactivity between members of the group. These groups are termed **cross-reactive groups (CREGs).** Thus, for example, the B7-CREG includes HLA-B7, -Bw22 (subsequently split into -Bw54, -Bw55, and -Bw56), -B27, -B40 (subsequently split into -Bw60 and -Bw61), and -Bw42. For at least 3 of the CREGs (B5-, B7-, and B15/B17-CREG), the basis for the cross-reactivity is a public HLA antigen common to all members of the CREG. It is assumed that the cross-reactivity between members of other CREGs will also be explained by the presence of public antigens.

Organization of the Class II Region

The organization of the class II region (also called the HLA-D region) has recently been clarified (Fig 4–8). It contains 3 distinct subregions, DR, DQ, and DP, each of which contains multiple

Table 4-3. Private B-locus antigens associated with the public HLA-Bw4 and HLA-Bw6 antigens.[1]

Bw4
B5, B13, B17, B27, B37 B38(16), B44(12), Bw47, B49(21), B51(5), Bw52(5), Bw53, Bw57(17), Bw58(17), Bw59, Bw63(15), Bw77(15)

Bw6
B7, B8, B14, B18, Bw22, B35, B39(16), B40, Bw41, Bw42, B45(12), Bw46, Bw48, Bw50(21), Bw54(22), Bw55(22), Bw56(22), Bw60(40), Bw61(40), Bw62(15), Bw64(14), Bw65(14), Bw67, Bw70, Bw71(w70), Bw72(w70), Bw73, Bw75(15), Bw76(15)

[1]Numbers in parentheses indicate parent HLA molecules from which these antigens split (see text and Table 4–4).

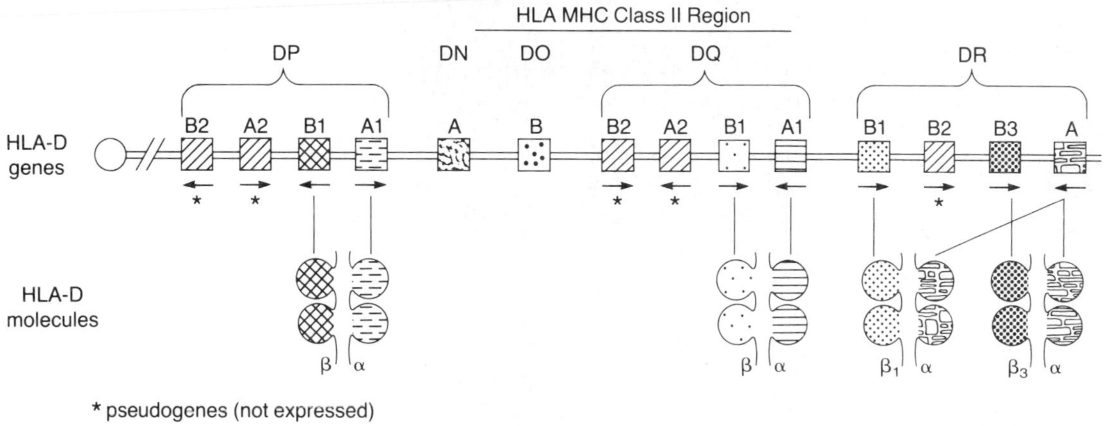

Figure 4–8. The HLA-D region and the molecules it encodes. The organization of the genes within each of the 3 defined subregions, DP, DQ, and DR is shown. Genes encoding α chains or genes with homologous nucleotide sequences are designated A, whereas genes encoding β chains or genes with homologous nucleotide sequences are designated B. The number of DRB genes depends on the DR type. DRB2, DQA2, DQB2, DPA2, and DPB2 genes are pseudogenes. The A gene of DN and the B gene of DO are not currently known to be transcribed in vivo. Pairs of class II genes that determine class II molecules are shown. The direction of transcription (5′ to 3′) is given under the genes (arrows). Most haplotypes determine four distinct class II molecules.

genetic loci. There are also 2 newly discovered subregions, termed DN (formerly DZ) and DO, each of which contains a single genetic locus. It should be recalled that each class II HLA molecule consists of 2 distinct chains, termed α and β, that form a heterodimer. Both the α and β chains of a given class II molecule are determined by genes within the corresponding subregion. For example, the HLA-DQα and -DQβ chains are both determined by genes within the DQ subregion (Fig 4–8).

Class II genes that determine α chains, as well as genes with related sequences, are designated by the letter "A," while class II genes that determine β chains, and genes with related sequences, are designated by the letter "B." If 2 or more A or B genes are present within a given subregion, they are designated by a number following the letter, eg, HLA-DRB1 and -DRB3, and HLA-DQA1 and -DQA2.

A. HLA-DR Subregion: The DR subregion contains a single HLA-DRA gene. The number of DRB genes varies with the DR type, but the most common configuration has 3 DRB genes, designated DRB1, DRB2, and DRB3 (or DRB4). (A given DR subregion will contain DRB3 or DRB4, but not both.) DRB2 is a pseudogene; ie, it is not expressed. The product of the DRA gene, the DRα chain, can combine individually with the products of both the DRB1 and the DRB3 (or DRB4) genes, the DRβ1 and the DRβ3 (or DRβ4) chains, to produce 2 distinct DR molecules,

DRαβ1 and DRαβ3 (or DRαβ4). The DRα chain is virtually nonpolymorphic, whereas the DRβ chains are highly polymorphic; thus, the DRβ chain is responsible for determining the DR antigen or DR type. The DRαβ1 molecules bear the DR specificities DR1–DRw18 (see Table 4–2), whereas the DRαβ3 molecules bear the DRw52 specificity and the DRαβ4 molecule bears DRw53. DRw52 and DRw53 are generally associated with particular subsets of DR specificities DR1–DRw18 (Table 4–5).

B. HLA-DQ Subregion: The DQ subregion contains 2 sets of genes: DQA1 and DQB1, and DQA2 and DQB2. DQA2 and DQB2 are pseudogenes. As products of the DQA1 and DQB1 genes, the DQα and DQβ chains combine to form the DQαβ molecule. In contrast to the DR molecules, both the DQα and β chains are polymorphic. However, it appears that the DQβ chain is the major determinant of the DQ type or antigen. The DQαβ molecules bear DQ specificities DQw1–DQw9. Because each individual has 2 DQ

Table 4–5. HLA-DRw52- and HLADRw53-associated DR antigens.

DRw52
DR3, DR5, DRw6, DRw8, DRw11(5), DRw12(5), DRw13(w6), DRw14(w6), DRw17(3), DRw18(3)
DRw53
DR4, DR7, DR9

subregions, one on each of the two chromosomes 6, and because DQ genes are codominantly expressed (see below), the fact that both the α and β chains of the DQ molecule are polymorphic allows individuals who are DQ heterozygotes (ie, who have 2 different DQA1 genes and 2 different DQB1 genes) to actually express 4 distinct DQ molecules by cis- and trans-pairing (Fig 4–9). cis-Pairing refers to the association of the α and β chains determined by genes on the same chromosome, and trans-pairing refers to the pairing of α and β chains encoded, respectively, by genes on opposite chromosomes. The molecules formed by trans-pairing are also called **hybrid molecules** and may be important in HLA-disease associations (see below).

C. HLA-DP Subregion: The HLA-DP subregion also contains 2 sets of genes: HLA-DPA1 and -DPB1, and HLA-DPA2 and -DPB2. HLA-DPA2 and -DPB2 are pseudogenes. The HLA-DPA1 and -DPB1 genes determine the DPα and β chains, respectively, which combine to form the DPαβ molecule. The DPα chain displays limited polymorphism (2 forms have been described to date), whereas the DPβ chain is highly polymorphic and appears to determine the DP antigen or type. Because both DPα and β chains display polymorphism, cis- and trans-pairing can occur, resulting in the expression of 4 distinct DP molecules in DP heterozygotes. The DP molecules bear DP antigens DPw1–DPw6.

D. Other Class II Subregions: The DN subregion contains a single HLA-DNA gene, and the DO subregion contains a single HLA-DOB gene. Neither of these genes has been found to be expressed in vivo, although expression has been induced in vitro. No function for these genes is presently known. It should be noted that there are no specific class II genes encoding the HLA-D antigens. The HLA-D antigens are defined by a cellular reaction termed the **mixed leukocyte reaction.** It is now thought that the antigenic determinants recognized during this reaction are actually antigenic epitopes present on the HLA-DR, -DQ, and possibly the -DP molecules. The highest correlation appears to be between the HLA-D and-DR antigens (Table 4–6).

Class III MHC Antigens

The complement components (see also Chapter 14) determined by the complement loci in the class III region also display polymorphism. There are 4 alleles determining the 4 alternative forms of properdin factor B (BF) that can be distinguished by their electrophoretic mobility: a common fast form (BF*F), a common slow form (BF*S), a rare fast form (BF*F1), and a rare slow form (BF*S1). There are C2 alleles determining the 2 common forms of C2 (C2*C and C2*A) and a rare deficiency allele (C2*QO). The C4 locus has actually been duplicated, so that there are 2 distinct C4 genetic loci, designated C4A (formerly Rogers), which determines the electrophoretically more acidic group of C4 components; and C4B (formerly Chido), which determines the electrophoretically more basic group of C4 components. There are 7 common structural alleles and one deficiency allele at the C4A locus and 3 common

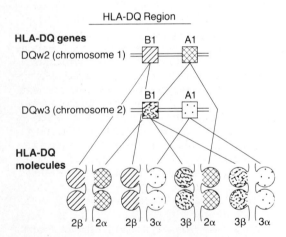

HLA-DQ Region

HLA-DQ genes

DQw2 (chromosome 1)

DQw3 (chromosome 2)

HLA-DQ molecules

2β 2α 2β 3α 3β 2α 3β 3α

Figure 4–9. cis- and trans-pairing of HLA-DQα and β chains. Both DQα and Dβ chains are polymorphic. An individual who is heterozygous at both the DQA1 locus and DQB1 locus will have 2 different DQα chains and 2 different DQβ chains. Either of the α chains can pair with either of the β chains to give 4 different DQ αβ molecules. The middle 2 molecules, which contain an α chain and a β chain encoded by DQ subregions on different chromosomes, are termed hybrid molecules and result from trans-pairing (see text). The specific class II HLA antigens, DQw2 and DQw3, are used for illustrative purposes. The outer molecules 2βα and 3βα are formed by cis-pairing (see text).The B2 and A2 pseudogenes are omitted from the chromosome.

Table 4-6. HLA-DR and -D associations.

DR Antigen	Associated D Antigen(s)
DR1	Dw1, Dw20
DRw15(2)	Dw2, Dw12
DR216(2)	Dw21, Dw22
DR3	Dw3
DR4	Dw4, Dw10, Dw13, Dw14, Dw15
DRw11(5)	Dw5
DRw13(w6)	Dw6, Dw18, Dw19
DRw14(w6)	Dw9, Dw16
DR7	Dw7, Dw11, Dw17
DRw8	Dw8
DR9	Dw23
DRw52	Dw24, Dw25, Dw26

Table 4-7. Common alleles at the HLA-linked complement loci.

BF	C2	C4A	C4B
BF*F	C2*C	C4A*1	C4B*1
BF*S	C2*A	C4A*2	C4B*2
BF*F1	C2*QO	C4A*3	C4B*3
BF*S1		C4A*4	C4B*QO
		C4A*5	
		C4A*5	
		C4A*6	
		C4A*7	
		C4A*QO	

structural alleles and one deficiency allele at the C4B locus. Table 4–7 presents a listing of the known common alleles at each of the HLA-linked complement loci.

Haplotype, Codominance, & Inheritance

Because of their close linkage, the combination of alleles at each locus on a single chromosome is usually inherited as a unit. This unit is referred to as the **haplotype.** Because individuals inherit one chromosome from each parent, each individual has 2 HLA haplotypes. All HLA genes are co-dominant, so both alleles at a given HLA locus are expressed, and 2 complete sets of HLA antigens, one from each parent, can be detected on cells. Based upon mendelian inheritance, there is a 25% chance that 2 siblings will share both haplotypes, a 50% chance that they will share one haplotype, and a 25% chance that they will share no haplotype and thereby be completely HLA-incompatible (Fig 4–10).

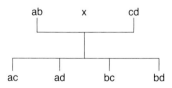

Figure 4-10. Inheritance of HLA haplotypes. A haplotype is the combination of alleles at each locus on a single chromosome that is inherited as a unit. Haplotype designations in the figure are given as a, b, c, and d. The maternal haplotypes are a and b, and the paternal haplotypes are c and d. Offspring of this mating (ab × cd) inherit one of the 2 possible haplotypes from each parent and so will have haplotypes ad, ab, bc, and bd. There is a 25% chance that 2 offspring will be HLA-identical (eg, ac and ac), a 25% chance that they will be totally HLA-nonidentical (eg, ac and bd), and a 50% chance that they will be HLA-semi-identical (eg, ac and ad).

Linkage Disequilibrium

Because human matings are random, the frequency of finding a given allele at one HLA locus with a given allele at a second HLA locus should simply be the product of the frequencies of each allele in the population. However, certain combinations of alleles are found with a frequency far exceeding that expected. This phenomenon is known as **linkage disequilibrium** and is quantitated as the difference (Δ) between the observed and expected frequencies.

As an example, the HLA-B8 allele and the HLA-DR3 allele are found in the North American white population with frequencies of 0.09 and 0.12, respectively. Thus, the expected frequency with which the HLA-B8-DR3 haplotype should be found is 0.09 × 0.12, or 0.0108. However, this haplotype is found with a frequency of approximately 0.0740, almost 7 times the expected frequency, for a Δ of 0.0740 − 0.0108 = 0.0632. Table 4–8 lists some common examples of linkage disequilibrium. Several hypotheses have been offered in an attempt to explain the phenomenon of linkage disequilibrium, including (1) a selective advantage of a given haplotype, (2) migration and admixture of 2 populations, (3) inbreeding, and (4) random drift of the gene pool.

IMMUNE RESPONSE GENES

Immune response (Ir) genes were originally described in animal models as genes that determine whether an individual can respond immunologically to a particular foreign antigen. Classic genetic techniques mapped the Ir genes to the vicinity of the class II MHC genes, and it was postulated that the respective class II molecules were in fact the protein products of Ir genes.

An extrapolation of the crystal structure of the class I molecules to the class II molecules and an understanding of the antigen-binding site of class

Table 4-8. Examples of linkage disequilibrium in Caucasians.

Haplotypes	Δ ($\times$ 10³)[1]
HLA-A1, B8	53.2
HLA-A2, B44	14.8
HLA-B27, Cw1	9.0
HLA-B27, Cw2	19.9
HLA-B7, DR2	36.8
HLA-B8, DR3	61.3
HLA-DR2, DQw1	93.6
HLA-DR3, DQw2	37.4
HLA-DR4, DQw3	87.5

[1]Δ is the difference between observed and expected frequencies of the haplotype that results from linkage disequilibrum.

II molecules have in essence confirmed this postulate and established the mechanism by which class II molecules can mediate the effect of Ir genes.

The variation of the antigen-binding site among different class II molecules and hence the variation in the ability of a given class II molecule to bind a given antigenic peptide fragment predict that only certain class II molecules can present particular antigens. These variations also account for the observation that only certain individuals, ie, those who inherit the appropriate class II genes, can respond to a given foreign substance.

Multiple examples of Ir gene effects in humans are known. Two of the most striking are the IgE antibody response to short ragweed antigen Amb a V (Ra5), which is highly associated with HLA-DR2; and the IgE antibody response to short ragweed antigen Amb a VI (Ra6), which is highly associated with HLA-DR5. Although currently unproved, it is thought that peptides derived from the ragweed antigens bind to these class II molecules.

HLA & DISEASE

Diseases associated with HLA antigens have several common characteristics. In general, these diseases (1) have unknown cause and unknown pathophysiologic mechanism, (2) have a hereditary pattern of distribution but weak penetrance and thus do not have an absolute association with a given HLA antigen, (3) are associated with immunologic abnormalities, and (4) have little or no effect on reproduction.

Methods Demonstrating HLA-Disease Associations

Both population and family studies have been used to demonstrate the relationship between marker genes within the HLA complex and various disease states. These 2 types of studies yield different types of information. Population studies determine the statistical associations to be made between a particular HLA marker gene and a particular disease. Such associations cannot be interpreted as proof of genetic linkage between a disease susceptibility gene and the HLA marker gene, because association does not necessarily indicate genetic linkage, nor does linkage necessarily indicate association. For example, if a disease susceptibility gene is on a chromosome other than chromosome 6 and therefore not linked to HLA, but the presence of a particular HLA antigen is necessary for the phenotypic expression of that disease susceptibility gene, then an HLA-disease association would be established.

Conversely, a gene such as phosphoglucomutase 3 (PGM_3) is on chromosome 6 and therefore

linked to HLA, but no HLA-specific association of disease with PGM_3 is found. In contrast to population studies, family studies can demonstrate linkage between a disease susceptibility gene and the HLA marker. Because population studies are easier to perform, most of the data on HLA and disease derive from this type of study.

Expressions of Risk in HLA-Disease Associations

The association of a particular disease with a particular HLA antigen is quantitated by calculating the relative risk (RR). This can be defined as the chance an individual with the disease-associated HLA antigen has of developing the disease compared with an individual who lacks that antigen. It is calculated by using the following formula:

$$RR = \frac{p^+ \times c^-}{p^- \times c^+}$$

where p^+ = the number of patients possessing the particular HLA, antigen

c^- = the number of controls lacking the particular HLA, antigen

p^- = the number of patients lacking the particular HLA, antigen and

c^+ = the number of controls possessing the particular HLA antigen

The higher (above 1) the relative risk, the more frequent is the antigen within the patient population.

In contrast, the absolute risk (AR) is the chance an individual who possesses the disease-associated HLA antigen has of actually developing the disease. It is calculated by the following formula:

$$AR = \frac{p^+}{c^+} \times P$$

where p^+ and c^+ are as above for the relative risk, and P = prevalence of the disease in the general population.

Ankylosing Spondylitis as Prototype Disease Associated With HLA-B27

The prototype of HLA-disease associations, ankylosing spondylitis with HLA-B27, can be used to illustrate these concepts. Ninety percent of Caucasian patients with ankylosing spondylitis in the United States possess HLA-B27, compared with approximately 9% of Caucasian controls. The relative risk is therefore p^+c^-/p^-c^+ = (90 × 91)/(10 × 9) = 91. Thus, an HLA-B27-positive individual has 91 times the risk that an HLA-B27-negative individual has of developing the disease. The prevalence of clinically apparent severe ankylosing spondylitis is approximately 0.4%. The absolute risk is calculated as $90/9 \times 0.004 = 0.04$. Therefore, of 100 HLA-B27-positive individuals, only 4 will actually develop clinically severe ankylosing spondylitis.

Because there is usually a significant difference in the frequency of a given antigen among different racial groups, it is always necessary to compare a patient group with a control population of the same race. Thus, for example, HLA-B27 is found in 48% of black patients with ankylosing spondylitis in the USA, compared with 2% of black controls in the USA, yielding a relative risk of 37 for this population.

Multiple Genetic & Disease Associations

In some cases, a disease may be associated with antigens determined by 2 different HLA loci. The actual association is frequently only with one antigen, but an apparent association with the second antigen is seen because of the phenomenon of linkage disequilibrium between the genes determining the 2 antigens (see above). The actual or primary association can usually be ascertained by statistically testing each antigen for disease association in the absence of the influence of the second antigen.

Antigens determined by almost all HLA loci have human disease associations. Thus, for example, idiopathic hemochromatosis has been associated with HLA-A3, ankylosing spondylitis with HLA-B27, rheumatoid arthritis with HLA-DR4, Sjögren's syndrome with DRw52, insulin-dependent diabetes mellitus with DQw8, celiac disease with a DP restriction fragment length polymorphism, and systemic lupus erythematosus with complement-deficient haplotypes. Selected HLA-disease associations are presented in Table 4–9.

The majority of diseases have been associated with class II antigens, and this association almost certainly reflects the role of the class II molecules in presenting processed antigenic fragments to CD4 T lymphocytes. Of interest is that several documented or presumed autoimmune diseases have been found to be associated with HLA-DR3 (Table 4–10). Most recently, specific class II region restriction endonuclease fragments have been associated with particular diseases.

Hypotheses To Explain HLA-Disease Associations

Several hypotheses, including the 5 discussed below, have been advanced to explain HLA-disease associations. Four of these apply equally to HLA class I and class II antigens, and one applies only to class II molecules.

The first 4 hypotheses will be illustrated by using the example of ankylosing spondylitis and

Table 4–9. Selected HLA-disease associations in Caucasian patients.

Disease	Antigen	Approximate RR
Ankylosing spondylitis	B27	81.8
Reiter's syndrome	B27	40.4
Acute anterior uveitis	B27	7.98
Rheumatoid arthritis	DR4	6.4
Juvenile rheumatoid arthritis Seropositive	DR4 Dw4 Dw14 Dw4/Dw14	7.2 25.8 47 116
Pauciarticular	DR5	2.9
Systemic lupus erythematosus (Caucasian patients)	DR2 DR3 C4A Null C4A deletion	3.0 2.7 5.4 5.5
Behçet's disease	B5	3.3
Sjögren's syndrome	DR3	5.6
Graves' disease	DR3	3.8
Insulin-dependent diabetes mellitus	DR4 DR3 DR3/4 DR2 DQw8	6.3 3.3 33 .25 31.8

HLA-B27. It should be immediately emphasized that these examples are purely speculative and that, except where noted, there is no evidence to support this speculation.

A. HLA Molecules Are Receptors of Etiologic Agents: Particular HLA molecules may act as receptors for etiologic agents such as viruses, toxins, or other foreign substances. Support for this hypothesis comes from the observation that other cell surface molecules act as receptors for viruses; eg, CD4 acts as a receptor for human immunodeficiency virus (HIV). If, for example, HLA-B27 is the receptor for a virus that causes ankylosing spondylitis, B27-positive indi-

Table 4–10. Diseases of known or presumed autoimmunity associated with HLA-DR3.

Systemic lupus erythematosus
Sicca syndrome
Myasthenia gravis
Dermatitis herpetiformis
Insulin-dependent diabetes mellitus
Graves' disease
Idiopathic Addison's disease
Celiac disease
Autoimmune chronic active hepatitis

viduals will be at increased risk for ankylosing spondylitis but can develop the disease only if they are exposed to the virus.

B. HLA Is Selective for Antigenic Peptides: The antigen-binding groove of only particular HLA molecules can accept the processed antigenic peptide fragment that is ultimately responsible for causing disease. If HLA-B27 is the only class I molecule that can accept a particular etiologic peptide for presentation to a CD8 T cell, only individuals with B27 will be predisposed to disease.

C. T Cell Receptor Determines Disease Predisposition: The T cell antigen receptor is actually responsible for disease predisposition, but because T cell recognition is restricted by an HLA molecule, and apparent association is seen between the disease and HLA. Suppose that all B27-positive individuals can form a particular B27-processed antigen complex but that only certain of these individuals possess B27-restricted T lymphocytes with the appropriate T cell receptor to recognize this complex. If the recognition of this complex by these T cells leads to ankylosing spondylitis, then only the individuals with these particular T cells can develop the disease. Although the antigen receptors on the T cells are ultimately responsible for the development of disease, an apparent association with HLA-B27 is observed because of the HLA-B27 restriction of these T cells.

D. Causative Agents Mimic HLA Molecules: The disease-associated HLA antigen is immunologically similar to the causative agent for the disease. This molecular mimicry hypothesis involves 2 alternatives. The first holds that because of the similarity between the causative agent and the HLA antigen, the etiologic agent is regarded as self, no immune response is mounted, and the causative agent produces disease without any interference from the host immune system. The second alternative suggests that the causative agent is regarded as foreign, and a vigorous immune response is mounted against the etiologic agent. Because of the similarity of the agent and the HLA antigen, the immune response is turned against the HLA antigen and this "autoimmune" response then produces disease. This theory has gained support from the following observations. HLA-B27 has been associated with Reiter's disease as well as ankylosing spondylitis. Reiter's disease in a B27-positive individual follows bouts of dysentery caused by certain strains of *Shigella flexneri*. These disease-producing *Shigella* strains contain a plasmid that encodes a protein with a stretch of 5 amino acids identical to a stretch of 5 amino acids in HLA-B27. Because only B27-positive individuals share this structural and immunologic similarity with the etiologic organism, only

these individuals are predisposed to disease according to the molecular mimicry hypothesis.

E. Expression of Class II MHC Molecules Is Aberrant: The last hypothesis relates only to diseases associated with class II HLA molecules. It postulates that the induction of class II expression on the surface of cells that do not normally express class II molecules is responsible for disease. Tissue-specific molecules on the surface of cells are constantly undergoing turnover and degradation. If the cells do not express class II molecules, degradation of the molecules to potentially antigenic peptides has no consequences. However, if these cells are induced to express class II molecules, the degradation of the tissue-specific molecules could lead to "antigen processing." A peptide fragment from the tissue-specific molecule would be bound by the antigen-binding site of the class II molecule, thereby forming an immunogenic complex and initiating an immunologic response against the tissue-specific molecule. If only certain class II molecules (eg, HLA-DR3) can bind these tissue-specific molecular fragments, then disease associations with HLA will be seen. Such a scenario has been postulated for the form of hyperthyroidism known as Graves' disease, in which antibodies directed against the receptor for thyroid-stimulating hormone are present and which is associated with HLA-DR3.

Other Diseases With Strong HLA Associations

The associations of insulin-dependent diabetes mellitus and rheumatoid arthritis with HLA are particularly instructive regarding several points.

A. Insulin-Dependent Diabetes Mellitus: This disease is negatively associated with HLA-DR2 (RR = 0.25), so that the presence of HLA-DR2 is protective against the development of disease. In contrast, the disease is positively associated with HLA-DR3 (RR = 3.3) and HLA-DR4 (RR = 6.3) but is even more highly associated with HLA-DR3/DR4 heterozygosity (RR = 33). Thus, there is something about this heterozygous state that particularly predisposes to insulin-dependent diabetes mellitus.

HLA-DR4 is in linkage disequilibrium with DQw3, and HLA-DR3 is in linkage disequilibrium with DQw2. Thus, the majority of HLA-DR3/DR4 heterozygotes will also be HLA-DQw2/DQw3 heterozygotes. Because both the DQα and β chains are polymorphic, DQw2/DQw3 heterozygotes will possess 2 hybrid molecules—DQw2αDQw3β and DQw3αDQw2β—not detected in other individuals (Fig 4–8). It is possible that one of these hybrid molecules is actually responsible for predisposition to disease.

HLA-DQw3 has recently been "split" into DQw7 (formerly DQw3.1) and DQw8 (formerly

DQw3.2). Further analysis has indicated that insulin-dependent diabetes mellitus is highly positively associated with HLA-DQw8 but negatively associated with HLA-DQw7. Sequence analysis has revealed that the HLA-DQw8 β chain has an alanine residue at position 57, whereas the HLA-DQw7 β chain has an aspartic acid at this position. Additional sequence data indicate that DQβ chains found in other haplotypes positively associated with insulin-dependent diabetes mellitus lack an aspartic acid at position 57, whereas DQβ chains present in haplotypes negatively associated with the disease possess this aspartic acid. Thus, a single amino acid appears to be crucial in the predisposition to this disease. Similar findings can be anticipated with respect to other diseases.

B. Rheumatoid Arthritis: Rheumatoid arthritis is highly associated with HLA-DR4 and particularly with 2 of the 5 subtypes of HLA-DR4, termed Dw4 and Dw14 (Table 4–5). In addition, it is associated with DR1. Sequence analysis indicates that the β chains of the Dw14 subtype of DR4 and DR1 share identical amino acid sequences from residues 67–78 in a highly polymorphic region of the molecule that is found in the α helix of the antigen-binding site.

This finding suggests that particular regions (eg, residues 67–78) or "antigenic epitopes" of molecules rather than entire molecules are responsible for predisposition to disease. It has been further proposed that such regions may be transferred between distinct HLA molecules by a mechanism termed **gene conversion.** Gene conversion, although not well defined mechanistically, is thought to be similar to recombination, but genetic information is transferred only in one direction. This observation of shared epitopes may also be one explanation for the lack of absolute associations between HLA and disease.

It should be emphasized that HLA-associated diseases are a heterogeneous group, that different mechanisms may be operating in different HLA-associated diseases, and that more than one mechanism may be operating concurrently to produce disease. Further studies are necessary to clarify these issues.

SUMMARY

The HLA complex contains a number of genes that are crucial in the initiation, regulation, and implementation of an immune response. It is the most highly polymorphic complex known in mammalian species. It contains the HLA-A, -B, and -C genes, which encode the class I HLA molecules, and the HLA-DR, -DQ, and -DP subregions, which encode the class II HLA molecules.

The class I and II HLA molecules are each 2-chain structures. The HLA-encoded class I α chain has 3 extracellular domains and is associated with a non-HLA-encoded chain, β_2-microglobulin. The class II α and β chains are both encoded by the HLA complex, and each contains 2 extracellular domains.

The demonstrated structure of the class I molecule and the presumed structure of the class II molecule indicate that the interactive portion of the molecules consists of a β-pleated sheet platform upon which rest 2 α helices. These 2 α helices form the sides and the β-pleated sheet forms the floor of a cleft or groove that is the antigen-binding site. Processed antigenic peptide fragments can fit into this groove. Because most of the polymorphism of the class I and II molecules is localized to the α helices and the portion of the β-pleated sheet that is the floor of the groove, the antigen-binding site varies from one HLA molecule to another. This observation explains why different HLA molecules bind different antigenic fragments; it also explains Ir gene effects and HLA-disease associations.

The class I molecules have a ubiquitous tissue distribution and present processed antigenic peptide fragments to CD8 (predominantly cytotoxic) T lymphocytes, whereas class II molecules have a distribution limited to immunocompetent cells and present processed antigenic peptide fragments to CD4 (predominantly helper) T lymphocytes.

Because of their role in the immune response, many HLA antigens have been associated with predisposition to particular diseases; the majority of such associations involve class II HLA antigens. The magnitude of the association is quantitated by the relative risk. Although very little is known about the etiology or pathogenesis of the HLA-associated diseases, several models have been proposed to explain the mechanism by which the HLA molecules may be involved. Recent evidence suggests that single amino acid changes in crucial regions of an HLA molecule can alter disease predisposition and that regions of identical amino acid sequence (epitopes) found on different HLA molecules may be responsible for disease predisposition.

REFERENCES

General

Dupont B (Editor): *Histocompatibility Testing 1987.* Vol 1 of: *Immunobiology of HLA.* Springer-Verlag, 1989.

Dupont B (editor): *Immunogenetics and Histocom-*

patibility. Vol. 2 of: *Immunobiology of HLA*. Springer-Verlag, 1989.

McDevitt HO: The HLA system and its relation to disease. *Hosp Pract* (July 15) 1985;**20**:57.

Schwartz, BD et al (editors): Workshop on the immunogenetics of the rheumatic diseases. *Am J Med* 1988;**85(Suppl 6A)**:1. [Entire issue.]

Nomenclature & Genetic Organization of the HLA System

Bohme J et al: HLA-DR beta genes vary in number between different DR specificities, whereas the number of DQ beta genes is constant. *J Immunol* 1985;**135**:2149.

Carroll MC et al: A molecular map of the human major histocompatibility complex class III region linking complement genes C4, C2, and factor B. *Nature* 1984;**307**:237.

HLA Nomenclature Committee: Nomenclature for factors of the HLA system, 1987 *Immunogenetics* 1988;**28**:391.

Möller G (editor): Molecular genetics of class I and II MHC antigens. (2 parts.) *Immunol Rev* 1985;**84**:1 and **85**:1. [Entire issues.]

Spies T et al: Structural organization of the DR subregion of the human major histocompatibility complex. *Proc Natl Acad Sci USA* 1985;**82**:5165.

Trowsdale J, Campbell RD: Physical map of the human HLA region. *Immunol Today* 1988;**9**:34.

Structure, Tissue Distribution, & Function

Babbitt BP et al: Binding of immunogenic peptides to Ia histocompatibility molecules. *Nature* 1985;**317**:359.

Bjorkman PJ et al: Structure of the human class I histocompatibility antigen, HLA-A2. *Nature* 1987;**329**:506.

Brown JH et al: A hypothetical model of the foreign antigen-binding site of class II histocompatibility molecules. *Nature* 1988;**332**:845.

Buss S, Sette A, Grey HM: The interaction between protein-derived immunogenic peptides and Ia. *Immunol Rev* 1987;**98**:116.

Marrack P, Kappler J: T cells can distinguish between allogeneic major histocompatibility complex products on different cell types. *Nature* 1988;**332**:840.

McMichael AJ et al: HLA restriction of cell-mediated lysis of influenza virus-infected human cells. *Nature* 1977;**270**:524.

Möller G (editor): Structure and function of HLA-DR. *Immunol Rev* 1982;**66**:1. [Entire issue.]

Ir Genes

Marsh DG, Meyers DA, Bias WB: The epidemiology and genetics of atopic allergy. *N Engl J Med* 1981;**305**:1551.

HLA & Disease

Möller G (editor): HLA and disease susceptibility. *Immunol Rev* 198;**70**:1. [Entire issue.]

Tiwari JL, Terasaki PI (editors): *HLA and Disease Associations*. Springer-Verlag, 1985.

Todd JA, Bell JI, McDevitt HO: HLA-DQ beta gene contributes to susceptibility and resistance to insulin-dependent diabetes mellitus. *Nature* 1987;**329**:599.

Cells of the Immune Response: Lymphocytes & Mononuclear Phagocytes

5

Lewis Lanier, PhD

Lymphocytes and **mononuclear phagocytes** play a central role in the immune response. These cell types are responsible for both innate and acquired immunity against bacterial and viral pathogens. In addition to cell-mediated immune functions, they are the source of a vast array of secreted proteins that influence the growth and development of many body tissues. Moreover, in addition to their beneficial role in protection against microbial pathogens, these cells may adversely affect normal body tissues during the course of certain autoimmune diseases. In this chapter, an overview of the functions of various types of lymphocytes and mononuclear phagocytes is presented.

Leukocytes (white blood cells) are a heterogeneous group of cells that mediate immune responses. Leukocytes are found predominantly in the blood, bone marrow, and lymphoid organs (eg, spleen, thymus, tonsils, and lymph nodes), as well as in epithelium and elsewhere. Classification of leukocytes was first based on morphologic criteria, principally nuclear size and shape and histochemical staining characteristics of the cytoplasm. Three major cell types were distinguished: **granulocytes, lymphocytes,** and **monocytes** (Fig 5-1).

Granulocytes (10-15 μm in diameter), also referred to as polymorphonuclear leukocytes, have a multilobular nucleus and abundant granules in the cytoplasm. Three subtypes of granulocytes exist: **neutrophils, basophils,** and **eosinophils.** When stained with Giemsa dye, the granules of neutrophils appear blue-gray, those of basophils blue, and those of eosinophils red. Lymphocytes are small (7-12 μm in diameter) mononuclear spherical cells typically containing very little cytoplasm that stains pale blue with Giemsa dye. Monocytes (10-30 μm in diameter) are also mononuclear; they have a characteristic kidney-shaped nucleus and more cytoplasm than lymphocytes do.

Blood monocytes differentiate when stimulated by various substances into **macrophages.** Like monocytes, macrophages are mononuclear cells, but they also possess more abundant cytoplasm with predominant intracellular vacuoles and granules and are pleomorphic. Certain types of macrophages, called **histiocytes,** are resident in spleen, lung (alveolar macrophages), liver (Kupffer's cells), skin (Langerhans cells), and other tissues.

I. LYMPHOCYTES

Although morphologic and biophysical properties have provided a useful classification for the major groups of leukocytes, these groups do not consist of homogeneous populations. Monoclonal antibodies directed against cell surface antigens have demonstrated identifying heterogeneity, particularly within lymphocytes. On the basis of expression of cell surface markers, 3 distinct lineages of lymphocytes have been identified: T cells, B cells, and natural killer (NK) cells. Moreover, the presence or absence of certain cell surface markers has been used to delineate stages of differentiation, states of cellular activation, and functionally distinct subsets of lymphocytes.

A series of International Human Leukocyte Differentiation Antigen Workshops has established a unified nomenclature for the most commonly studied cell surface antigens (Table 5-1).

T cells, B cells, and NK cells are distinguished primarily by their antigen receptors and by certain characteristic cell surface markers called clusters of differentiation (CD; Fig 5-2). T cells recognize antigens by a membrane structure called the CD3/T cell antigen receptor complex (the CD3/TCR complex), whereas B cells recognize antigens by using surface immunoglobulin molecules. (The structure and function of the CD3/TCR complex are discussed in Chapter 6.) Although the recogni-

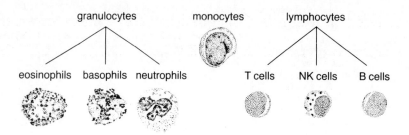

Figure 5-1. Classification of leukocytes.

Table 5-1. Leukocyte differentiation antigen nomenclature.

CD[1]	MW	Predominant Leukocyte (Function)	Frequently Used Antibodies
1a	49,000	Thymocytes, Langerhans cells	αLeu 6, T6
1b	45,000	Thymocytes, Langerhans cells	
1c	43,000	Thymocytes, Langerhans cells	
2	50,000	T and NK cells	αLeu 5, T11
2R	50,000	Activation-related epitope of CD2	T11-3, 9.1
3	20,000–30,000	T cells (T cell-antigen receptor complex)	αLeu 4, T3
4	60,000	T cell subset (class II MHC interaction, HIV receptor)	αLeu 3, T4
5	67,000	T cells and B subset	αLeu 1, T1
6	120,000	T cells	T12
7	40,000	T and NK cells, platelets	αLeu 9, 3A1
8α	32,000	T and NK subsets (class I MHC interaction)	αLeu 2, T8
8β		T subset	
9	24,000	Pre-B, monocytes, platelets	
10	100,000	Pre-B cells, cALL[3] (enkephalinase)	αCALLA,J5
11a	180,000	Leukocytes (cellular adhesion)	αLFA-1α
11b	160,000	Myeloid cells, NK cells, T subset (complement receptor type 3)	αCR3, OKM1
11c	150,000	Myeloid cells, NK cells, T subset (complement receptor type 4)	αLeuM5
12		Monocytes, granulocytes, platelets	
13	150,000	Granulocytes, monocytes (aminopeptidase N)	
14	53,000	Monocytes	αLeuM3, Mo2
15	CHO[4]	Granulocytes	αLeuM1
16	50,000–70,000	NK cells, granulocytes, T subset (IgG-Fc receptor type III)	αLeu 11,3G8
17	Lipid	Granulocytes, monocytes, platelets (lactoceramide)	
18	95,000	Leukocytes (β subunit of CD11a, b, c)	αLFA-1β
19	95,000	B cells	αLeu 12, B4
20	35,000	B cells	αLeu 16,B1
21	140,000	B cells (complement receptor type 2)	αCR2, B2
22	135,000	B cells	αLeu 14
23α	45,000	B cells (IgE-Fc receptor type II)	αLeu 20
23β	45,000	B cells, monocytes, eosinophils, T subset	
24	65,000, 55,000, 65,000	B cells, granulocytes	
25	55,000	Activated lymphocytes, monocytes (low-affinity IL-2 receptor)	αIL2-R, TAC-1
26	130,000	T cells (dipeptidyl peptidase IV)	5.9, Ta1
27	55,000	T cells, plasma cells	
28	44,000	T cell subset	9.3
29	135,000	Leukocytes, platelets	4B4, VLA-β
30	120,000	Activated B, T cells	
31	130,000–140,000	Monocytes, granulocytes, platelets gpLLa[5]	
32	40,000	Monocytes, granulocytes, platelets, B cells (IgC-Fc receptor type II)	
33	67,000	Myeloid leukemia	
34	115,000	Hematopoietic stem cells	αHPCA-1
35	220,000	Granulocytes, monocytes (complement receptor type 1)	
36	85,000	Monocytes, platelets	
37	40,000–45,000	B cells	
38	45,000	Subsets of leukocytes	αLeu 17, OKT10
39	80,000	B cells, macrophages	
40	50,000	B cells	

Table 5-1 (cont'd). Leukocyte differentiation antigen nomenclature.

CD[1]	MW	Predominant Leukocyte (Function)	Frequently Used Antibodies
41a	125,000	Platelets gpIIb/IIIa	
41b		Platelets gpIIb	
42a	145,000	Platelets gpIX	
42b		Platelets gpIb	
43	95,000	T cells, granulocytes	
44	65,000–85,000	Leukocytes (homing receptor)	Hermes
45	180,000–220,000	Leukocytes	HLE-1
45R	220,000	T subset, NK cells, B cells	αLeu 18, 2H4
45R0	180,000	T subset, activated T	UCHL-1
46	55,000–66,000	Leukocytes, platelets	
47	47,000–52,000	Leukocytes, platelets	
48	41,000	Leukocytes	
w[6]49a	210,000	Leukocytes, platelets (cell adhesion)	VLA-1α
w49b	165,000	Leukocytes, platelets (cell adhesion)	VLA-2
w49c	135,000	Leukocytes, platelets (cell adhesion)	VLA-3
w49d	150,000	Leukocytes, platelets (cell adhesion)	VLA-4
w49e	135,000	Leukocytes, platelets (cell adhesion)	VLA-5
w49f	120,000	Leukocytes, platelets (cell adhesion)	VLA-6
w50	140,000/108,000	Leukocytes	
w51	120,000	Leukocytes, platelets (vitronectin receptor α chain)	
w52	25,000–30,000	Leukocytes	CAMPATH-1
53	32,000–40,000	Leukocytes	
54	85,000	Activated B and T, macrophages (CD11/CD18 ligand, rhinovirus receptor)	ICAM-1
55	73,000	Leukocytes (delayed accelerating factor)	
56	140,000–200,000	NK cells, T subset	αLeu 19, NKH1
57	CHO	T and NK subsets	αLeu 7
58	45,000–60,000	Leukocytes (CD2 ligand)	LFA-3
59	18,000–20,000	Leukocytes, platelets	MEM-43
w60	120,000	T subset, platelets (GD3 ganglioside)	
61	114,000	Platelets gpIIIa	
62	150,000	Platelets	
63	53,000	Platelets	
64	75,000	Monocytes, macrophages (IgG Fc receptor type I)	
w65		Granulocytes, monocytes (fucoganglioside)	
66	180,000–200,000	Granulocytes	
67	100,000	Granulocytes	
68	110,000	Macrophages	
69	28,000–32,000	Activated lymphocytes	αLeu 23
w70		Activated lymphocytes	Ki-24
		Reed-Sternberg cells	
71	90,000	Proliferating cells (transferrin receptor)	
72	43,000/39,000	B cells	
73	69,000	B, T subset (ecto-5' nucleotidase)	
74	41,000, 35,000/33,000	B cells, monocytes (invariant chain)	
w75		B cells, T cell subset	
76	85,000/67,000	B cells, T cell subset, granulocytes	
77		Activated B cells	
w78		B cells	αLeu 21

[1]CD, cluster of differentiation.
[2]α, antibody to. . . .
[3]cALL, common acute lymphocytic leukemia.
[4]CHO carbohydrate antigen.
[5]gp, glycoprotein.
[6]w is the provisional (Workshop) designation.

tion structure(s) of NK cells has not been identified, these cells use neither T cell antigen receptors nor immunoglobulins. T, B, and NK cells mediate a vast array of cellular functions in immune responses. Their distribution in the body is given in Table 5-2.

T LYMPHOCYTES

Development of T Lymphocytes in the Thymus

T cells are the special lineage of lymphocytes that arise from maturation of stem cells in the thy-

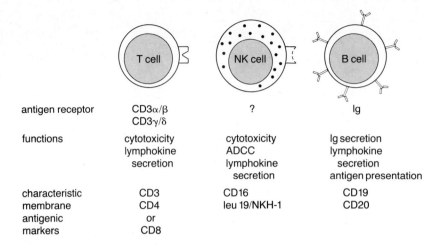

	T cell	NK cell	B cell
antigen receptor	CD3α/β CD3γ/δ	?	Ig
functions	cytotoxicity lymphokine secretion	cytotoxicity ADCC lymphokine secretion	Ig secretion lymphokine secretion antigen presentation
characteristic membrane antigenic markers	CD3 CD4 or CD8	CD16 leu 19/NKH-1	CD19 CD20

Figure 5–2. Lineages of lymphocytes.

mus; hence the name "T" cells. The central role of the thymus is the rearrangement and productive expression of the T cell receptor (TCR) genes and the subsequent selection of the antigen receptor repertoire that enables mature T cells to recognize foreign but not usually self antigens. Progenitor cells from either bone marrow or fetal liver enter the thymus and undergo stages of differentiation, resulting in the migration of mature T lymphocytes into the blood and peripheral lymphoid tissues (eg, spleen, lymph nodes, lymphatic system, and tonsils).

A complex series of changes in genotype and phenotype accompany the maturation of T cells in the thymus (Fig 5–3). The earliest recognizable thymocyte, the **pro-T cell,** can be identified by expression of certain antigens on the cell surface (eg, CD2 and CD7) and by the presence of CD3ε protein in the cytoplasm (but not on the cell surface). Pro-T cells differentiate into **pre-T cells** by rearrangement of δ-, γ-, and β-TCR genes. First, γ/δ-TCR-bearing cells arise from pre-T cells that productively rearrange and express γ- and δ-TCR genes. Pre-T cells destined to generate α/β-TCR-bearing T cells then rearrange α-TCR genes,

thereby deleting the δ-TCR genes between the Vα and Cα genes on the chromosome.

Thymocytes that express CD3/α/β-TCR on the cell surface and react with self antigens are usually deleted from the population by an unknown process. Other CD3/α/β-TCR-bearing thymocytes are "educated" to recognize antigenic peptides only when associated with self MHC proteins by a process that also has not yet been delineated. Most thymocytes fail in this selection process and die within the thymus; only a minority successfully differentiate into mature T lymphocytes and migrate to the peripheral lymphoid organs and blood. In peripheral blood, about 70% of lymphocytes are T cells.

Markers of Thymic Lymphocytes

Molecules other than the CD3/TCR complex are involved in thymic differentiation of T lymphocytes and can also be used as markers to identify stages of maturation (Fig 6–3). Pro-T cells express CD2 and CD7 on the cell surface; these immature thymocytes lack CD3, CD4, and CD8. As they mature, the majority of pro-T and pre-T lymphocytes begin to express CD1, CD4, and CD8 markers, usually within the thymic cortex.

Subsequently, these $CD4^+8^+$ immature thymocytes express low levels of the CD3 α/β-TCR complex and then undergo selection and "education." A proportion of the relatively immature $CD4^+8^+$ cells lose expression of either CD4 or CD8 to become $CD4^+8^-$ or $CD4^-8^+$; the amount of CD3/TCR on the cell surface is increased, and the CD1 molecule is lost. These more mature thymocytes are found predominantly in the cortex and have a phenotype similar to that of T cells in the periph-

Table 5–2. Distribution of lymphocytes.

Tissue	Percentage of Lymphocytes (normal range)		
	T cells	B cells	NK cells
Blood	65–75	5–10	5–15
Thymus	>95	<1	<1
Lymph node	70–80	10–20	<1
Spleen	20–30	40–50	1–5

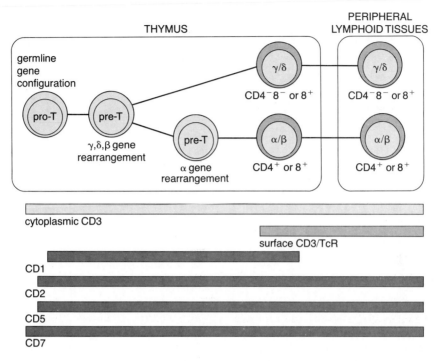

Figure 5–3. T lymphocyte differentiation. Bars below the model refer to synthesis of differentiation antigens at the different stages during T cell development depicted in the diagram above.

eral lymphoid tissues. They presumably represent the population from which truly mature α/β-TCR T cells arise. γ/δ-TCR-bearing thymocytes apparently do not follow this maturation pathway and do not coexpress CD4 and CD8 during differentiation. α/β-TCR- and γ/δ-TCR-bearing T cells probably then represent distinct lineages of T lymphocytes that arise from a common progenitor. Their precise relationship, however, has not been fully delineated. α/β-TCR-bearing T cells are the predominant T cell type in the thymus and peripheral lymphoid tissues after birth, constituting nearly all of both CD3 thymocytes and mature, peripheral T cells.

Function of T Cells in Immune Responses

T cells initiate the immune response, mediate antigen-specific effector responses, and regulate the activity of other leukocytes by secreting soluble factors. Effector functions of T cells include **cell-mediated cytotoxicity** and **cell-mediated immunity,** also known as delayed-type hypersensitivity (DTH). Augmentation of B and T cell activation and differentiation (ie, helper or amplifier function), suppression of an immune response (suppressor function), and secretion of potent cytokines, including gamma interferon and interleu-

kins (see Chapter 7), constitute the regulatory effects of T cells on many leukocytes as well as on other nonimmune cells in the body (Fig 5–4).

A correlation exists between the expression of membrane antigens and the functional activities of T cells. Mature T lymphocytes can be subdivided on the basis of expression of CD4 or CD8 antigens on the cell surface. CD4$^+$8$^-$ and CD4$^-$8$^+$ T cells represent some 70% and 25%, respectively, of the total T cell population in blood and peripheral lymphoid tissues. Minor subsets of T cells can express CD4$^-$8$^-$ or CD4$^+$8$^+$ phenotypes and account for the remaining 4% and 1%, respectively, of total mature T cells. CD4 and CD8 are membrane glycoproteins that bind to class II and class I major histocompatibility complex (MHC) antigens, respectively.

Recognition of Antigen by T Lymphocytes

T cells usually do not react with intact protein antigens, but rather bind to antigens that are processed into small peptides and bound to major histocompatibility complex (MHC) antigens on the cell surface of an antigen-presenting cell or target cell. Antigen-presenting cell (APC) is a general term to describe any cell (including monocytes, macrophages, B cells, dendritic cells, and some T

Subsets of Mature Peripheral T Lymphocytes

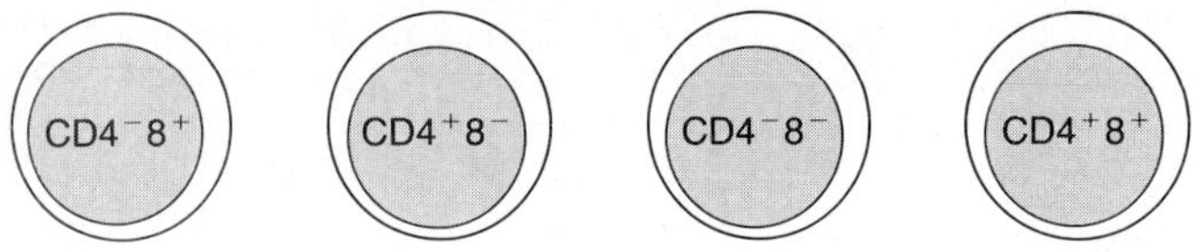

	$CD4^-8^+$	$CD4^+8^-$	$CD4^-8^-$	$CD4^+8^+$
MHC restriction	class I	class II	?	?
predominant function	cytotoxicity	help	cytotoxicity	?
frequency (% of T lymphocytes) in peripheral tissues	~25%	~70%	~4%	~1%
predominant antigen receptor	α/β	α/β	γ/δ	α/β

Figure 5–4. Functional roles of T lymphocytes.

cells) that can internalize and degrade a protein antigen into peptide fragments and then present these peptides on the cell surface membrane bound to self MHC antigens. Both class I (HLA-A, -B, -C) and class II (HLA-DR, -DP, -DQ) structures bind peptides for interaction with α/β-TCR. Natural ligands for the γ/δ-TCR have not been defined, but it is likely that these receptors will also bind peptide antigens. The CD3/TCR complex on the cell surface of T cells binds to the peptide/MHC on the APC. This interaction generates an activation signal for the T cells. The initial phase of signal transduction results in activation of phosphodiesterases that hydrolyze phospholipid phosphatidylinositol bisphosphate to generate diacylglycerol and inositol triphosphate, which is subsequently metabolized to inositol bisphosphate, inositol phosphate, and inositol. Inositol triphosphate rapidly increases intracellular free Ca^{2+} levels, and diacylglycerol stimulates protein kinase C activity. These early activation events are necessary, but not sufficient, for the subsequent induction of lymphokine secretion and proliferation. Usually, a cosignal is required. In some cases, cytokines produced by the APC (eg, interleukin-1 from monocytes) may provide cofactors that result in production of lymphokines and growth factors by T cells and, ultimately, cellular proliferation. The mechanism of these cosignals in T cell activation is not well understood.

Antigen-driven proliferation is an important feature of the immune system. Given the extent of the antigen receptor repertoire, only a few T cells in the total population will specifically react with any given antigen prior to immunization; however, exposure to antigen, usually in conjunction with other cofactors or cytokines that facilitate

the process (eg, IL-1), results in preferential clonal proliferation and expansion of these specific effectors. A consequence of exposure to antigen is the generation of memory T cells. Memory T cells are capable of self-renewal, resulting in the generation of cells that rapidly respond to reexposure to the antigen, following years or even decades after the primary stimulation (eg, tetanus immunization). Although the mechanism of this process is unknown, it is an essential and unique aspect of the immune response.

Cytotoxic-Suppressor T Cells

CD4$^-$8$^+$ T cells mediate most antigen-specific cytotoxicity—the ability to kill other cells that are perceived as foreign, eg, virus-infected or allogeneic cells introduced into the host by transplantation. CD4$^-$8$^+$ T cells recognize peptide antigens bound to class I MHC molecules on the cell surface of the target. During viral infection, viral peptides bind to self MHC molecules within the cytoplasm of the virus-infected target cell and are transported to the cell surface for recognition by cytotoxic T lymphocytes (CTL). In transplantation, allogeneic MHC molecules are themselves recognized as antigens by the CTL. Activated CTL destroy the target cell by a process that is not well-defined.

As a consequence of activation, CD4$^-$8$^+$ T cells also release **lymphokines** (eg, IL-2, gamma interferon), which can augment immune responses by other B and T lymphocytes. In addition to their cytotoxic function, CD4$^-$8$^+$ T cells can suppress immune responses, possibly by the release of soluble factors that interfere with the function of other immune cells. Because of these functions, the CD4$^-$8$^+$ T cell population is often referred to as the **T cytotoxic-suppressor subset (Tc/s).** This is an oversimplification, however, because cytotoxic and suppressive functions can also be mediated by other T cells, including the CD4$^+$8$^-$ and CD4$^-$8$^-$ T subsets. Moreover, whether suppression and cytotoxicity are mediated by independent cells within the CD4$^-$8$^+$ T population or, alternatively, represent functions mediated by the same cell has not been determined.

Helper T Cells

CD4$^+$8$^-$ T lymphocytes make up the subset referred to as the helper or helper/inducer T (TH or TH/I) cells because of their ability to augment B cell responses and to amplify the cell-mediated responses effected by CD4$^-$8$^+$ T cells. Under certain circumstances, CD4$^+$8$^-$ T cells can also mediate cytotoxicity and immune suppression. CD4$^+$8$^-$ T lymphocytes usually recognize peptide antigens that are bound to class II MHC glycoproteins present on the surface of an antigen-presenting cell. After exposure to peptide-MHC, CD4$^+$8$^-$ T cells are activated and proliferate.

Activated CD4$^+$8$^-$ T cells secrete soluble factors that influence effector functions mediated by other leukocytes. For example, antigen-stimulated CD4$^+$8$^-$ cells secrete IL-2, which, in turn serves as a growth factor for antigen-independent polyclonal proliferation of other T cells and augments cytotoxic activity mediated by CTL and NK cells.

IL-4, also secreted by T cells activated by antigens, augments the growth of B cells and other T cells, enhances CTL function, and induces the expression of Fc receptors for IgE on B cells and monocytes. However, IL-4 can also inhibit the activation of B and NK cells by IL-2. Many other cytokines (eg, IL-2, -3, -4, -5, and -6, granulocyte macrophage colony-stimulating factor (GM-CSF), tumor necrosis factor (TNF), and gamma interferon) are produced by antigen-specific stimulation of CD4$^+$8$^-$ T lymphocytes (see Chapter 7). Thus, the CD4$^+$8$^-$ T cells provide regulatory factors that either augment or suppress functions mediated by the entire immune system.

Minor T Cell Subsets

The role of the minor CD4$^-$8$^-$ and CD4$^+$8$^+$ T subsets is less clear. Culture of mature CD4$^+$8$^-$ T cells in IL-4 induces the expression of CD8 on the cell surface, suggesting a possible explanation for in vivo CD4$^+$8$^+$ cells. The physiologic consequence of this process is unknown, but it may permit cells to interact with both class I and II MHC antigens, thus facilitating immune responses. Unlike the majority of CD4$^+$8$^-$, CD4$^-$8$^+$, and CD4$^+$8$^+$ T lymphocytes that express an α/β-TCR, most CD4$^-$8$^-$ T cells possess a γ/δ-TCR. Although the natural antigens recognized by CD4$^-$8$^-$ γ/δ-TCR T cells have not been identi-

fied, these cells can mediate cell-mediated cytotoxicity and secrete cytokines such as IL-2, IL-4, and gamma interferon after activation.

Relationship of Cell Surface Markers With Stages of Differentiation or Activation

Lymphoid tissues contain a diverse collection of T cells that differ in terms of stage of differentiation, prior exposure to antigen, and state of activation as reflected by the heterogeneity of their cell surface marker expression within the T cell population in these tissues. It was previously thought that expression of different antigenic phenotypes reflected the existence of distinct lineages of T cells with unique functions; however, recent studies indicate that these phenotypes relate to the state of differentiation or state of activation of the cells (Fig 5–5).

Activation of T lymphocytes via either antigen-specific or antigen-independent (eg, cytokine, mitogen) stimulation alters the phenotype of the cells. Expression of new cell surface markers is induced, some markers are lost, and the amounts of other markers may be increased or decreased. For example, deliberate activation of T cells by stimulation of the CD3/TCR complex induces de novo synthesis of class II MHC antigens; the early activation antigen, CD69; and receptors for IL-2 (CD25) and transferrin. Activation increases the amount of CD2, CD18, CD26, CD29, CD38, CD44, CD45RO, CD54, and CD58 on the cell surface and results in down-regulation of CD45R antigens. Thus, the antigenic phenotype of T cells appears to reflect the stage of differentiation or activation rather than identifying a unique lineage within the T cell population. (ie. CD markers)

B LYMPHOCYTES

Immunoglobulin as Antigen Receptor

B cells express **immunoglobulin** on the cell surface membrane. Immunoglobulin is responsible for binding of antigen, subsequent cellular activation, and the secretion of soluble immunoglobulin into serum and tissues. Unlike the TCR, which usually recognizes only peptide antigens bound to MHC molecules, immunoglobulins on B cells are able to bind directly and with high affinity to intact antigens, including glycoproteins, glycolipids, polysaccharides, peptides, and virtually any immunogenic molecule.

Immunoglobulins are glycoproteins composed of 2 disulfide-bonded **heavy (H) chain** subunits, each of which is linked by interchain disulfide bonds to a **light (L) chain,** forming a tetramolecular complex. In humans, 2 L chain genes, desig-

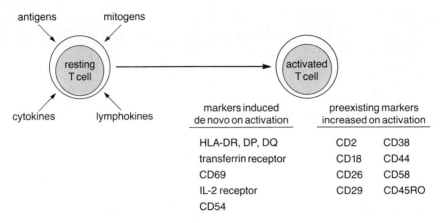

Figure 5-5. Phenotypes of resting and activated T lymphocytes.

nated κ and λ, are on chromosomes 2 and 22, respectively; the H chain locus is present on chromosome 14. Like the T cell antigen receptor, immunoglobulin H and L chains are composed of variable (V), joining (J), and constant (C) genes that rearrange during B cell development. H genes also possess diversity (D) elements. The human H chain locus contains several C region elements: μ, δ, $\gamma1-\delta4$, ϵ, $\alpha1$, and $\alpha2$. Numerous (>100) V_H and V_L genes and a high rate of V-region somatic mutation allow for an extensive repertoire of antigen recognition that is expanded further by junctional diversity.

Isotype Switching of Immunoglobulin in B Cells

B cells initially express a single RNA transcript containing both μ and δ segments that are processed into separate μ and δ H chain mRNA by alternative splicing, allowing a single B cell to express both IgM and IgD with an identical V region and hence the same antigenic specificity. Although a single B cell expresses a unique immunoglobulin V_H and V_L throughout its life, as a consequence of maturation the V/J segment may be "switched" to other 3' C region elements by somatic recombination, with resulting deletion of the intervening genetic material including the μ and δ C segments. This allows for the generation of immunoglobulin with identical specificity (V regions) but diverse effector functions contributed by the different H chain isotypes. These C region elements differ with respect to binding of complement components, interaction with Fc receptors, and transfer of immunoglobulin across membranes (eg, placenta).

Differentiation of B Cells

B lymphocytes arise from progenitor cells in the bone marrow. B cells rearrange immunoglobulin genes during the early stages of maturation (Fig 5-6). During this process, the pre-B cells first rearrange immunoglobulin heavy chain genes and then rearrange light chain genes. When functional H and L chains are both synthesized, immunoglobulin is expressed on the cell surface. These immunoglobulin-expressing cells are referred to as **virgin B cells** because they possess competent immunoglobulin on the membrane but have not yet interacted with antigen. At this stage, B cells migrate from the bone marrow into the blood and peripheral lymphoid tissues.

The stages of B cell maturation are reflected by changes in the expression of several cell surface differentiation antigens (Fig 5-6). After interaction of antigen with surface immunoglobulin, B cells are activated and ultimately mature into **plasma cells,** which are responsible for production of large quantities of immunoglobulin, which is secreted. After the same exposure to antigen, some B cells live for years and are thus referred to as **memory B cells.** These cells are responsible for the rapid **recall responses** observed after reexposure to antigens previously recognized by the immune system.

Activation & Function of B Cells

Antigen-specific activation of B cells occurs after binding of antigen to membrane immunoglobulin independent of the action of APC. A second signal is provided by soluble factors released from monocytes or T cells. This results in activation via the phosphatidylinositol pathway and

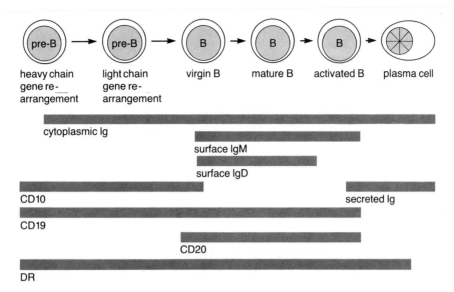

Figure 5-6. B lymphocyte differentiation. Bars below the model refer to synthesis of differentiation antigens at the different stages during B cell development depicted in the diagram above.

subsequent clonal expansion similar to activation of T cells. Two general types of antigen have been described: **T cell-independent antigens** and **T cell-dependent antigens.** B cells encountering T cell–independent antigens are capable of proliferation and immunoglobulin secretion in the absence of TH cells. These antigens are often carbohydrates or antigens expressing multiple repeating determinants that permit extensive cross-linking of the surface immunoglobulin on the B cells.

In contrast, response to T cell-dependent antigens requires interaction between B and T cells for subsequent immunoglobulin production. TH cells recognize the antigen and produce several soluble mediators, including IL-4 and -5 and other cytokines that augment or help B cells to respond. Depending upon the nature of the antigen and the availability of T cell-generated cytokines, immunoglobulin **isotype switching** occurs.

Plasma Cells & Memory B Cells

When provided with the appropriate factors, B cells ultimately differentiate into plasma cells, which secrete large amounts of soluble immunoglobulin into the serum or tissue. In the plasma cell, the immunoglobulin RNA transcripts are truncated by mRNA splicing to delete the transmembrane segment of the molecule, permitting immunoglobulin secretion rather than attachment to the cell membrane. After primary exposure to antigen, memory B cells are generated. In addition to producing immunoglobulin, B cells also may secrete certain cytokines (eg, IL-6) that affect the growth and differentiation of B cells and other lymphocytes.

NATURAL KILLER (NK) CELLS

Phenotypic Characteristics of NK Cells

NK cells are a subset of lymphocytes that arise from a precursor cell in the bone marrow. Mature NK cells are present in blood, bone marrow, and spleen but are infrequent in the lymph nodes or thymus. The exact developmental relationship of NK cells to T and B lymphocytes is unknown. However, NK cells are clearly a distinct lineage; children with **severe combined immunodeficiency disease (SCID),** a disorder that prevents the development of mature B and T lymphocytes, possess normal mature NK cells. Moreover, NK cells rearrange neither immunoglobulin nor T cell antigen receptor genes. NK cells can be identified by the presence of certain characteristic differentiation antigens (Fig 5-7). All NK cells express CD56 and CD16 but lack expression of the CD3/TCR. Most mature NK cells are large granular lymphocytes (LGL), as are some T cells. In normal individuals, NK cells make up 10–15% of lymphocytes in peripheral blood and 1–2% of lymphocytes in spleen.

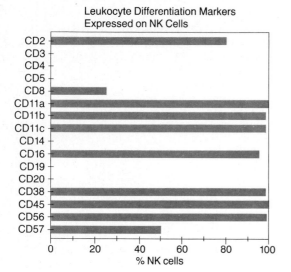

Leukocyte Differentiation Markers
Expressed on NK Cells

Figure 5–7. Antigens expressed on NK cells.

Function of NK Cells

NK cells were originally defined by their ability to kill certain tumor cells (referred to as **NK activity**) without deliberate tumor cell immunization of the host. Unlike most CTL, NK cells recognize and kill both autologous (self) and allogeneic tumors without requiring recognition of MHC antigens on the target cell. This **MHC-unrestricted cytotoxicity** is not confined to NK cells, however; a small subset of T lymphocytes can also mediate this function. It has been suggested that this NK activity may be important in immune surveillance by preventing metastasis of tumors through the blood, although this remains controversial.

The most important role of NK cells is probably in defense against viral infection. NK cells kill virus-infected host cells but not normal uninfected cells. In very rare cases, NK cells are absent; these patients have been reported to be particularly susceptible to certain viral infections, such as cytomegalovirus infection and varicella. Because NK cells do not require prior exposure to the antigen to respond, they may provide the initial antiviral defense during the latent period before development of antibodies and antigen-specific CTL.

Unlike T and B lymphocytes, NK cells do not possess antigen specificity and do not acquire immune memory after an initial exposure to a virus-infected or tumor cell. The membrane receptors on NK cells responsible for recognition of tumor and virus-infected cells have not yet been identified.

Antibody-Dependent Cellular Cytotoxicity (ADCC)

In addition to NK activity, NK cells mediate **antibody-dependent cellular cytotoxicity (ADCC)**, the mechanism whereby a cytotoxic effector cell can kill an antibody-coated target cell. Binding and signal transduction occur through a cell surface receptor that is located on the cytotoxic effector cells and that binds the Fc region of immunoglobulin. The effector cells mediating ADCC were formerly referred to as "K (killer cells)"; however, it now appears that a unique "K cell" does not exist. Rather, most ADCC in peripheral blood is mediated by NK cells and a small subset of T lymphocytes that express CD16, an Fc receptor that preferentially binds complexes of human IgG1 and IgG3. Thus, ADCC provides a mechanism for NK cells to use the antigen-binding specificity of antibodies to direct their killing activity.

NK Cell Activation by Cytokines

Resting NK cells isolated from normal individuals kill only a limited range of tumors (the K562 erythroleukemia is the prototype "NK-sensitive" tumor); however, NK cells can be activated by certain cytokines to increase their cytotoxic activity and proliferate. For example, after a few hours of exposure to IL-2 in tissue culture, NK cells acquire the capacity to kill essentially all tumor cell types without damaging most normal tissues. This phenomenon is called **lymphokine-activated killer (LAK)** activity. Although some T lymphocytes can also mediate this activity, NK cells are responsible for most of it.

In addition to increasing cytotoxic activity, IL-2 acts as a growth factor and directly induces the proliferation of NK cells. Patients treated with IL-2 demonstrate an elevated level of NK cells in peripheral blood, and these circulating IL-2-activated NK cells are capable of killing a broad spectrum of tumor cell types. The cytotoxic activity of NK cells can also be increased by alpha interferon and, to a lesser extent, by gamma interferon. Interferons are frequently induced during viral infection, so they may play a role in the antiviral immunity mediated by NK cells.

Other Functioning NK Cells

NK cells mediate a variety of immune factors other than cytotoxicity. After appropriate stimulation (eg, interaction with certain tumors, virus-infected cells, bacterial products, lymphokines, or immunoglobulin complexes), NK cells secrete several cytokines, including gamma interferon, TNF, serine esterases, GM-CSF. These cytokines can influence the function of other mature lymphocytes and monocytes in peripheral lymphoid tissues and affect the development of immature hematopoietic cells in bone marrow. They can either augment or suppress the function and development of these cell types, depending on the circumstances.

II. MONOCYTES & MACROPHAGES

DIFFERENTIATION & PHENOTYPE

Monocytes and macrophages develop from immature hematopoietic progenitor cells in the bone marrow. These progenitor cells can give rise to erythrocytes, granulocytes, megakaryocytes, or monocytes, depending upon the signals provided by CSF or certain interleukins.

The monocyte progenitor is the monoblast, which develops into a promonocyte and then a monocyte in the bone marrow. Mature monocytes enter the circulation, and a proportion exit from the blood and develop into resident macrophages in the spleen, lymph nodes, liver, lung, thymus, peritoneum, nervous system, skin, and other tissues.

MONOCYTE IDENTIFICATION

Monocytes and macrophages can be identified by morphology, expression of certain cell surface differentiation antigens, and the presence of characteristic enzymes in the cytoplasm. Human monocytes and macrophages express class II MHC antigens (HLA-DR, -DP, and -DQ), gamma interferon receptor, aminopeptidase N (CD13), receptors for complement components (complement receptor types 1 [CD35], 3 [CD11b], and 4 [CD11c]), and receptors for the Fc region of IgG (IgG-Fc receptor types I (CD64) and II (CD32)). Mature monocytes express high levels of a relatively monocyte-specific antigen, CD14; however, expression of this antigen is lost when the monocytes differentiate into macrophages. Histocytochemical studies have shown that monocytes and macrophages possess nonspecific esterases, lysozyme, alkaline phosphodiesterase, and peroxidase and that the amount and intracellular localization of these substances change during monocyte-macrophage differentiation and activation.

FUNCTION OF MONOCYTES & MACROPHAGES

The term "macrophage" originated from the observation that these cells engulf and ingest for-

eign matter, a process designated **phagocytosis** (ingestion of small soluble substances is called **pinocytosis**). A major role of monocytes and macrophages in an inflammatory response is to eliminate bacteria and other pathogens by this process (see Chapters 11 and 12).

IMMUNE RESPONSES & MONOCYTES

Monocytes and macrophages can serve as APC for T lymphocytes by ingesting and degrading foreign antigen in phagolysosomes into peptides that bind to MHC glycoproteins for presentation on the cell surface. Because human monocytes and macrophages express both class I (HLA-A, -B, and -C) and class II (HLA-DR, -DP, and -DQ) MHC glycoproteins, they are able to present antigen to CD8 and CD4 T lymphocytes, respectively. Activated lymphocytes, in turn, secrete factors that affect monocyte and macrophage function and differentiation.

Monocyte and macrophage development is affected by the secretion of cytokines (CSF), lymphokines (IL-2, IL-3, and IL-4), and interferons by activated T lymphocytes. For example, gamma interferon produced by activated T cells stimulates and increases the amount of MHC glycoproteins on monocytes and macrophages, allowing for more efficient antigen presentation.

Cytokines produced by monocytes and macrophages similarly affect the response of lymphocytes. Prostaglandin E, for example, inhibits lymphocyte function and proliferation, whereas IL-1 acts as a potent cosignal with antigen for activation and proliferation of T lymphocytes. Thus, monocytes and macrophages are of central importance in initiation and regulation of immune responses, as well as being major sources of secretory proteins for many tissues and organs.

SUMMARY

The immune system contains several cell types, including lymphocytes, mononuclear phagocytes (monocytes, macrophages), and granulocytes. These cells mediate distinct immune functions and secrete a great variety of soluble substances that regulate the immune system as well as inflammation and functions in other tissues and organs.

Three distinct types of lymphocytes exist: T cells, B cells, and NK cells. T and B cells can recognize more than 10^{11} different antigens by using their membrane glycoprotein receptors, the T cell antigen receptor and immunoglobulin, respectively. These receptors are generated by somatic recombination of genetic elements during T and B cell development in the thymus and bone marrow, respectively.

Immunoglobulin on B cells directly binds many types of antigens, including proteins, carbohydrates, lipids, and small quantities of chemicals. In contrast, T cell antigen receptors bind only peptide antigens that are bound to class I or II MHC molecules or APC. Binding of antigen receptors of either B or T cells results in activation and proliferation and in the release of soluble factors that inhibit or augment other aspects of the immune response.

Subsets of T cells interact with antigen bound to either class I (HLA-A, -B, and -C) or class II (HLA-DR, -DP, and -DQ) MHC structures. CD8 T cells usually react with peptide class I MHC complexes and are principally mediators of cellular cytotoxicity or killing. CD4 T cells react with peptide-class II MHC complexes and are the predominant mediators of lymphokine secretion, which augments or suppresses the response of other lymphocytes.

An important and probably unique feature of B and T lymphocytes is immunologic memory, whereby they remember prior exposure to antigen and respond rapidly after reexposure to the same antigen.

The third type of lymphocyte, the NK cell, does not have immunologic memory and does not express an antigen receptor resulting from gene rearrangement. NK cells recognize and kill virus-infected cells and certain tumors by an unknown process. Unlike T lymphocytes, NK cells do not require the presence of MHC glycoproteins on the target to recognize and kill a virus-infected cell or tumor.

Lymphocytes and mononuclear phagocytes act in concert to respond rapidly to eliminate the foreign antigen and then to regulate the response after the antigen has been eliminated.

REFERENCES

Lymphocytes

Allison JP, Lanier LL: Structure, function, and serology of the T-cell antigen receptor complex. *Annu Rev Immunol* 1987;**5**:503.

Clevers H et al: The T cell receptor/CD3 complex: a dynamic protein ensemble. *Annu Rev Immunol* 1988;**6**:629.

Kishimoto T, Hirano T: Molecular regulation of B lymphocyte response. *Annu Rev Immunol* 1988;**6**:485.

McMichael AJ et al (editors): *Leucocyte Typing IV.* Oxford Univ Press, 1989.

Miyajima A et al: Coordinate regulation of immune and inflammatory responses by T cell-derived lymphokines. *FASEB J* 1988;**2**:2462.

Sanders ME, Makgoba MW, Shaw S: Human naive and memory T cells: reinterpretation of helper-inducer and suppressor-inducer subsets. *Immunol Today* 1988;**9**:195.

Trinchieri G: Biology of natural killer cells. *Adv Immunol* 1989;**47**:187.

Monocytes & Macrophages

Clark SC, Kamen R: The human hematopoietic colony-stimulating factors. *Science* 1987;**236**:1229.

Hamilton TA, Adams DO: Molecular mechanisms of signal transduction in macrophages. *Immunol Today* 1987;**8**:151.

Werb Z et al: Secreted proteins of resting and activated macrophages. In: *Handbook of Experimental Immunology,* 4th ed. Vol 2. Weir DM et al (editors). Blackwell, 1986.

The T Cell Receptor

6

Joan Goverman, PhD and Jane R. Parnes, MD

T and B lymphocytes are responsible for the ability to recognize an invasion of foreign materials or antigens in the body. These cells are capable of recognizing an almost limitless variety of foreign cells and substances and, at the same time, exhibiting exquisite specificity. For example, a person immunized against smallpox can resist infection by smallpox but not by other viruses. T cells are specially suited for dealing with infections within the cells of the host; in contrast, B cells recognize free or soluble antigen through cell surface–bound immunoglobulin with no requirement except antigen-receptor complementarity. To carry out this function, T cells have unique properties for antigen recognition.

T cells recognize antigen only when it is presented on the cell surface of an antigen-presenting cell (APC), where it must be associated with polymorphic cell surface polypeptides encoded within the major histocompatibility complex (MHC). The requirement for simultaneous recognition of MHC molecules with antigen provides a mechanism for ensuring that T cells come into action only when they touch another cell. This is important because T cells regulate or kill other cells through cell-to-cell contacts, unlike B cells, whose secreted antibodies act at a distance. T cells are said to be self-MHC-restricted because they recognize antigen only when it is associated with self as opposed to nonself MHC proteins. The actual ligand of the T cell receptor (TCR) is composed of a small fragment of a foreign antigen complexed to some of the polymorphic residues within an MHC molecule (Fig 6–1). The receptor appears to contact portions of both the antigen peptide fragment and the MHC. The TCR is assisted in binding its ligand by accessory molecules, CD4 or CD8, which are expressed on the T cell surface and also bind MHC molecules. However, these accessory molecules appear to bind to a nonpolymorphic region of the MHC molecule, whereas the TCR interacts with both polymorphic residues of MHC proteins and antigenic determinants. Thus, TCRs exhibit a tremendous amount of di-

versity to correspond to the wide array of antigens encountered in the life span of the host. The molecular structure of the TCR and the mechanisms used in generating diversity are the subject of this chapter. Correlations of TCR genes with particular diseases and approaches toward treating these diseases through immunotherapy are briefly discussed.

STRUCTURE & DIVERSITY OF THE T CELL RECEPTOR

The TCR is a disulfide-linked heterodimer composed of α and β glycoprotein chains (MW 40,000–50,000). Both chains are composed of 2 domains: the amino-terminal portion consists of a region of variable amino acid sequence (V region) and the carboxy-terminal portion consists of a region of constant amino acid sequence (C region) (Fig 6–2). The region domains associate with each other to form an antigen-binding "pocket," whereas the C region domains anchor the receptor to the T cell membrane and presumably participate in initiating the effector function of the cell. The TCR is noncovalently associated on the cell surface with CD3, a complex of at least 5 polypeptides that may participate in mediating activation signals. CD3 is functionally important because it is required for the expression of the TCR on the cell surface. T cells, in fact, can be activated directly by antibodies specific for the CD3 complex.

Like immunoglobulin genes, the genes that encode the TCR α and β chains are formed from the joining together of separate genetic elements. The sequence encoding the V region of the α chain is formed from a V and a J (joining) gene segment, whereas that encoding the V region of the β chain is formed from a V, a D (diversity), and a J gene segment (Fig 6–3). These gene segments rearrange during T cell ontogeny within the thymus by deletion of intervening DNA to form a contiguous V gene. As with immunoglobulin gene rearrangement, this process is dependent upon the presence

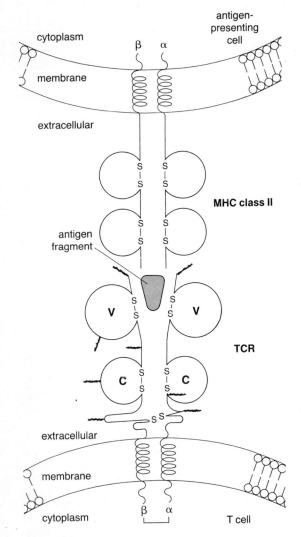

cytoplasm

β α

antigen-
presenting
cell

membrane

extracellular

MHC class II

antigen
fragment

V   V

TCR

C   C

extracellular

membrane

cytoplasm

β α

T cell

Figure 6–1. Complex of antigen fragment and class II MHC molecule forming the ligand of the TCR. See the legend to Fig 6–2 for an explanation of structural details of the TCR.

but closely linked clusters, in each of which the C region gene is preceded by a series of J segments and one D segment (Fig 6–3). The number of possible $V_\alpha J_\alpha$ and $V_\beta D_\beta J_\beta$ combinations therefore provides for the enormous diversity generated by the rearrangement process. In addition, there are 2 mechanisms directly linked to rearrangement that generate even more diversity. First, the endpoints of the rearranging gene segments are flexible, causing variation in the amino acid sequence between the joining gene segments. Second, nucleotides can be either deleted or added randomly (N region diversity) at the junctions of rearranging gene segments. These mechanisms, together with the random pairing of α and β chains, account for much of the diversity potential of the TCR repertoire. In contrast to immunoglobulin genes, TCR genes do not appear to diversify by means of somatic mutation of the rearranged genes.

Determination of the molecular structure of the TCR has yielded several insights into the nature of the dual specificity for antigen and MHC. Extensive analysis of T cells with defined specificity has shown that there is no absolute correlation between V gene usage and recognition of either antigen or MHC determinants. Thus, the TCR is not composed of separate binding sites for antigen and MHC but, rather, appears to recognize its ligand as a single antigenic complex, much like an antibody. The phenomenon of self MHC restriction is most probably a result of developmental influences of the thymus during T cell ontogeny rather than of germline-encoded, unique structural properties of the receptor.

A second receptor present on the surface of early thymocytes and a small subset of peripheral T cells has been characterized. It is also a disulfide-linked heterodimer composed of a γ and δ chain. These chains also consist of V and C regions and are encoded by rearranging gene segments. The diversity potential of the γ/δ receptor appears to be limited relative to that of the α/β receptor. The function of cells expressing the γ/δ receptor and the ligand for the receptor are unknown, although many demonstrate non-MHC-restricted killing of target cells.

When an α/β-TCR on a CD4 lymphocyte binds to its specific peptide antigen-class II MHC molecule combination on an APC, a trimolecular complex is formed that transmits a signal to the CD4 lymphocyte. The signal initiates a series of biochemical reactions within the cell, resulting in subsequent biologic responses (Fig 6–4). The critical biochemical events are (1) hydrolysis of phosphatidylinositol biphosphate to form inositol triphosphate and diacylglycerol, (2) influx of Ca^{2+} into the cell cytoplasm, and (3) activation of protein kinase C. Ca^{2+} and protein kinase C act as second messengers, probably in conjunction with other

of specific DNA sequences adjacent to the rearranging gene segments. Sequences encoding the V region are joined to those encoding the C region after transcription by means of mRNA splicing. The rearrangement of gene segments to form the TCR gene allows for the generation of the enormous diversity of receptors. There are at least 50 V_α gene segments and an estimated 100 or more J_α gene segments for encoding of the α chain. Similarly, for the β chain there are at least 60 V gene segments, two D gene segments, and 13 J gene segments. There are also 2 closely related C region genes for β, and these are located in 2 separate

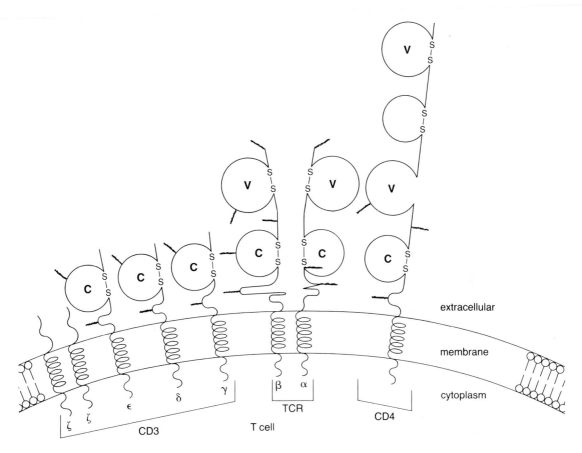

Figure 6-2. Structure of TCR α and β polypeptides. The variable (V) and constant (C) domains and positions of disulfide bonds (SS) are shown. The sites of N-linked glycosylation are marked ($\sim\!\sim\!\sim$). The transmembrane region is shown ($\ell\ell\ell\ell$) traversing the plasma membrane. The polypeptide chains of the adjacent CD3 and CD4 molecules are also shown.

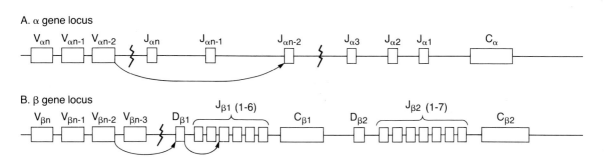

Figure 6-3. Organization of the TCR genes. **A:** α chain gene organization. Only a few of the multiple V and J gene segments are shown. The arrow indicates one potential rearrangement between a V and a J segment. **B:** β chain gene organization. A few of the multiple V gene segments are shown. All D and J gene segments are indicated. One potential rearrangement is illustrated. The $D_{\beta 1}$ gene segment could also rearrange to a J in the $J_{\beta 2}$ gene cluster. In both panels the jagged lines indicate separation of the DNA on either side by very large distances.

7

Cytokines

Joost J. Oppenheim, MD, Francis W. Ruscetti, PhD, & Connie Faltynek, PhD

Over the past 25 years, an important group of peptide mediators has been detected, characterized, and purified. These mediators, termed **cytokines,** function as up- and down-regulators of immunologic, inflammatory, and reparative host responses to injury. Many of these hormone-like polypeptides are secreted in the course of immunologic and inflammatory responses. Cytokines produced by lymphocytes are called **lymphokines,** whereas the peptides produced by monocytes or macrophages are called **monokines.** Cytokines function as intercellular signals that regulate local and, at times, systemic inflammatory responses. Cytokines are distinct from endocrine hormones since they are produced by a number of cells rather than by specialized glands. Cytokines are not usually present in serum and generally act in a paracrine (ie, locally near the producing cells) or autocrine (ie, directly on the producing cells) rather than in an endocrine manner on distant target cells. Cytokines modulate reactions of the host to foreign antigens or injurious agents by regulating the growth, mobility, and differentiation of leukocytes and other cells.

Although some transformed lymphocyte, macrophage, keratinocyte, and fibroblast cell lines spontaneously secrete cytokines into the culture medium, normal resting cells and most cell lines must be stimulated to produce cytokines. T or B lymphocytes obtained from immunized donors can be specifically activated by antigens to produce lymphokines. Many cytokines are simultaneously produced by activated cells and are difficult to isolate from one another. Now that many of the genes encoding the cytokines have been cloned, it is clear that there are multiple dissimilar and genetically unrelated cytokines.

Cytokines generally are synthesized and secreted peptides or glycoproteins with molecular weights (MW) ranging from 6000 to 60,000. They are extremely potent compounds that act at concentrations of 10^{-10}–10^{-15} mol/L to stimulate target cell functions following specific ligand-receptor interactions. This high specific activity has facilitated cytokine detection by bioassays, but the small quantities produced have impeded their purification. Nevertheless, characterization of cytokines has progressed at a phenomenal rate because of recent technologic developments: (1) the use of cell clones that produce large amounts of limited numbers of cytokines; (2) the development of high-performance liquid chromatography (HPLC) techniques; (3) the availability of monoclonal antibodies for neutralization and detection; (4) immunoaffinity purification; and, especially, (5) the use of gene cloning techniques.

A single purified cytokine can have multiple effects on the growth and differentiation of many cell types. Consequently, cytokines may exhibit considerable overlap in their biologic effects on lymphoid, myeloid, and connective tissue target cells. In addition, biologically distinct cytokines may have similar effects by initiating the production of a cascade of identical cytokines or of one another.

This chapter will focus on a discussion of the more pivotal cytokines that amplify the afferent and efferent limbs of the immune and inflammatory responses: IL-1 to IL-8, tumor necrosis factor (TNF), interferons (IFN), colony-stimulating factors (CSF), and other growth and chemotactic factors (Table 7–1).

INTERLEUKIN-1 (IL-1)

IL-1 consists of 2 distinct peptides that have a multiplicity of immunologic, inflammatory, and reparative activities. These include effects on lymphoid and nonlymphoid cells (Fig 7–1). In 1972, a **lymphocyte-activating factor (LAF),** which was mitogenic for murine thymocytes, was discovered in the supernatant of cultures of adherent human peripheral blood cells and murine splenocytes. Human LAF was also *comitogenic* in that it synergistically enhanced the proliferative

Table 7-1. Characteristic properties of cytokines.

Cytokine	MW	Principal Cell Sources	Primary Type of Activity	Preeminent Effects
IL-1	17,500	Macrophages and others (see Table 7–2)	Immunoaugmentation.	Inflammatory and hemato-poietic
IL-2	15,500	T lymphocytes and LGL	T and B cell growth factor.	Activates T and NK cells
IL-3	14,000–28,000	T lymphocytes	Hematopoietic growth factor.	Promotes growth of early mye-loid progenitor cells
IL-4	20,000	TH cells	T and B cell growth factor; promotes IgE reactions.	Promotes IgE switch and mast cell growth
IL-5	18,000	TH cells	Stimulates B cells and eosinophils	Promotes IgA switch and eo-sinophilia
IL-6	22,000–30,000	Fibroblasts and others	Hybridoma growth fac-tor; augments inflam-mation.	Growth factor for B cells and polyclonal immunoglobulin production
IL-7	25,000	Stromal cells	Lymphopoietin.	Generates pre-B and pre-T cells and is lymphocyte growth factor
IL-8	8,800	Macrophages and others	Chemoattracts neutro-phils and T lympho-cytes.	Regulates lymphocyte homing and neutrophil infiltration
G-CSF	18,000–22,000	Monocytes and others	Myeloid growth factor.	Generates neutrophils
M-CSF	18,000–26,000	Monocytes and others	Macrophage growth factor.	Generates macrophages
GM-CSF	14,000–38,000	T cells and others	Monomyelocytic growth factor.	Myelopoiesis
IFN α IFN β IFN γ	18,000–20,000 25,000 20,000–25,000	Leukocytes Fibroblasts T lymphocytes and NK cells	Antiviral, antiprolifera-tive, and immunomo-dulating.	Stimulates macrophages and NK cells Induce cell membrane anti-gens (eg, MHC)
TNFα LT = TNFβ	17,000 18,000	Macrophages and others T lymphocytes	Inflammatory, immu-noenhancing, and tu-moricidal.	Vascular thromboses and tu-mor necrosis
TGFβ	25,000	Platelets, bone, and others	Fibroplasia and immu-nosuppression.	Wound healing and bone re-modeling

response of murine thymocytes to lectins such as concanavalin A (Con A) or phytohemagglutinin (PHA).

In 1974, it was reported that cultured human monocytes also secreted a **B cell–activating factor (BAF)** that stimulated antibody production by T cell-depleted murine splenocytes. Subsequent analyses revealed that the biochemical properties of LAF and BAF were similar and that they also resembled the structure of pyrogenic macrophage-derived factors called **endogenous pyrogens.** In 1979, these factors were all renamed interleukin-1 (IL-1). IL-1 is detected by bioassays of its comito-genic effect on thymocytes, IL-1-reactive cell lines, or, more recently, by enzyme-linked immu-nosorbent assay (ELISA).

IL-1 Producers & Inducers

IL-1 is produced by 11 types of macrophages, irrespective of their tissue of origin, as well as by keratinocytes, dendritic cells, astrocytes, micro-glial cells, normal B lymphocytes, cultured T cell clones, fibroblasts, neutrophils, endothelial cells, and smooth muscle cells. However, IL-1-like fac-tors are produced by virtually all nucleated cell types. Although a number of cell lines produce low levels of IL-1 constitutively, most normal cells must be stimulated by a variety of agents to pro-

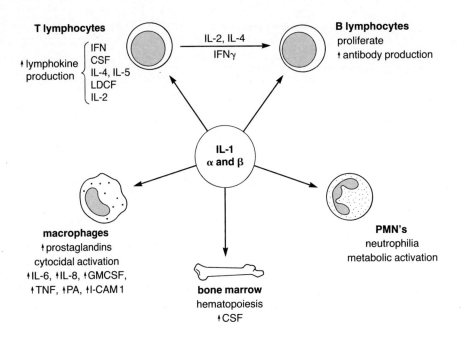

T lymphocytes

↑ lymphokine
production

{ IFN
CSF
IL-4, IL-5
LDCF
IL-2

IL-2, IL-4
IFNγ

B lymphocytes
proliferate
↑ antibody production

**IL-1
α and β**

macrophages
↑ prostaglandins
cytocidal activation
↑IL-6, ↑IL-8, ↑GMCSF,
↑TNF, ↑PA, ↑I-CAM 1

bone marrow
hematopoiesis
↑CSF

PMN's
neutrophilia
metabolic activation

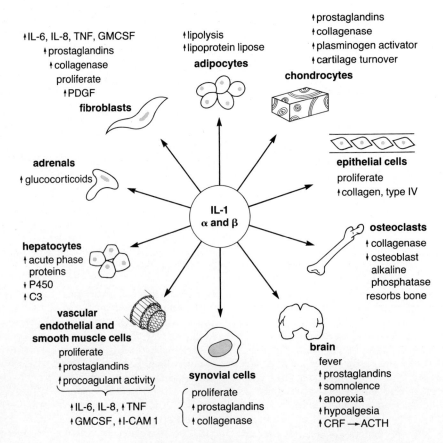

↑IL-6, IL-8, TNF, GMCSF
↑ prostaglandins
↑ collagenase
proliferate
↑PDGF
fibroblasts

↑ lipolysis
↑ lipoprotein lipose
adipocytes

↑ prostaglandins
↑ collagenase
↑ plasminogen activator
↑ cartilage turnover
chondrocytes

adrenals
↑ glucocorticoids

epithelial cells
proliferate
↑collagen, type IV

**IL-1
α and β**

hepatocytes
↑ acute phase
proteins
↓ P450
↑ C3

osteoclasts
↑ collagenase
↓ osteoblast
alkaline
phosphatase
resorbs bone

**vascular
endothelial and
smooth muscle cells**
proliferate
↑ prostaglandins
↑ procoagulant activity

↑IL-6, IL-8, ↑ TNF
↑GMCSF, ↑I-CAM 1

synovial cells
{ proliferate
↑ prostaglandins
↑ collagenase

brain
fever
↑ prostaglandins
↑ somnolence
↑ anorexia
↑ hypoalgesia
↑ CRF → ACTH

Figure 7–1. a: Actions of IL-1 on hematopoietic and lymphoid tissues. **b:** Actions of IL-1 on nonlymphoid tissues.

duce IL-1. IL-1 production by these cells is stimulated by diverse agents, including adjuvants such as lipopolysaccharide (LPS) and muramyl dipeptide (MDP), injurious ultraviolet irradiation, urate or silicate particles, aluminum hydroxide, and microorganisms. Agents that activate lymphocytes can stimulate macrophages to produce IL-1 either by direct contact between the cells, which is genetically controlled by class II major histocompatibility complex (MHC) molecules (see Chapter 4), or by producing lymphokines such as TNF, CSF, or IFN γ which stimulate macrophages.

The nature of the stimulant determines whether IL-1 accumulates predominantly at intracellular sites or is released into the extracellular environment. Latex particles, LPS, and zymosan, for example, stimulate increases in both the intracellular and extracellular levels of IL-1, whereas silica particles and phorbol myristate acetate (PMA) predominantly stimulate the extracellular release of IL-1. The intrinsic cellular factors that regulate the release of IL-1 are unidentified, but cell injury appears to be one cause.

IL-1 is found in some tissues in the absence of noxious stimuli. For example, amniotic fluid and urine contain significant levels of IL-1, and IL-1β. mRNA expression and production occur in the skin and adult brain. At the time of the luteal phase of the menstrual cycle and during strenuous exercise, IL-1 levels are elevated in human plasma.

Specific antagonists of IL-1 production are of considerable therapeutic interest because IL-1 is implicated in chronic inflammatory diseases. Corticosteroids, already in wide use as anti-inflammatory agents, inhibit IL-1 production by macrophages. Prostaglandins, which are themselves mediators of inflammation, appear to inhibit the release of IL-1 from macrophages. Thus, prostaglandin E_2 (PGE$_2$), for example, a product of the cyclooxygenase pathway, exerts a negative effect on IL-1 production. Conversely, inhibitors of the lipoxygenase pathway reduce the amount of IL-1 released, and leukotrienes appear to stimulate IL-1 production (see Chapter 13).

Structure-Function Studies of IL-1

IL-1 exists in 2 molecular forms called IL-1α and IL-1β. Two distinct IL-1 genes coding for IL-1α and IL-1β have been identified in all species to date (Table 7–2). Human IL-1α and IL-1β, which exhibit 45% homology at the nucleotide level and only 26% homology at the amino acid level, are antigenically distinct. Despite this, the potency and activities of IL-1α and IL-1β are virtually identical, and they bind with equal affinity to the same cell surface receptors. Many cell types express both IL-1 genes, but ratios of IL-1α to IL-1β can vary widely; eg, human monocytes produce predominantly IL-1β, whereas keratinocytes produce largely IL-1α.

IL-1α and IL-1β are initially translated as propeptides (MW 31,000) that are enzymatically processed to yield a soluble form (MW 17,000) at

Table 7-2. Properties of human inflammatory cytokines.

Property	IL-1	TNF
Chromosome	2	6
Proform	271 amino acids (IL-1α), 269 amino acids (IL-1β)	236 amino acids (TNFα), 204 amino acids (TNFβ)
Mature form	159 amino acids (IL-1α), 153 amino acids (IL-1β)	157 amino acids (TNFα), 171 amino acids (TFNβ)
Cell sources	Macrophages, keratinocytes, endothelial cells, fibroblasts, astrocytes, B and T cells	Macrophages, T and B lymphocytes, Keratinocytes, Fibroblasts, endothelial cells, astrocytes (TNFα); T lymphocytes (TH1 subset), EBV B cell lines (TNFβ)
Receptor	60–80-kDa glycoprotein $K_d = 10^{-10}$ mol/L 50–5000 sites/cell	80-kDa glycoprotein $K_d = 10^{-10}$ mol/L 1000–10,000 sites/cell
In vivo effects	Local neutrophilic infiltration Delayed-type hypersensitivity Fibroplasia and angiogenesis Endogenous pyrogen Acute-phase reactants Neutrophilia Radioprotection Adjuvant and antimicrobial agent	Local neutrophilic infiltration Schwartzman reaction and necrosis of tumors Endogenous pyrogen Acute-phase reactants Cachexia, neutrophilia Radioprotection Adjuvant Angiogenesis

or beyond the outer cell membrane, which then acts extracellularly. Biologically active IL-1α, but not IL-1β, has been detected on the surface of cells and can thus participate in interactions during cell-to-cell contact.

Receptors for IL-1

IL-1 acts on target cells via high-affinity receptors on the plasma membrane. The numbers of such receptors vary from about 100 on T cells to a few thousand on fibroblasts, but the affinity is relatively constant ($K_d = 10^{-10}$ mol/L), suggesting that most cell types have a common IL-1 receptor. The extracellular piece of the IL-1 receptor belongs to the immunoglobulin gene superfamily. There are a 21-amino-acid transmembrane region and a 217-amino-acid cytoplasmic tail. Expression of IL-1 receptors on the cell surface is down-regulated by internalization following binding of IL-1. In contrast, both glucocorticoids and prostaglandins increase the expression of functional IL-1 receptors on some human cell types, eg, fibroblasts and B cells, but not on T cells, monocytes, or neutrophils. The critical intracellular events following binding of IL-1 to its receptor are still unidentified, although elevated levels of diacylglycerol, cyclic AMP (cAMP), G proteins, and ornithine decarboxylase have been detected in some cell types.

Inhibitors of Activities of IL-1

IL-1 activity can be regulated by endogenous factors that affect cytokine production by modulating either receptor expression or signal transduction after receptors are triggered. Potent nonspecific antagonism to the actions of IL-1 is attributed to transforming growth factor β (TGFβ), corticosteroids, and α melanocyte-stimulating hormone (αMSH). An inhibitory factor in urine of myelogenous leukemia patients specifically competes with IL-1 binding to receptors for IL-1. Pharmacologic inhibition of IL-1 activity (eg, by corticosteroids) may be useful in controlling some inflammatory reactions.

Immunologic & Inflammatory Effects of IL-1 & TNF

TNF also consists of 2 distinct peptides with multiple immunologic and local as well as systemic inflammatory activities. These also include effects on lymphoid and nonlymphoid cells (Fig 7-2). TNFα was first described as an activity in serum that induces hemorrhagic necrosis in certain tumors in vivo and was later independently discovered as **cachectin,** a circulating mediator of wasting during parasitic disease. TNFα is produced by activated macrophages and other cells and has a broad spectrum of biologic actions on many immune and nonimmune target cells. **Lym-**

photoxin, which is primarily a product of T lymphocytes, has also been called TNFβ. TNFα and TNFβ bind to the same receptor on target cells and consequently have the same biologic activities.

TNFα & TNFβ Genes & Their Products

The gene for human TNFα is located within or near the MHC genes on the short arm of chromosome 6, closely linked to the gene for TNFβ (Table 7-2). The degree of homology between TNFα and TNFβ is 46% at the nucleotide level and 28% at the amino acid level. The precursor form of TNFα consists of 236 amino acids. Prior to or during secretion, 79 N-terminal amino acids are enzymatically removed from the pro form to yield the MW-17,400 soluble mature TNFα. Although TNFα and the MW-20,000 TNFβ do not cross-react immunologically, they bind equally well to the same receptors. Since tumor cell killing by formaldehyde-fixed and activated macrophages can be blocked by monoclonal antibodies to TNFα, an active membrane-associated form of TNFα has been proposed.

TNF Inducers & Producers

Many cell types can produce TNFα. Monocyte-macrophages produce TNFα in response to PMA, LPS, Sendai virus, MDP, tumor cells, mycoplasmas, or BCG (bacilla Calmette-Guérin) (Table 7-2). Lymphocytes can be stimulated by antigens or mitogens to produce TNFβ, but lymphocytes and natural killer (NK) cells can also produce some TNFα. A number of endogenous mediators are also active inducers of TNF; these include IL-3 (for mast cells), IL-1, TNF itself, GM-CSF, CSF-1, leukotriene B_4 (LTB$_4$), platelet-activating factor (PAF), and IFN γ in conjunction with LPS (for macrophages) (see Table 7-1 for abbreviations).

Receptors for TNF

Between 1000 and 10,000 high-affinity receptors for TNF per cell have been observed on various cells (K_d is approximately 2×10^{-10}–6×10^{-10} mol/L). Cross-linking studies revealed TNF-binding structures of MW 60,000–80,000 on human cells. The action of TNF is considerably augmented by IFN γ on several target cell types, at least in part by increasing TNF receptor expression. The intracellular effects of TNF are still largely unknown.

Immunologic Activities of IL-1 & TNF

The multifaceted effects of the major "broad-spectrum" inflammatory mediators, namely IL-1 and TNF, can be reviewed together. Although the high-affinity receptors for IL-1 and TNF, which

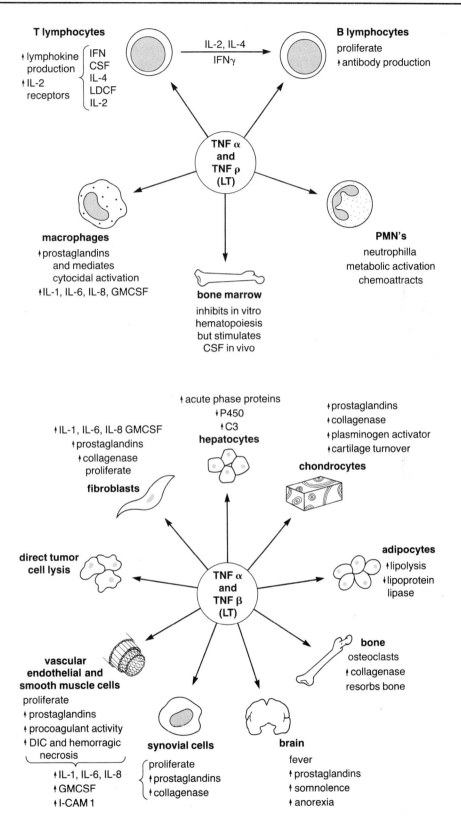

Figure 7-2. *a:* Effects of TNFα and β (LT) on hematopoietic and lymphoid tissues. *b:* Effects of TNFα and β on nonlymphoid tissues.

have been detected on virtually all nucleated cell types, are structurally completely unrelated, these 2 cytokines show a remarkably high degree of overlap in their in vitro immunologic and nonimmunologic activities (Table 7–3). Although the in vivo effects of IL-1 and TNF also exhibit some similarities, TNF has more in vivo toxic, vascular occlusive, and antitumor effects, whereas IL-1 is more protective against lethal mediation and is a greater mobilizer of bone turnover (Table 7–3). Differences in the rate and site of in vivo production, as well as half-life and distribution, may account for the differences in these in vivo effects.

IL-1 augments immunologically mediated inflammatory reactions. It promotes the proliferation of T lymphocytes by enhancing the produc-

Table 7–3. Comparison of target cells and actions of IL-1 and TNF/LT.

Target Cells or Tissues	Effects	IL-1α, β	TNF/LT
T lymphocytes	Enhance IL-2 receptor expression	+	+
	Induce lymphokine production	+ +	+
	Act as thymocyte comitogen	+ +	+
B lymphocytes	Enhance antibody production	+	+
	Promote B cell proliferation	+	+
Neuroendocrine cells	Release CRF to Pituitary ACTH adrenal cortico-steroids	+	−
	Induce prostaglandin-mediated fever	+	+
	Induce somnolence and anorexia	+	+
Neutrophils	Act as chemoattractants	−	+
	Increase adhesiveness, phagocytosis, ADCC, oxygen intermediates	−	±
	Cause degranulation and enzyme release		
Monocytes and macrophages	Act as chemoattractant	−	±
	Induce prostaglandins, IL-1, IL-6, GM-CSF, and IL-8	+	+
	Coactivate to cytocidal state	+	+ +
Endothelial cells and vascular smooth muscle	Increase adhesiveness (I-CAM1)	+	+ +
	Induce procoagulant activity, IL-1, IL-6, GMC-SF, plasminogen activator inhibitor, prostaglandins, and MHC	+	+ +
	Act as mitogenic and angiogenic agents	+	+ +
Osteoblasts	Decrease alkaline phosphate levels	+ +	+
Osteoclasts	Cause bone resorption (increase collagenase)	+	+
Chondrocytes	Increase cartilage turnover	+	+
Fibroblasts/synovial cells	Act as mitogen agents and express oncogenes	+	+
	Induce prostaglandins, IL-1, IL-6 collagenase, GM-CSF, and IL-8	+	+
Hepatocytes	Induce some acute-phase reactants	+	+
	Decreased cytochrome P450 and Increase C3	+	+
	Increase Plasma Cu, decrease Plasma Fe + Zn	+	+
Hematopoietic cells	Inhibit some precursor cell proliferation and differentiation	−	+
	Stimulate precursor cells	+	−
Tumor cells and virus-infected cells	Selectively act as cytostatic/cytocidal agents	+	+ +
Adipocytes	Decrease lipoprotein lipase levels	+	+ +
	Increase lipolysis	+	+ +
Epithelial cells	Act as mitogenic agents	+	N.D.[1]
	Secrete collagen type IV	+	N.D.
Pancreatic β Cells	Modulate insulin levels	+	−
Dendritic Cells	Increase T cell activation	+	N.D.

[1]N.D., No reported data.

tion of T lymphocyte-derived lymphokines such as IL-2 and IL-2 receptors on T cells. In addition, IL-1 augments the capacity of accessory antigen-presenting cells (APC) to activate T cell-dependent immune responses. Although the immunologic effects of TNF are not as well established as those of IL-1, TNF also is comitogenic for thymocytes and induces IL-2 receptors. Both IL-1 and TNF have been shown to augment B cell proliferation, surface immunoglobulin receptor expression, and antibody production. Injection of either IL-1 or TNF together with an antigen has an adjuvant effect on T cell-dependent antibody responses.

Inflammatory Activities
of IL-1 & TNF

TNF has more potent in vitro effects than IL-1 on neutrophils, monocytes, and endothelial cells. Higher concentrations (approximately 1000 U/ml) of TNF, but not of IL-1, are chemotactic for neutrophils, and TNF activates the neutrophil respiratory burst and degranulation. Similarly, TNF (but not IL-1) is said to be chemotactic in vitro for monocytes. However, both IL-1 and TNF can augment the capacity of monocytes to produce other inflammatory mediators such as prostaglandins, IL- 6, and the neutrophil-attracting peptide, which has been renamed IL-8. In addition, IL-1 and, to an even greater degree, TNF increase the adhesiveness of endothelial cells by inducing the expression of cell membrane adhesion molecules such as intrinsic cell adhesion molecule type 1 (I CAM-1). These differences may account for the greater vascular and in vivo antitumor effects of TNF.

Injection of IL-1 induces local acute inflammatory responses that begin within 1 hour and peak within 3–4 hours. Initially, neutrophils adhere to endothelial cells and marginate along blood vessel walls. This is followed by neutrophil infiltration and edema from extravasation of fluids into the tissues. In contrast, slow release of IL-1 from ethylene vinyl acetate copolymer disks implanted into a subcutaneous site results in delayed-type hypersensitivity (DTH) granuloma formation with considerable mononuclear cell infiltration, fibrosis, and new blood vessel formation. Intradermal injections of TNF also produce acute inflammation with neutrophil infiltration.

Both IL-1 and TNF are mitogenic for endothelial cells and have in vivo angiogenic activity. TNF and, to a lesser degree, IL-1 stimulate endothelial cells and to produce prostaglandins, IL-6, and procoagulant factor (tissue factor III), which has the capacity to initiate the clotting cascade. These local coagulation and inflammatory effects block the blood supply and may account for the unique capacity of TNF to cause infarcts and hemorrhagic necrosis of tumors, the property that led to the initial discovery of TNF.

The hemorrhagic Shwartzman reaction has been attributed to TNF because endotoxin shock can be blocked by the administration of antiserum to TNF. The Shwartzman reaction is a usually fatal disseminated intravascular coagulopathy (DIC) that occurs after systemic exposure to endotoxin followed within 24 hours by a second dose of intravenous endotoxin. Repeated injections of IL-1 are reported to yield local Shwartzman reactions. Low doses of IL-1 act synergistically with TNF to induce the hemorrhagic shock of a Shwartzman reaction.

Neuroendocrine Effects
of IL-1 & TNF

IL-1 and TNF act alone and together to induce a number of other systemic inflammatory reactions such as hypothalamus-mediated fever and hepatocyte-mediated acute-phase responses. IL-1, but not TNF, has been reported to stimulate the hypothalamus to produce corticotropin-releasing factor (CRF), which stimulates the release of adrenocorticotropic hormone (ACTH) from the pituitary; this, in turn, induces the production of glucocorticoids by the adrenals. IL-1 thereby initiates a negative regulatory feedback loop, since glucocorticoids suppress the production of both IL-1 and TNF. In addition, TNF as well as IL-1 can induce IL-6, which, in turn, stimulates the production of ACTH, potentially elevating the plasma levels of glucocorticoids.

Glucocorticoids have the capacity to increase IL-1 receptor (IL- 1R) expression, but not TNF receptor expression, on human B lymphocytes. The capacity of glucocorticoids to increase IL-1R expression on B cells suggests that IL-1 may participate in the reported capacity of these steroids to act as polyclonal B lymphocyte activators in vitro and in vivo. This paradoxical up-regulation of IL-1R on B lymphocytes by otherwise immunosuppressive steroids may serve to further suppress inflammation by diverting the immune response from cellular immunity. Thus, steroids seem to favor humoral immunity at the expense of cell-mediated immunity, thereby diminishing inflammation.

Connective Tissue Effects
of IL-1 & TNF

Both IL-1 and TNF stimulate alkaline phosphatase activity in osteoblasts, induce osteoclasts to resorb bone and chondrocytes to increase cartilage turnover, and activate proliferation by fibroblasts and synovial cells. Increased levels of IL-1 and TNF are found in inflammatory joint fluids. Fibrosis and thickening of tissues in joints can be mediated by these cytokines.

Effects of IL-1 & TNF on Hematopoiesis

IL-1 is identical to hematopoietin-1, a factor that synergizes with CSF to stimulate early bone marrow hematopoietic progenitor cells to form giant colonies with high proliferative potential (HPP colonies). In addition, IL-1 induces the production by bone marrow stromal cells of a number of the hematopoietic CSF as well as receptors for CSF-1. TNF also actively induces CSF production by bone marrow stromal cells and macrophages but does not promote HPP colonies. Both TNF and IL-1 administration induce a considerable bone marrow-derived neutrophilia. TNFα, if given 1 day prior to lethal radiation, is radioprotective. However, IL-1 is more effective as a radioprotective agent at lower concentrations than TNFα. Furthermore, IL-1 and TNF show additive or synergistic radioprotective effects, suggesting that their mechanisms of action differ.

Other Activities of IL-1 & TNF

IL-1 stimulates epithelial-cell proliferation and function, eg, production of collagen type IV, whereas the effect of TNF on epithelial cells is unknown. IL-1, but not TNF, selectively affects pancreatic β cells and causes changes in plasma insulin levels. Both TNF and IL-1 exhibit indirect antiviral effects that are mediated in part by the induction of IFN β. TNF and LT are cytostatic and cytocidal for a number of tumor cells in vitro. TNF is cytocidal for a wider variety of tumor cells and kills them more rapidly than does IL-1. The hallmark of the cachectin (or wasting) activity of TNF is probably related to the ability of TNF to increase lipoprotein lipase activity and hence lysis of fat cells. However, IL-1 is also reported to have this capability.

Overall, the considerable overlap in the broad spectrum of activities of these cytokines results in a rather perplexing redundancy in intercellular communications. The redundancy provides alternative pathways for mobilizing host reactions in emergencies, and it enhances efficiency, since IL-1 and TNF exhibit many synergistic interactions. This results in an enormous amplification of the effects of relatively small amounts of these cytokines when both are produced.

INTERLEUKIN-2

IL-2 is an MW-15,400 peptide consisting of 133 amino acids and an essential internal disulfide bond. It exerts numerous immunologic effects by stimulating proliferation and lymphokine production by T cells, B cells, and NK cells. In 1976, a polypeptide hormone, initially called **T cell growth factor (TCGF)**, was found to stimulate human T cell proliferation and to enable T cells to grow continuously in culture. The discovery of TCGF not only made it possible to study the factors involved in T lymphocyte growth but also provided a valuable tool for studying cellular and humoral immunity in vitro. The ability to propagate and develop clones from single normal T cells that maintained their specific immunologic functions has greatly facilitated biochemical and molecular studies of the development, properties, and regulation of immunocompetent T cells.

Molecular Properties of IL-2

Human, primate, and mouse IL-2 have been purified to homogeneity. IL-2 is a single protein (MW 15,000), but the presence of variable amounts of carbohydrate results in higher-MW forms of IL-2. Because recombinant IL-2, which lacks carbohydrate groups, is as active as natural IL-2, carbohydrates are not necessary for IL-2 activity.

Molecular studies with cloned complementary DNA (cDNA) from various human sources and other species indicate that there is only a single gene for IL-2 and that it is located on human chromosome 4. There is little or no homology between the sequence of IL-2 and other sequenced growth factors.

Receptors for IL-2

An initial signal, the antigen, is presented on accessory cells to T cells. This step is required to activate lymphocytes to maximally respond to IL-2. Resting T lymphocytes do not proliferate in response to the same low concentrations (10–20 pmol) of IL-2 that result in maximal proliferation of such antigen-activated T cells. Consequently, antigens and lectins such as PHA are mitogenic for T cells because they cause some T cells both to produce IL-2 and to become maximally responsive to IL-2. This IL-2-responsive state is based on the development of lymphocyte membrane IL-2 receptors that satisfy all the criteria of hormone receptors: (1) a high-affinity binding constant of about 10^{-12} mol/L; (2) binding that is saturable at 20 minutes at 37 °C; and (3) specificity of ligands for target cells. There is a close correlation between the concentration of IL-2 causing lymphocyte proliferation and the concentration that lead to significant IL-2 binding.

A monoclonal antibody, designated **anti-Tac** (for a *T C*ell *A*ctivation antigen that specifically recognizes the the alpha chain of the human IL-2 receptor) suppresses IL-2 mediated proliferation of previously activated T cell lines and blocks activation of peripheral blood lymphocytes by antigens or lectins. The IL-2 receptor was characterized by radioisotopically labeling IL-2 receptor-bearing cell lines followed by immunoprecipitation of IL-2 receptor with anti-Tac. The molecule is a glycoprotein of MW 55,000–60,000.

Characterization of Another IL-2-Binding Protein Distinct From Tac

Several different leukemia cell lines or clones of these cell lines bind IL-2 in the absence of any detectable cell surface Tac antigen via another IL-2-binding protein (MW 75,000). In fact, 3 IL-2-binding affinities have now been identified: The Tac antigen (p55) binds IL-2 with a K_d of 10^{-8} mol/L; the MW-75,000 protein (p75) binds with an intermediate-affinity K_d of 10^{-9} mol/L, and a third receptor binds with a high-affinity K_d of 10^{-11} mol/L and is a complex of the other 2 proteins. A number of studies suggest that p75 can function alone and transmit a biologic signal in response to binding IL-2. The sole function of the Tac moiety seems to be the formation of high-affinity IL-2 receptors by complexing with p75, called the beta chain of the IL-2 receptor thereby increasing the sensitivity and rapidity of the lymphocytic response (Table 7–4). The precise nature of the complex between these 2 IL-2-binding proteins is unknown. In a hypothetic model of this complex, p75 has an intracytoplasmic domain responsible for signaling, and one molecule of IL-2 binds to one molecule of both binding proteins.

IL-2 Production & Detection

Freshly isolated resting T cells do not express IL-2 mRNA, nor do they contain IL-2 protein. The production of IL-2 by normal T lymphocytes requires that cells be activated by antigens or poly-clonal T cell activators. Other pathways of T cell and thymocyte activation, such as ligand binding to CD2 surface receptors, also stimulate IL-2 production.

Studies of isolated subpopulations of lymphocytes and thymocytes show that antigens induce IL-2 from CD4 helper T (TH) cells. However, potent polyclonal mitogens and class I MHC alloantigens can stimulate the CD8 T lymphocytes to produce IL-2. Medullary thymocytes stimulated with T cell mitogens secrete low levels of IL-2. In addition, a subset of large granular lymphocytes (LGL) that bear the CD2 and CD6 markers and are related to NK cells can be induced by lectins such as PHA or by CSF and IFN γ to produce IL-2.

The assay of IL-2 uses tritiated thymidine incorporation to measure the growth-supporting effects on IL-2-dependent human or murine cytotoxic T cell lines. Human IL-2 is active on mouse cells; therefore, the murine cell line CTLL has been most widely used. The precise IL-2 concentration in an experimental sample is determined by comparison with a standard containing a known amount of IL-2. There is a radioimmunoassay for IL-2, but it is less sensitive than the bioassay and the antibodies used can react to inert IL-2, giving potentially false values. A radioreceptor assay in which purified IL-2 receptors are used is being developed.

Intracellular Regulation of IL-2 Production

After activation of T cells, de novo transcription and translation precede the appearance of secreted IL-2. In normal human lymphocytes stimulated with PHA, IL-2 mRNA accumulates at 4 hours, reaches a peak at 12 hours, and sharply declines thereafter. The rapid shutoff of IL-2 mRNA production, together with its short half-life (1–2 hours) in vivo, ensures that IL-2 production is very transient. Removal of the activating signal leads to a decay in IL-2 mRNA levels owing to a cessation of transcription. It has recently been demonstrated that the A + T- rich region of the 3′ untranslated mRNA for inducible cytokines such as IL-2 imparts instability to mRNA and shortens its half-life. The rapid decline in IL-2 mRNA that is always seen in activated normal cells, despite persistent stimulation and transcription of the gene, suggests that repressive protein(s) is also induced. This intricate control mechanism, which ensures the transience of IL-2 mRNA, is important in the regulation of immune reactivity by ensuring the decay of IL-2 after antigen is removed from the reaction.

Role of IL-2 in T Cell Activation

The induction of lymphocyte proliferation involves 2 steps (Fig 7–3). The first step, called **com-**

Table 7–4. Properties of the human IL-2 receptor.

High-Affinity Complex
1. Composed of 2 heterologous subunits
2. Transiently expressed
3. Internalized by IL-2, induced by antigen, IL-2, TNF, and IL-4
4. Conveys protein-kinase C activation, [Ca2+], and pH changes
5. Enhances cell-mediated functions (eg, lymphokine production)
6. Signals S-phase progression

P75
1. Participates in high-affinity complex
2. Responsible for internalization of complex
3. Present alone on a few resting T cells and LGL
4. At high IL-2 doses, yields signal transduction and gene activation

p55
1. Participates in high-affinity complex
2. Transient expression increased by IL-2
3. Induced by IL-2, TNF, IL-4, and IL-6
4. No signal transduction
5. No defined function by itself

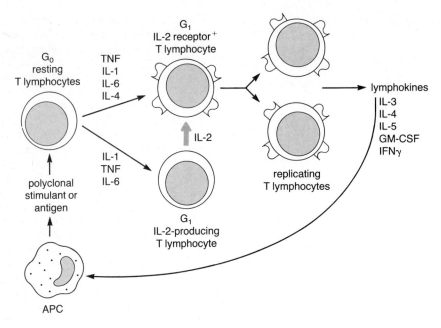

Figure 7–3. Lymphocyte activation and role of interleukins.

petence, is initiated by an exogenous signal delivered to the quiescent T cell by mitogen or antigen. This leads to partial activation of the T cell, resulting in an increase in size, induction of transcription of certain genes, and passage from the G_0 phase to the early G_1 phase in the cell cycle. However, the first signal by itself is not sufficient to stimulate growth. A second, endogenous, signal is needed to induce cell cycle progression, with transition to the S phase and ultimately to cell division. In the second step, the binding of IL-2 to its high-affinity receptor is required for progression of the T cell through the cell cycle. Both anti-IL-2 and anti-Tac antibodies can inhibit this T cell growth. T cells are unique in that both IL-2 and its receptor are synthesized de novo following initial activation.

Lymphocytes express maximal levels of high-affinity IL-2 receptors for only a brief period following exposure to specific antigen. The subsequent decline in receptor expression is unusual because it occurs independently of the presence of IL-2, indicating that there is another mechanism of receptor regulation besides IL-2-mediated receptor down-regulation. It also means that there is only a finite period for immune T cell clones to expand. Consequently, T lymphocyte proliferation ceases and the cells arrest in the G_1 phase, even in the presence of saturating concentrations of IL-2. Readdition of antigen causes the reappearance of optimal numbers of IL-2 receptors on

the lymphocytes, enabling cells to again grow in response to IL-2. These events can be repeated; they describe the cyclical nature of normal T cell growth in vivo and underscore the constant need for stimuli (ie, antigens) to induce IL-2 receptors necessary for continuous proliferation of T cell clones in vitro.

IL-2-Induced Cytokine Production

The addition of IL-2 to purified activated T cells promotes several cellular functions besides proliferation (Table 7–5). T lymphocytes activated by IL-2 produce other lymphokines including IFN γ; lymphotoxin; B cell growth and differentiation factors such as IL-4, IL-6, BCGF, and BCDF; hematopoietic growth factors such as IL-3, IL-5, and GM-CSF; and TGF β. IL-2-activated T cells can also exhibit enhanced cytotoxicity. These various functions are amplified even further by the capacity of IL-2 to clonally expand the pool of antigen-reactive cells. A model for the development of immune reactivity of T cells incorporates the concept that an initial signal is required for IL-2 production and IL-2 receptor expression (Fig 7–3).

T Cell Clones & Lines
Dependent on IL-2

IL-2 preferentially supports the growth of CD8 Tc cells, but CD4 TH cells and a few CD8 Ts cell lines also have been grown. In addition to the ca-

Table 7-5. Properties of human IL-2.

Origin
1. Activated peripheral T cells
2. Activated medullary thymocytes
3. Activated subset of LGL

Target Cell Specificity for Proliferative Stimulus
1. Activated mature T cell subsets
2. Activated LGL
3. Activated B cells

Biologic Effects
1. Binds to specific receptors on T cells, B cells, and monocytes
2. Promotes entry into the S phase, except monocytes
3. Stimulates lymphokine secretion
4. Enhances macrophage cytocidal state
5. Augments immunoglobulin production
6. Activates natural killer activity of LGL

Biochemical properties
1. MW 15,400
2. 133 amino acids
3. Isoelectric point 8.0

pacity of these cloned cells to release IL-2, they appear to cooperate with histocompatible adherent cells in the presence of specific antigen to release a variety of other lymphokines.

The continuous IL-2-dependent lymphocyte lines developed from normal cells that have been used for IL-2 bioassays (such as the widely used CTLL-2 line) are actually cell variants that spontaneously express high levels of receptors for IL-2. Successive generations of cells constitutively express IL-2 binding sites and therefore need only IL-2 to grow. CTLL is used for bioassays because it responds only to IL-2, unlike cell lines that respond to other growth factors such as IL-4. In the absence of IL-2, these cells cease to proliferate, and they die within 12–24 hours.

Interactions of IL-2 With Non-T Cells

Freshly isolated large granular lymphocytes (LGL), which exhibit antigen-nonspecific NK cell activity, do not express the MW-55,000 Tac antigen (a part of the IL-2 receptor). Nevertheless, they can be stimulated by IL-2 to proliferate, to produce other lymphokines, and to exhibit enhanced NK activity. This response to IL-2 requires the expression of the p75 IL-2-binding protein on the unstimulated LGL. After in vitro incubation, LGL also begin to express both p55 Tac antigen and the high-affinity IL-2 receptor complex.

High-affinity receptors for IL-2 have also been found on B lymphoblasts. Activated normal as well as some transformed B lymphoblasts, but not resting B cells, express about 30% as many Tac antigen receptors for IL-2 as do activated T cells. IL-2 can induce both increased antibody production and proliferation by purified normal B lymphocytes but at higher (2- to 3-fold) doses of IL-2.

Monocytes and macrophages also normally express a low density of the p55 Tac antigen. In mice, myeloid precursors, mast cells, and monocytes possess only low-affinity receptors for IL-2. Activation of macrophages by IFN γ or LPS, however, results in the development of high-affinity IL-2 receptors consisting of p75 and the p55 Tac antigen. Addition of IL-2 to these activated macrophages results in the activation of the Tac, GM-CSF, and G-CSF genes and also augments the tumoricidal activities of these macrophages.

In Vivo Effects of IL-2

Intravenously injected recombinant IL-2 is rapidly cleared from the circulation of humans, with a half-life of 3–22 minutes. Part of the clearance may be due to absorption by activated T cells, but the kidneys constitute the main clearance site. However, ligation of renal arteries prolongs the serum half-life only transiently, and only breakdown products of IL-2 are recovered in the urine, suggesting the existence of alternative clearance sites for IL-2. Based on the molarity of IL-2 required to half-maximally bind receptors, 15,000–25,000 units must be given intravenously to human subjects to obtain effects on the immune system. Continuous intravenous infusion results in sustained high levels of IL-2. These high doses of recombinant IL-2 have elicited multiple toxic side effects. One of the most important of these is the "vascular leak syndrome," wherein infusion of recombinant IL-2 leads to a rapid accumulation of extracellular fluid and hence to ascites and pulmonary edema. IL-2 stimulates the production of cytokines capable of activating endothelial cells, leading to vascular permeability. High levels of IL-2 elevate the serum levels of ACTH and cortisol; this elevation leads to immunosuppressive effects. Intraperitoneal and subcutaneous injections of IL-2 lead to more prolonged serum concentrations of >2 U/mL at about 2 and 6 hours, respectively, so that these routes of administration permit the use of lower doses with less toxic side effects.

Toxins (eg, diphtheria toxin) fused to growth factors (eg, IL-2) have exciting therapeutic potential for deletion of antigen-reactive T cells. IL-2 toxin has been shown to be very selective and to have potent toxic effects (50% maximum effective dose (ED_{50}) of 10–50 pmol) against a number of cell lines, particularly human T-cell lymphotrophic virus type I (HTLV-I)- associated cells in vitro. Such a toxin could be used in treatment of acute T cell leukemia and other IL-2-bearing neoplasias.

INTERLEUKIN-4 & -5

This section addresses IL-4 and IL-5, 2 other lymphokines with TCGF and BCGF activities; however, IL-3, which acts as a multi-CSF, will be discussed subsequently with the other hematopoietic CSF.

Cloned murine CD4 TH lymphocyte lines can be separated into 2 distinct subsets based on their capacity to produce lymphokines. Only the murine TH1 subset secretes IL-2, IFN γ, and lymphotoxin (TNFβ), whereas the TH2 subset and mast cells secrete IL-4 and IL-5. The properties of these lymphokines are shown in Table 7-6. The human analogues of these TH subsets have not yet been identified.

IL-4

IL-4 (Fig 7-4) was initially detected and its gene was cloned by using its B cell growth activity for assay. IL-4, formerly designated BCGF-I, is mitogenic for B cells that have previously been activated by T cell–dependent antigens, T cell–independent antigens, or anti-immunoglobulin antisera. IL-4 synergizes with IL-2 to stimulate B cell growth. Although it is not a growth factor for resting B cells, IL-4 induces rapid increases in B cell surface expression of class II MHC antigens and Fc receptors for IgE. It is also a major regulator of immunoglobulin isotype expression. IL-4 induces IgE and IgG1 production and decreases IgG2b and IgG3 production by LPS- stimulated B cells. Thus, IL-4 promotes immunoglobulin iso-

type switching to the C-ϵ and C-γ 1 genes and therefore may be important in the etiology of atopic allergies.

Like other cytokines, IL-4 also acts on nonlymphoid cells. It is mitogenic for T lymphocytes and supports the growth of mast cell lines. Furthermore, IL-4 costimulates, with CSF, the growth of hematopoietic precursors and induces the differentiation of more mature myeloid cells. It is a potent activator of macrophage cytocidal functions and induces the expression of cell surface class II MHC antigens on macrophages as well as B lymphocytes.

IL-5

IL-5 (Fig 7-4) was first detected and its gene was later cloned on the basis of its T cell-replacing activity (TRF) and B cell growth activity (BCGF-II) for the BCl-1 lymphoma line. Recombinant murine IL-5 has been shown to promote the growth of activated B cells and to combine with IL-2 to promote B cell proliferation. IL-5 promotes antibody production by B cells, particularly of the IgA isotype. Thus, IL-5 favors isotype switching to the C-α gene. IL-5 has modest mitogenic effects on T cells. In addition, it induces the differentiation of bone marrow precursors into eosinophils and supports the growth of eosinophilic cell lines and induction of TC.

Therefore, by producing IL-4 and IL-5, murine TH2 cells promote IgE and IgA production as well as mast cell and eosinophil growth and differentiation. This suggests that TH2 cells participate preferentially in the development of antibodies for atopic reactions and for host defense against parasitic diseases. In contrast, the lymphokines produced by TH1 cells selectively engage in host defense against viral, microbial, and neoplastic diseases, since IL-2, interferons, and TNFβ promote macrophage activities such as cytotoxicity and phagocytosis, mediate DTH reactions, and

Table 7-6. Properties of IL-4 and IL-5

Property	IL-4	IL-5
Size of mature form	20 kDa	18 kDa
Cell sources	TH cells, mast cells	TH cells
Cell targets and activities	Acts as comitogen for B cells Enhances Ia and FcRε expression on B cells Promotes switch to IgG1 and IgE (decreases IgG2b and IgG3) Acts as mast cell stimulant Comitogen for thymocytes Activates macrophages Stimulates hematopoiesis	Acts as costimulant of B cell proliferation and differentiation Enhances IL-2 receptor expression Promotes switch to IgA Stimulates BCl-1 growth Stimulates eosinophils Acts as comitogen for thymocytes
Size of receptors	60 kDa	46.5 kDa

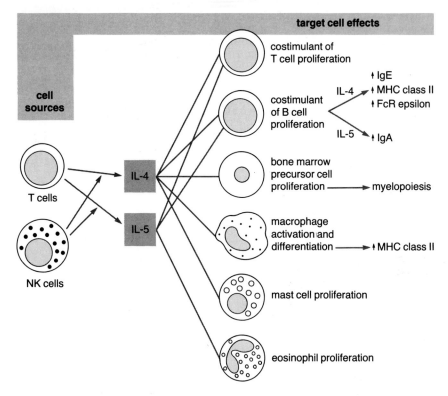

Figure 7-4. Cell sources and target cell effects of IL-4 and IL-5.

favor IgG1a production. In fact, IFN γ and IL-4 generally have opposing effects on immunoglobulin production; IFN γ will favor the production of IgG3 at the expense of IL-4 induction of IgG or IgE. The homologous subpopulations of TH1 and TH2 cells and their products remain to be identified in humans.

INTERLEUKIN-6

Properties of IL-6

IL-6 was initially called IFN β_2 on the basis of its presumed antiviral activity and its cross-reactivity with some antisera to IFN β. However, more recent studies show that IL-6 has little or no antiviral activity and therefore should not be considered an interferon. IL-6 is a cytokine with multiple biologic activities on a variety of cells (Table 7–7). Cloning of the genes coding for molecules expressing these various biologic activities revealed that the protein product of a single gene possesses all these activities. This substance is now most commonly called IL-6.

The gene for IL-6 is located on human chromosome 7. The reported MW of IL-6 ranges between 22,000 and 30,000, owing in part to differential glycosylation and phosphorylation of a single protein. IL-6 can be produced by many cells, including T and B lymphocytes, monocytes, endothelial cells, epithelial cells, and fibroblasts. A variety of stimuli including TNF, IL-1, platelet-derived growth factor, antigens, mitogens, and bacterial endotoxin (LPS) induce the production of IL-6.

IL-6 Receptor

There is a wide range of IL-6-responsive target cells that bear specific high-affinity IL-6 receptors. These include Epstein-Barr virus (EBV)-transformed B cell lines, plasma cell lines, myelomonocytic cell lines, and normal resting T lymphocytes. IL-6 receptors are present on activated but not resting B cells, which accounts for the ability of IL-6 to induce differentiation of preactivated but not resting B cells. Reported dissociation constants (K_d) are in the range of 10^{-10}–10^{-12} mol/L, and there are 10^2–10^4 receptors per cell.

The gene encoding the IL-6 receptor has been cloned and has a domain similar to one in the immunoglobulin gene superfamily. Unlike the receptors for many growth factors, the IL-6 receptor does not have a tyrosine kinase domain.

Table 7-7. Properties of IL-6.

Property	IL-6
Chromosome	7
MW of mature form	22,000–30,000
Cell sources	T and B lymphocytes, monocytes, endothelial cells, epithelial cells, fibroblasts
Cell targets and activities	Acts as cofactor for immunoglobulin secretion by B cells Acts as growth factor for myelomas, hybridomas, and plasmacytomas Stimulates hepatocytes to produce acute-phase proteins Acts as comitogen for thymocytes and T cells inhibits growth of some carcinoma and non-B-cell leukemia and lymphoma cell lines Has differentiation effects on myelomonocytic cell lines and on normal hematopoietic precursor cells Stimulates pituitary ACTH and adrenal glucocorticoids

Activities of IL-6

IL-6, as a B cell stimulatory factor, is a differentiation or maturation agent that promotes the ability of activated cells of the B cell lineage to secrete immunoglobulins. IL-6 is also a growth factor for hybridomas, plasmacytomas, and EBV-transformed peripheral blood B cells. Recently, it has been demonstrated that freshly isolated human myeloma cells both produce IL-6 and express IL-6 receptors. Moreover, anti-IL-6 antibodies inhibit the growth of the myeloma cells in vitro, suggesting that IL-6 may function as an autocrine signal in the process of uncontrolled proliferation during myeloma.

In contrast to these stimulating properties, IL-6 performs antiproliferative activities for carcinoma and non-B-cell leukemia and lymphoma cell lines. In vivo administration of IL-6 increases neutrophil counts. It also has differentiation effects on myelomonocytic cell lines and on normal hematopoietic precursor cells, and it augments colony formation by hematopoietic cells.

In the acute inflammatory response to infection or trauma, the liver responds by altering the synthesis of several plasma proteins known as acute-phase proteins. IL-6, as a **hepatocyte-stimulating factor (HSF),** induces the synthesis of acute-phase proteins, including C-reactive protein, α_1-antichymotrypsin, α_1-acid glycoprotein, fibrinogen, and C3 while inhibiting the synthesis of proteins such as prealbumin and albumin. The expression of some of these acute-phase proteins is also modulated by IL-1 or TNF, which combine synergistically with the HSF activity of IL-6. In addition, administration of high doses of IL-6 also produces fever by stimulating the hypothalamic fever center; IL-6 is therefore an endogenous pyrogen.

IL-6, as a T cell-activating factor or T cell costimulant, can provide, at least in part, the second (antigen-nonspecific) signal that is required in addition to antigen or mitogen for T cell activation. IL-6 has been shown to augment proliferation of thymocytes and monocyte-depleted preparations of peripheral blood T lymphocytes stimulated with suboptimal doses of PHA via both IL-2-dependent and IL-2-independent pathways. It enhances both IL-2 production and expression of receptors for IL-2.

As is apparent, IL-1, TNF, and IL-6 have some overlapping biologic activities (Tables 7–1 and 7–2). Since IL-1 and TNF are potent inducers of IL-6, it will be of interest to determine which biologic activities ascribed to IL-1 or TNF are actually mediated by IL-6.

INTERLEUKIN-7

IL-7, an MW-25,000 cytokine that acts predominantly on T and B lymphocyte progenitors, has recently been identified. Murine and human IL-7 have both been purified, and the genes have been cloned and expressed. IL-7 is produced by stromal cells of the bone marrow. It stimulates pre-B cells and is a costimulant of early thymocytes. Therefore, it can be considered a lymphopoietin. In addition, it is a costimulant together with polyclonal lectins of mature T cells but not of mature B cells. In vivo administration of IL-7 to mice stimulates predominantly B cell hyperplasia of the spleen and lymph nodes. However, IL-7 also promotes in vivo recovery from cyclophosphamide toxicity by stimulating myeloid precursors and megakaryocytes to produce colony-forming units and platelets. Consequently, IL-7 also appears to have hematopoietic activities.

INTERFERONS

In 1957, it was discovered that a soluble factor produced by cells exposed to inactive virus was able to transfer "interference" of viral replication to fresh cells. It was therefore named "interferon" the interferons have since been shown to be a large family of secreted proteins having antiviral activity. Moreover, they also have potent antiproliferative and immunomodulatory activities. The interferons are produced by most cells of vertebrate species in response to viral infection or other selected stimuli.

Assays for Interferon

The commonly used assays for interferon are antiviral bioassays that measure inhibition either of virus production or of the cytopathic effect of virus on cultured cell lines. The more recent development of radioimmunoassays or other ligand-binding tests has facilitated the quantification and identification of interferons.

Interferon Types & Induction

Many proteins with various degrees of structural homology have the property of inducing an antiviral state in target cells and therefore are, by definition, interferons. The interferons can be divided into antigenically distinct types and classified according to their primary cell of origin or according to the stimulus for induction, as shown in Table 7–8.

A. Type I Interferons (IFN α and IFN β): These are induced by viral infections or artificially by a double-stranded RNA such as poly(I·C). Most type I interferons are characterized by being stable at pH 2.0. IFN α, which is produced primarily by leukocytes, consists of multiple subspecies that are antigenically related. One human IFN α gene family has at least 14 functional nonallelic members. The amino acid sequences of these human IFN α subspecies are about 80% homologous. A second family of IFN α genes has also been identified in the human genome. The antigenically distinct IFN β is the major interferon synthesized by nonleukocytic cells, including fibroblasts, although it can also be produced by leukocytes. The amino acid sequence of IFN β is approximately 30% homologous with that of the IFN α family.

B. Type II Interferon (IFN γ or Immune Interferon): This is produced during immune reactions by antigen-, mitogen-, or lectin-stimulated T lymphocytes or by LGL with NK activity. Type II interferon is labile at pH 2.0, a property often used as a simple method of identification.

Although the reasons for the genetic diversity of the interferons in humans are unknown, different interferons are not equally potent in each of their diverse activities, and the various types of interferon may be differentially active on different cell types and at different times in various organs or tissues.

Activities of Interferons

The interferons induce an antiviral state that protects the target cells against most types of viruses (Fig 7–5). In addition, the interferons have potent cellular effects (Table 7–9), primarily inhibition of cell proliferation. Interferons can either inhibit or enhance cell differentiation, depending on the cell type and the dose of interferon. The interferons are also potent immunomodulatory agents and play important roles in normal host defense.

Immunomodulatory Effects of Interferon

The immunomodulatory activities of interferon are mediated by its effects on the cells responsible for host defense, ie, macrophages, T and B lymphocytes, and LGL with NK activity.

A. Activation of Macrophages: The interferons increase bactericidal and tumoricidal capabilities of macrophages and augment their accessory cell functions. The interferons possess the activities described as **macrophage-activating factor (MAF)** and **monocyte migration inhibitory factor (MIF),** although other proteins may also have these activities.

Table 7–8. Classification of human interferons.

Interferon	Principal Cellular Source	Inducing Stimulus	MW of Natural Monomeric Form	Chromosome Number	
				IFN	Receptor
Type I					
IFN α	Leukocytes	Virus or double-stranded RNA	18,000–20,000	9	21
IFN β	Fibroblasts	Virus or double-stranded RNA	23,000	9	21
Type II (Immune)					
IFN γ	T lymphocytes, LGL	Antigen or mitogen	20,000–25,000	12	6

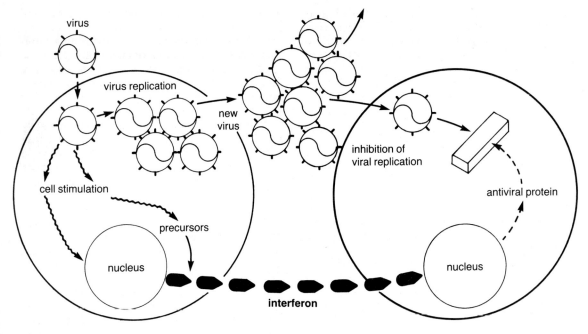

Figure 7-5. Schematic representation of interferon activity.

Macrophages that have been activated in vitro by IFN α show morphologic evidence of maturation such as enlargement, increased spreading, pseudopod formation, and vacuolization beginning in vitro at 1 hour and peaking in 48–72 hours. The activation of macrophages by IFN α, β, or γ is accompanied by increased expression of receptors for the Fc portion of immunoglobulins

Table 7-9. Effects of interferons on cellular functions.

Inhibit
Cell proliferation
Tumor growth
Fibroblast-adipocyte differentiation

Enhance
Promyelocytic and monoblastic leukemic cell differentiation
Phagocytosis by macrophages
Accessory cell functions of macrophages (IFN γ > IFN α, β)
Endotoxin-induced IL-1 secretion by macrophages (IFN γ > α, β)
Generation of CTL
Activity of NK cells
Expression of class I and II MHC antigens and Fc receptors

Mixed Effects
Erythroleukemic cell differentiation
Production of antibodies
Cell-mediated immune phenomena

(FcR). This increase in FcR expression promotes both increased phagocytosis of immune complexes and increased capacity of the macrophages to lyse antibody-coated bacteria, parasites, and tumor cells by ADCC, in which antibody molecules couple macrophages to target cells by binding to their FcR and antigenic sites, respectively.

The induction of antigen-specific, T lymphocyte-mediated immune responses requires "presentation" of antigen in conjunction with a class II MHC antigen by an accessory cell to a TH cell. IFN γ and, to a much lesser degree, IFN α and β maintain the expression of class II MHC antigen on the surface of macrophages as well as on other cell types. In addition, IFN γ can boost the level of class II antigen expression above resting levels. Owing at least in part to increased expression of class II MHC antigen, macrophages pretreated with IFN γ thus exhibit significantly enhanced accessory cell functions, which enable them to activate T lymphocytes more effectively.

B. Effects of Interferon on Lymphocytes: Interferon can either augment or suppress cellular and humoral immunity, depending on the dose, time of administration, and genetic makeup of the recipient. In general, in vivo administration of interferon or interferon inducers before or concomitant with antigenic sensitization has considerable inhibitory effects, whereas administration of interferon after antigenic sensitization augments both cellular and humoral immune responses. The latter observation is probably of greater physiologic relevance, since IFN γ is produced in vivo relatively late in the normal course of an immune response. The inhibitory and stimulatory effects of all the interferons can also be demonstrated in vitro. For example, higher preexposure doses of interferon or simultaneous addition of interferon suppresses lymphocyte proliferation and in vitro antibody production, whereas low doses of interferon or late addition can enhance lymphocyte proliferation and antibody production. IFN α, β, and γ also have both positive and negative effects on such cell-mediated immunologic phenomena as delayed hypersensitivity, graft-versus-host response, and mixed leukocyte reactions.

The mechanisms by which interferons augment cellular and humoral immunity are complex and are partly based on increased class II MHC antigen expression, increased class I antigens on CTL targets, increased production of other cytokines such as IL-1, and direct effects on T and B cell differentiation. The immunosuppressive effects of interferons may be due in part to their antigrowth activity.

C. Effects of Interferon on NK Cell Activity: NK cell activity is mediated by the cytotoxic effects of LGL in the absence of prior sensitization against virus-infected cells, certain tumor cell lines, and normal hematopoietic cells. Both in vitro and in vivo administration of IFN α or β or interferon inducers enhance the NK cell activities of LGL. Paradoxically, pretreatment of some target cells with interferon makes them less susceptible to NK cytolysis, again emphasizing the complexities of the actions of the interferons in the immune system.

Molecular Mechanisms of Action of Interferon

In contrast to antibodies that react with and neutralize viruses directly, the interferons establish an antiviral state and act as antiproliferative and immunodulatory agents by inducing the synthesis of cellular proteins and altering the metabolism of target cells. In this regard, the interferons are similar in their mechanism of action to polypeptide hormones and growth factors.

A. Interferon Receptors: The initial event in the action of the interferons is their binding to specific receptors on the cell surface. All type I interferons can bind to a single type of interferon receptor, whereas type II interferon binds to a different receptor. Most cell types respond to interferon, and interferon receptors are therefore present on most cells. The binding of the interferons to their receptors is primarily of high affinity, with K_d in the range of 10^{-10}–10^{-11} mol/L. The binding is saturable, with up to 7000 type I and 13,000 type II interferon receptors per cell on

some cultured cell lines. However, some cells express far fewer interferon receptors; eg, small resting T lymphocytes have only 250 IFN α and 500 IFN γ high-affinity receptors per cell.

The type II interferon receptor was recently purified, monoclonal antibodies were prepared, and the cDNA for the receptor was cloned. Current evidence suggests that a single type of IFN γ-binding protein exists; however, other species-specific proteins besides the IFN γ-binding protein are required for the response to IFN γ. To date, the type I interferon receptor has not been purified to homogeneity, nor has its gene been cloned.

After the binding of the interferons to cell surface receptors, the interferon-receptor complexes cluster in coated pits and are internalized by receptor-mediated endocytosis. At least part of the internalized interferon is degraded in lysosomes. The biochemical events that transduce the signal from the cell surface interferon receptor to the rest of the cell to produce the various biologic responses to interferon are not defined. There is evidence for a role for protein kinase C in some of the actions of the interferons; however, nuclear receptors for the interferons have been described, and the results of several studies have suggested that signals for some of the responses to the interferons may be generated following ligand internalization.

B. Interferon-Induced mRNAs and Proteins: The interferons exert their biologic effects by modulating the synthesis of several specific mRNAs and proteins. Interferon-induced proteins include, among others, the MHC antigens and 2 enzymes: a protein kinase and 2'-5' oligo(A) (2-5A) synthetase. The protein kinase phosphorylates the small subunit of protein synthesis initiation factor type 2. After activation by double-stranded RNA, the 2-5A synthetase synthesizes small 2'-5' oligoadenylates that bind to and activate a latent endoribonuclease. Therefore, 2 enzymes participate in the antiviral and perhaps antimitogenic effects of the interferons. Several lines of evidence indicate that there are different but intersecting biochemical pathways for the establishment of the different biologic responses to type I and II interferons.

In Vivo Role of Interferon in Disease States

Interferon activity cannot normally be detected in tissues or serum but appears rapidly during viral infections. Interferon also transiently appears in the sera of animals with a systemic hypersensitivity reaction following intravenous administration of a large dose of a relevant antigen. It has been detected in the sera of some patients with clinically active autoimmune diseases including systemic lupus erythematosus, rheumatoid arthritis, scleroderma, and Sjögren's syndrome. The serum interferon activity from systemic lupus erythematosus patients has been identified as a mixture of IFN γ and IFN α.

Interferon plays a protective role in viral diseases, since addition of interferon or interferon inducers can halt the development of viral diseases. Moreover, anti-interferon antibodies exacerbate viral infections. Interferons are protective as antiviral agents even in immunodeficient subjects; however, the effects of interferon are not all beneficial. Overexpression or inappropriate expression of IFN α or β has been shown to have deleterious effects in mice. The interferon component of the host antiviral response, in excess, may cause aberrant autoimmune states or self-destructive host inflammatory responses.

HEMATOPOIETIC COLONY-STIMULATING FACTORS

Colony-stimulating factors (CSF) are the cytokines that stimulate a limited number of pluripotent stem cells, present predominantly in the bone marrow, to produce large numbers of platelets, erythrocytes, neutrophils, monocytes, eosinophils, and basophils, most of which are short-lived in the blood. The CSF were named according to the type of target cells that form colonies in soft agar. Consequently, IL-3, otherwise known as **multi-CSF,** acts on pluripotent stem cells to produce all types of hematopoietic cells. GM-CSF acts on a bipotential stem cell (the colony forming unit in culture (CFU-C)) to produce mononuclear phagocytes and granulocytes; G-CSF principally causes granulocyte precursor proliferation; M-CSF is a mononuclear phagocyte progenitor growth factor; and erythropoietin is a stimulator of erythroid development. However, in vivo administration of purified recombinant CSF frequently leads to effects that extend beyond the known in vitro activities of these cytokines; presumably this is based on their capacity to produce a cascade of other cytokines and to stimulate the functional activities of leukocytes (Table 7–10). In addition to maintaining homeostasis, these cytokines marshall bone marrow responses to environmental stress such as infection or trauma. For example, in defense against microorganisms, the number of granulocytes increases from 10^9 per day to as many as 2×10^{11}.

Both progenitors and mature progeny of lymphoid and myeloid cells require stimulation by several hemopoietins for proliferation and differentiation. The various CSF have totally unrelated protein sequences and apparently use distinct receptors, although these distinct receptors may be functionally linked on the target cell populations. Despite these differences, these growth factors have many overlapping functions and induce quite similar biologic responses in some cells, particularly in the production of mature granulocytes and macrophages (Table 7–10). The significance of this overlapping system is not entirely clear. It may be a fail-safe system, or the differences in cellular sources of these proteins may reflect different roles in steady-state maintenance or immune amplification of hematopoiesis.

A number of other cytokines have recently been found to influence hematopoiesis. They include IL-1, TNF, IL-4, IL-5, IL-6, and IL-7 and are discussed above. Whether these cytokines act directly or indirectly (by stimulating the production of CSF or receptors for CSF) must be defined. Overall, the hematopoietic growth factors alone or in combination are not just mitogenic stimuli but have 4 distinct actions on target cells: (1) enhanced survival, (2) growth stimulation, (3) dif-

Table 7-10. Human hematopoietic growth factors.

Name	Protein Size (kDa)	Cellular Sources	Cells Stimulated
G-CSF	18–22	Monocytes, fibroblasts	Neutrophils
GM-CSF	14–38	T cells, endothelial cells, fibroblasts, monocytes	Neutrophils, monocytes, eosinophils, erythroid cells, megakaryocytes
IL-3 (Multi-CSF)	14–28	T cells	Neutrophils, monocytes, eosinophils, basophils, erythroid cells, megakaryocytes
M-CSF	18–26[1] 35–45[1]	Monocytes, T and B cells Fibroblasts, endothelial cells, epithelial cells	Megakaryocytes
Erythropoietin	30–34	Kidney cells	Erythroid cells

[1]Protein is dimeric.

ferentiation commitment, and (4) functional activation of end-stage cells.

Immune amplification of leukocyte development may be controlled primarily at the level of cytokine production. Some of the genes encoding these hematopoietins are not normally expressed. IL-2, IL- 3, IL-4, and IL-5 are produced only when T lymphocytes are stimulated by specific antigens such as microbial proteins. G-CSF and GM-CSF are produced by both fibroblasts and endothelial cells after stimulation by products of activated macrophages such as IL-1 and TNF. Activated macrophages can also produce their own hematopoietins.

Biologic Activities of the CSF

It is not clear how the wide array of hematopoietic cells develop from a single cell type. The majority of pluripotent stem cells are not actively going through the cell cycle. IL-6 and IL-1 have been implicated in stimulating the entry of these cells into the cell cycle, whereas other factors, such as TGFβ take the stem cells out of cycle. Furthermore, it is not clear what regulates the commitment of the stem cell to differentiate to a specific cell lineage. The evidence supports a random selection by hematopoietic factors, but other regulatory factors may be required.

Both IL-3 and GM-CSF support the development of multipotent colonies (colony forming units giving rise to granulocytes, erythrocytes,

monocytes, and megakaryocytes (CFU-GEMM)). although IL-3 seems to stimulate the more primitive progenitor cells. After treatment with 5-fluorouracil, IL-3-responsive cells are detectable earlier than GM-CSF-responsive cells. G-CSF, M-CSF, IL-5, and erythropoietin represent a class of molecules whose function is restricted to one specific lineage. For example, G-CSF stimulates the growth and differentiation of pure neutrophil colonies in semisolid media. In addition, it stimulates the functional activities of mature neutrophils by enhancing superoxide anion production, phagocytosis, and ADCC. Thus, G-CSF stimulation makes neutrophils much more efficient in killing bacteria.

Therapeutic Applications of CSF

New techniques in molecular biology have made possible the cloning and expression of the hematopoietin genes. This has provided large numbers of these molecules for study in the clinic. The preclinical studies of hematopoietins have revealed fewer toxic side effects than for agents such as TNF, IL-1, and IL-2. Thus, these molecules appear to have therapeutic potential in 2 areas: (1) stimulating production of blood cells in patients in whom one or more of the formed blood elements are abnormally low, and (2) boosting host defenses against microbial invasion. Hematopoietic dysfunction, such as granulocytopenia, is the major cause of death in cancer patients undergo-

Table 7-11. Properties of human TGFβ.

Property	TGFβ
Chromosome	Long arm of chromosome 19
Proform	391 amino acids
Mature Form	112 amino acids TGFβ1 or CIF-A, 25-kDa homodimer TGFβ2 or CIF-B, 25-kDa homodimer TGFβ1,2, 25-kDa heterodimer TGFβ3, 25-kDa homodimer
Cell sources	Platelets, placenta, kidney, bone, and T and B lymphocytes
Cell target and activities	Is chemotactic and mitogenic for fibroblasts Enhances collagen, fibronectin and collagenase synthesis Stimulates osteoclastic bone resorption Is mitogenic for osteoblasts Inhibits proliferation of endothelial cells, epithelial cells, smooth muscle cells, T and B lymphocytes, early hematopoietic stem cells, fetal hepatocytes, and keratinocytes Inhibits mixed leukocyte reaction, generation of CTL Suppresses NK and lymphocytic-activated killer cell development
Receptor	280 kDa with 65 K_d and 85 K_d chains Murine 3T3 fibroblasts express 80,000 receptors/cell; lymphocytes have only 250 receptors/cell.
In vivo effects	Enhances wound repair Causes angiogenesis and fibroplasia

ing chemotherapy or radiotherapy. Since there is no present method to elevate granulocyte counts, the ability of GM-CSF and G-CSF to stimulate the production and function of neutrophils could aid in the management of iatrogenic suppression of neutrophilic granulocytes. In addition, preclinical studies have shown that GM-CSF and G-CSF can protect against lethal bacterial septicemia, suggesting that these molecules would be therapeutic in bacterial infections. Eventually, combinations of the regulators will be used for maximal effectiveness

TGFβ

TGFβ was initially discovered as a cofactor with TGFα that promoted anchorage-independent growth of rat kidney fibroblasts and enabled them to grow in a non-contact-inhibited manner. Thus, TGFβ is a growth factor for fibroblasts and promotes wound healing. However, it has consider-able antiproliferative activity and acts as a negative regulator of immunity and hematopoiesis (Table 7–11). It is produced by many cell types, including activated macrophages and T lymphocytes. There are at least 3 forms of TGFβ (TGFβ1, 2, and 3). These 3 gene products react with the same high-affinity cell surface receptors that are expressed in widely varying numbers by many cell types.

TGFβ has antiproliferative effects on a wide variety of cell types, including epithelial cells, endothelial cells, smooth muscle cells, fetal hepatocytes, early myeloid progenitor cells, and T and B lymphocytes (Fig 7–6). TGFβ at 10^{-10}–10^{-12} mol/L blocks the proliferative effects of IL-2 on T and B cells, of BCGFs on B cells, and of IL-1 on thymocytes. In addition, TGFβ inhibits T cell-dependent polyclonal antibody production, mixed leukocyte reactions, and the in vitro generation of CTL. It also inhibits the induction of NK cell ac-

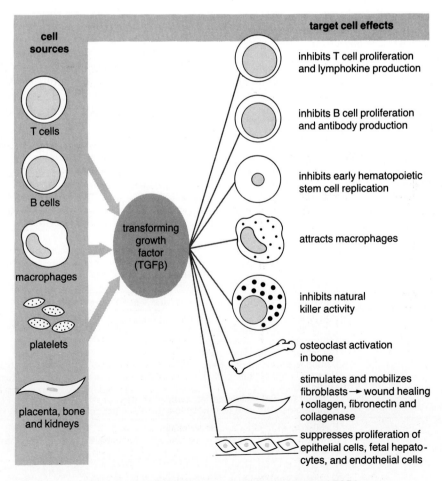

Figure 7–6. Cell sources and target cell effects of TGFβ.

tivities and the induction of lymphokine-activated killer cells by IL-2. Consequently, as a late product of activated T cells, TGFβ is unique in that it can act as a negative-feedback regulator that can dampen immunologically mediated inflammatory reactions.

SUMMARY

Exogenous as well as endogenous agents that induce or inhibit cytokine production or action can modulate immunologic reactions. Exogenous stimuli are of primary importance as inducers of endogenous cytokines. Most cytokines are produced by many cell types in response to noxious or physiologic stimuli, whereas lymphokines are produced only by lymphocytes and have largely immunoregulatory functions.

Lymphokines that are produced largely by T cells and by LGL, including IL-2, IL-4, IL-5, and IFN γ, act predominantly on lymphoid cells and are immunologically induced regulators of the immune response. However, IL-2, IL-4, and IL-5 can also modulate the function of a variety of other leukocytes such as macrophages, mast cells, and eosinophils, respectively; IFN γ also acts on a broad spectrum of cells in addition to lymphoid cells. In contrast, IL-3 is a lymphokine that acts as a hematopoietic growth factor. The other cytokines that modulate the activities of lymphoid and nonlymphoid cells are produced by many cell types and consist of IL-1, IL-6, IL-7, IL-8, TNF, IFN α, IFN β, and TGFβ. They presumably represent intercellular signals that enable connective tissues, skin, nervous system, and other tissues to communicate with the immune system.

Cytokines, in turn, regulate each other by competition, interaction, and mutual induction in a series of lymphokine cascades and circuits with positive or negative feedback effects. For example, cytokines such as IL-1 and IL-2 induce the production of other cytokines such as TNF and interferon. Furthermore, IL-1 and IL-2 induce each other reciprocally. Less well known, but perhaps equally important, are observations that even mesenchymal growth factors such as TGFβ can induce IL-1 production by macrophages.

In addition to cytokine regulation of cytokines, neuroendocrine hormonal peptides such as endorphins and corticosteroids, as well as products of the lipoxygenase and cyclooxygenase pathway, can have agonistic or antagonistic effects on some cytokine activities. The effects of cytokines can also be regulated at the level of cell membrane re-

ceptors. Agents that influence cytokine receptor expression modulate the activities of these mediators. Thus, a complex network of endogenous ligand-receptor interactions is involved in regulating host defense mechanisms. The therapeutic use of cytokines is still in its infancy. However, some disease states have already been shown to respond to interferon and IL-2. Agonists and antagonists of the cytokines and their receptors will probably play an important role in the eventual therapy of inflammatory, infectious, autoimmune, and neoplastic diseases.

REFERENCES

General

Aarden LA et al: Revised nomenclature for antigen-nonspecific T cell proliferation and helper factors. *J Immunol* 1979;**123**:2978.

Gillis S (editor): *Recombinant Lymphokines and Their Receptors*. Marcel Dekker, 1987.

Pick E (editor): *Lymphokines*. Vols 9–14. Academic Press, 1984–1987.

Interleukin-1

Dinarello CA: Biology of interleukin-1. *FASEB J* 1988;**2**:108.

Durum SK, Oppenheim JJ, Neta R: Role of interleukin-1. In: Oppenheim JJ, Shevach EM (editors): *Textbook of Immunophysiology*. Oxford University Press (in press).

Mizel SB: Interleukin-1 and T cell activation. *Immunol Today* 1987;**8**:330.

Neta R, Oppenheim JJ: Why should internists be interested in IL- 1? *Ann Intern Med* 1988.

Oppenheim JJ et al: There is more than one IL-1. *Immunol Today* 1986;**7**:45.

Tumor Necrosis Factor

Beutler B, Cerami A: Cachectin and tumor necrosis factor as two sides of the same biological coin. *Nature* 1986;**320**:584.

Beutler B et al: Control of cachectin (tumor necrosis factor) synthesis: mechanism of endotoxin resistance. *Science* 1986;**232**:977.

Carswell EA et al: An endotoxin-induced serum factor that causes necrosis of tumors. *Proc Natl Acad Sci USA* 1975;**72**:3666.

Le J, Vilcek J: TNF and IL-1: Cytokines with multiple overlapping biological activities. *Lab Invest* 1987;**56**:234.

Old LJ: Tumor necrosis factor (TNF). *Science* 1985;**230**:630.

Paul NL, Ruddle NH: Lymphotoxin. *Annu Rev Immunol* 1988;**6**:407.

Interleukin-2, -4, and - 5

Greene WC, Leonard WJ: The human IL-2 receptor. *Annu Rev Immunol* 1986;**4**:69.

Kishimoto T, Hirano T: Molecular regulation of B lymphocyte response. *Annu Rev Immunol* 1988;**6**:485.

Paul WE, Ohara J: B cell stimulatory factor-1/interleukin-4. *Annu Rev Immunol* 1987;**5**:429.

Rosenberg S, Lotze M: Cancer immunotherapy using IL-2 and IL-2- activated lymphocytes. *Annu Rev Immunol* 1985;**4**:681.

Smith K: The two-chain structure of high-affinity IL-2 receptors. *Immunol Today* 1987;**8**:11.

Smith KA: Interleukin-2: inception, impact and implications. *Science* 1988;**240**:1169.

Interferons

DeMaeyer E, DeMaeyer-Guignard J: *Interferons and Other Regulatory Cytokines.* Wiley, 1988.

Faltynek CR, Kung H-F: The biochemical mechanisms of action of the interferons. *Biofactors* 1988;**1**:277.

Friedman RM, Vogel SN: Interferons with special emphasis on the immune system. *Adv Immunol* 1983;**34**:97.

Pestka S et al: Interferons and their actions. *Annu Rev Biochem* 1987;**56**:727.

Taylor-Papadimitriou J: The effects of interferon in the growth and function of normal and malignant cells. In: *Interferons from Molecular Biology to Clinical Application.* Burke DC, Morris AG (editors). Cambridge University Press, 1983.

Vilcek J, DeMaeyer E (editors): *Interferon 2: Interferons and the Immune System.* Elsevier/North-Holland, 1984.

Interleukin-6

Billiau A: Interferon B2 as a promoter of growth and differentiation of B cells. *Immunol Today* 1987;**8**:84.

Kawano M et al: Autocrine generation and requirement of BSF-2/IL-6 for human multiple myelomas. *Nature* 1988;**332**:83.

Revel M: Interleukin-6. In: *Monokines and Other Non-Lymphocytic Cytokines.* Powanda M et al (editors). Liss, 1988.

Wong GC, Clark SC: Multiple actions of IL-6 within a cytokine network. *Immunol Today* 1988;**9**:137.

Hematopoietic Cytokines

Clark S, Kamen R: Human hematopoietic colony-stimulating factors. *Science* 1987;**236**:1229.

Golde D, Glasson J: Myeloid growth factors in inflammation. In: *Inflammation: Basic Principles & Clinical Correlates.* Gallin J, Goldstein I, Snyderman R (editors). Raven Press, 1988.

Ihle JN: Lymphokine regulation of hematopoietic development. In: *Textbook of Immunophysiology.* Oppenheim JJ, Shevach EM (editors). Oxford University Press (in press).

Metcalf D: Molecular biology and functions of granulocyte-macrophage colony-stimulating factors. *Blood* 1986;**67**:257.

Metcalf D: Role of colony-stimulating factors in resistance to acute infections. *Immunol Cell Biol* 1987;**65**:35.

Transforming Growth Factor β

Ellingsworth LR: Effect of growth factors on immunity and inflammation. In: *Textbook of Immunophysiology.* Oppenheim JJ, Shevach EM (editors). Oxford University Press (in press).

Sporn MB et al: TGFβ biological function and chemical structure. *Science* 1986;**233**:532.

Other Cytokines

Goodwin RG et al: Human interleukin-7: molecular cloning and growth factor activity on human and murine B-lineage cells. *Proc Natl Acad Sci USA* 1989;**86**:302.

Matsushima K et al: Molecular cloning of a human monocyte-derived neutrophil chemotactic factor (MDNCF) and the induction of MDNCF mRNA by IL-2 and TNF. *J Exp Med* 1988;**167**:1883.

Peveri P et al: A novel neutrophil-activating factor produced by human mononuclear phagocytes. *J Exp Med* 1988;**167**:1547.

Immunogenicity & Antigenic Specificity

8

Joel W. Goodman, PhD

Immunogenicity is a property that allows a substance to induce a detectable immune response (humoral or cellular or, most commonly, both) when introduced into an animal. Such substances are called "immunogens." The older term "antigen" now refers to agents that can react with antibodies evoked by immunogens, whether or not they are themselves immunogenic. It follows that all immunogens are also antigens, although the converse is not true. Low-molecular-weight compounds, including many drugs and antibiotics, are nonimmunogenic but, when coupled to immunogenic proteins, give conjugates that can raise antibodies against the low-molecular-weight component. This component can react with such an antibody by itself (see the section below on haptens) and thus is antigenic but not immunogenic.

The term **epitope** refers to the part of an antigen that combines with specific antibody or T cell receptor. The term "antigenic determinant" was previously used to connote what we now call an epitope. These terms are in contrast with the term "immunogenic determinant," which connotes immunogenicity, not merely antigenicity.

IMMUNOGENS

Chemical Nature of Immunogens

The most potent immunogens are macromolecular proteins, but polysaccharides, synthetic polypeptides, and other synthetic polymers such as polyvinylpyrrolidone are immunogenic under appropriate conditions (see below). Although pure nucleic acids or lipids have not been shown to be immunogenic, antibodies that react with them may be induced by immunization with nucleoproteins or lipoproteins. Antibodies reactive with DNA appear spontaneously in the serum of patients with systemic lupus erythematosus.

Requirements for Immunogenicity

Immunogenicity is not an inherent property of a molecule, as are its physicochemical characteristics, but is operationally dependent on the experimental conditions of the system. These include the immunogen, the mode of immunization, the organism being immunized, and the sensitivity of the methods used to detect a response. The factors that confer immunogenicity on molecules are complex and incompletely understood, but it is known that certain conditions must be satisfied in order for a molecule to be immunogenic.

A. Foreignness: The immune system somehow discriminates between "self" and "nonself," so that only molecules that are foreign to the animal are normally immunogenic. Thus, albumin isolated from the serum of a rabbit and injected back into the same or another rabbit will not generate the formation of antibody. Yet the same protein injected into other vertebrate animals is likely to evoke substantial amounts of antibody depending on the dose of antigen and the route and frequency of injection.

B. Molecular Size: Extremely small molecules such as amino acids or monosaccharides are not immunogenic, and it is generally accepted that a certain minimum size is necessary for immunogenicity. However, there is no specific threshold below which all substances are inert and above which all are active, but rather a gradient of immunogenicity with molecular size. In a few instances, substances with molecular weights of less than 1000 have proved to be immunogenic, but as a general rule molecules smaller than molecular weight 10,000 are only weakly immunogenic or not immunogenic at all. The most potent immunogens are macromolecular proteins with molecular weights greater than 100,000.

C. Chemical Complexity: A molecule must possess a certain degree of chemical complexity to be immunogenic. The principle has been illus-

MOST IMPORTANT

trated very clearly with synthetic polypeptides. Homopolymers consisting of repeating units of a single amino acid are poor immunogens regardless of size, whereas copolymers of 2 or—even better—3 amino acids may be quite active. Once again, it is difficult to establish a definite threshold, and the general rule is that immunogenicity increases with structural complexity. Aromatic amino acids contribute more to immunogenicity than nonaromatic residues, since relatively simple random polypeptides containing tyrosine are better antigens than the same polymers without tyrosine, and immunogenicity is proportionate to the tyrosine content of the molecule. Also, the attachment of tyrosine chains to the weak immunogen gelatin, which is poor in aromatic amino acids, markedly enhances its immunogenicity.

D. Genetic Constitution of the Animal: The ability to respond to a particular antigen is a function of the way the immune response is controlled genetically. It has been known for some time that pure polysaccharides are immunogenic when injected into mice and humans but not when injected into guinea pigs. Much additional information has accrued from the use of inbred strains of animals. As one of many examples, strain 2 guinea pigs respond readily in an easily detectable manner to poly-L-lysine, whereas strain 13 guinea pigs do not. The ability to respond is inherited as an autosomal dominant trait. Many analogous examples have been described in humans, and the genetic control of the human immune response is discussed in Chapter 4.

E. Method of Antigen Administration: Whether an antigen will induce an immune response depends on the dose and the mode of administration. A quantity of antigen that is ineffective when injected intravenously may evoke a copious antibody response if injected subcutaneously in adjuvant (see below). In general, once the threshold is exceeded, increasing doses lead to increasing—but less than proportionate—responses. However, excessive doses may not only fail to stimulate antibody formation; they can also establish a state of specific unresponsiveness or tolerance.

ADJUVANTS

The response to an immunogen can be enhanced if it is administered as a mixture with substances called **adjuvants**. Adjuvants function in one or more of the following ways: (1) by prolonging retention of the immunogen, (2) by increasing its effective size, or (3) by stimulating the influx of populations of macrophages and/or lymphocytes. A number of adjuvants have been used in experimental animals, the most potent being Freund's complete adjuvant (CFA), a water-in-oil emulsion containing killed mycobacteria. CFA presumably works by providing a depot for the immunogen and by stimulating macrophages and certain lymphocytes, but its very strong inflammatory effect precludes its use in humans. A muramyl dipeptide constituent of mycrobacterial cell walls has also been found to possess adjuvant activity. The most widely used adjuvant in humans is a suspension of aluminum hydroxide on which the immunogen is adsorbed (alum precipitate). This adjuvant increases the effective particle size of the immunogen, promoting its presentation to lymphocytes (see Chapter 5).

EPITOPES

Although strong immunogens are large molecules, only restricted portions of them are involved in actual binding with antibody combining sites. Such areas, which determine the specificity of antigen-antibody reactions, are designated epitopes (previously called antigenic determinants). The number of distinct determinants on an antigen molecule usually varies with its size and chemical complexity. Estimates of the number of epitopes on an antigen have been made on the basis of the number of antibody molecules bound per molecule of antigen. Such measurements provide minimum values, since steric hindrance may prevent simultaneous occupation of all sites. Furthermore, antibody populations from different animals are likely to vary in specificity, and variations also occur in specificities of a single individual at different times. This means that antibodies specific for all epitopes of an antigen molecule may not be present in a particular antiserum. Typical results for this approach are about 5 epitopes for hen egg albumin (MW 42,000) and as many as 40 for thyroglobulin (MW 700,000). However, it has been found that virtually any region on the exposed surface of a protein may serve as an epitope.

Size & Location of Epitopes

Antibody complementarity is directed against limited parts of the antigen molecule. Numerous studies with homopolymers of sugars or amino acids or multichain polymer-protein conjugates indicate that an epitope is of the order of 4-6 amino acid or sugar residues (Fig 8-1). The weight of evidence also indicates that the entire exposed surface of a protein may be antigenic. Therefore, large proteins express many potential epitopes. However, a given individual will make antibodies against only a small subset of the total. For exam-

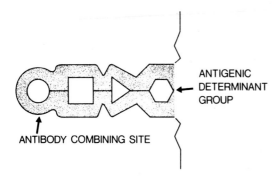

Figure 8–1. A view of the "lock-and-key" complementariness between an antigenic determinant group and an antibody combining site. The determinant can be considered to be composed of discrete subunits, which may be amino acids in a peptide chain or sugars in a saccharide chain. The antibody combining site is then composed of subsites, each of which can accommodate a discrete subunit of the antigenic determinant. (Reproduced, with permission, from Goodman JW: Antigenic determinants and antibody combining sites. In: *The Antigens.* Vol 3. Sela M [editor]. Academic Press, 1975.)

ple, as noted above, a given antiserum to hen egg albumin has specificity for no more than about 5 epitopes. Since the total number when comparing different antisera is much greater, there is obviously a selection of potential epitopes in any given immunization.

A cardinal factor in the selection of epitopes is exposure of the structure to the aqueous environment and therefore to the immune apparatus. The terminal side chains of polysaccharides represent the most potent epitope regions of that class of compounds. The principle has been demonstrated most vividly with multichain synthetic polypeptides having sequences of alanine on the outside and tyrosine-glutamic acid closer to the backbone, or the reverse (Fig 8–2). Antibodies to the former were largely alanine-specific, whereas the latter evoked antibodies with a predominant specificity for tyrosine-glutamic acid sequences. The most exposed region was preferred as the determinant in each instance. The same is generally true for globular proteins. A feature of proteins that correlates well with accessibility and has had predictive value for identifying epitopes is the **hydrophilicity** of local regions within the protein. The greater the average hydrophilicity, the higher the likelihood that the region will be antigenic.

In addition to accessibility, which is an intrinsic feature of the antigen, host factors play important roles in epitope selection and probably account for the different specificity patterns in antisera from different individuals. A large body of evidence attests to the genetic control of antibody specificity to a given antigen. Some of the earliest evidence accrued from a comparison of the specificity of anti-insulin antibodies from strain 2 and strain 13 guinea pigs, which are uniformly di-

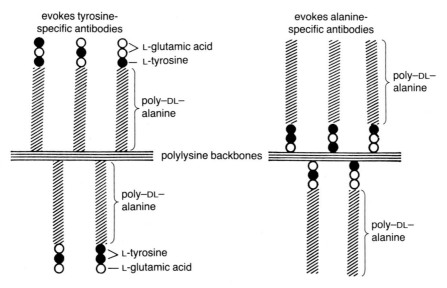

Figure 8–2. *Left:* A multichain copolymer in which L-tyrosine and L-glutamic acid residues are attached to multi-poly-DL-alanyl-poly-L-lysine(poly-[Tyr,Glu]-poly-DL-Ala-poly-Lys). *Right:* Copolymer in which tyrosine and glutamic acid are attached directly to the polylysine backbone with alanine peptides on the ends of the side chains. Horizontal lines: poly-L-lysine; diagonal hatching: poly-DL-alanine; closed circles; L-tyrosine; open circles: L-glutamic acid. (From Sela M: Antigenicity: Some molecular aspects. *Science* 1969;**166**:1365. Copyright© 1969 by the American Association for the Advancement of Science.)

rected against opposite ends of the insulin molecule. Outbred populations are more difficult to study, but the principle that genetic makeup strongly influences epitope selection has been clearly established (see Chapter 4).

Haptens

Much of our understanding of the specificity of antigen-antibody reactions derives from the pioneering studies of Karl Landsteiner in the early years of the 20th century with small, chemically defined substances which are not immunogenic but can react with antibodies of appropriate specificity. They are called haptens, from the Greek word *haptein,* "to fasten." Landsteiner covalently coupled the diazonium derivatives of a wide variety of aromatic amines to the lysine, tyrosine, and histidine residues of immunogenic proteins (Fig 8–3). The conjugated proteins raised antibody specific for the azo substituents, as demonstrated by the capacity of the free hapten to bind antibody. The conjugated hapten therefore becomes a partial or complete epitope. The total epitope may include amino acids in the protein to which the hapten is linked. The protein, called the **carrier,** has its set of native or integral epitopes as well as the new ones introduced by the conjugated hapten (Fig 8–4).

Although most haptens are small molecules, macromolecules may also function as haptens. The definition is based not on size but on immunogenicity.

The use of hapten-protein conjugates has spotlighted the remarkable diversity of immune mechanisms as well as the exquisite structural specificity of antigen-antibody reactions. Virtually any chemical entity may serve as an epitope if coupled to a suitably immunogenic carrier. Even antibodies with specificity for metal ions have been produced in this way.

Landsteiner's studies showed that antibody could distinguish between structurally similar haptens. In one series of experiments, antibodies raised to *m*-aminobenzenesulfonate were tested for their ability to bind with other isomers of the homologous hapten and related molecules in which the sulfonate group was replaced by arsonate or carboxylate groups (Table 8–1). As expected, the strongest reaction occurred with the homologous hapten. The compound with the sulfonate group in the *ortho* position was somewhat poorer than the *meta* isomer but distinctly better than the *para* isomer. The substitution of arsonate for sulfonate resulted in very weak binding with antibody. Although both substituents are negatively charged and have a tetrahedral structure, the arsonate group is bulkier because of the larger size of the arsenic atom and the additional hydrogen atom. The benzoate derivatives are also negatively charged, but the carboxylate ion has a planar rather than tetrahedral 3-dimensional configuration and shows even less affinity for the antisulfonate antibody.

The reaction of antibody with an antigen or hapten other than the one that induced its formation is called a **cross-reaction.** Thus, the reaction of anti-*m*-aminobenzenesulfonate with any of the other compounds in Table 8–1 is a cross-reaction. Cross-reactions almost invariably have a lower binding affinity than homologous reactions between antibody and its inducing antigen.

Studies of this kind have shown that antibody recognizes the overall 3-dimensional shape of the epitope group rather than any specific chemical property such as ionic charge. It is believed that epitopes and antibody combining sites possess a structural complementariness which may be figuratively visualized as a "lock-and-key" arrangement (Fig 8–1). The electron cloud box of the antibody site is contoured to match that of the

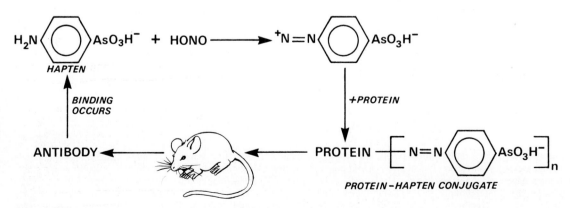

Figure 8–3. The preparation of hapten-protein conjugates and their capacity to induce the formation of antihapten antibody to the azophenylarsonate group in this example.

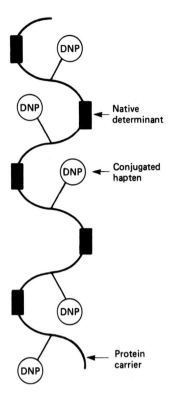

Figure 8-4. Diagrammatic illustration of a hapten-protein conjugate. The protein has several native or integral antigenic determinants denoted by thickened areas. The conjugated dinotrophenyl (DNP) hapten introduces new antigenic determinants.

Table 8-1. Effect of variation in hapten structure on strength of binding to *m*-aminobenzenesulfonate antibodies.

	ortho	meta	para
R = sulfonate	+ +	+ + +	±
R = arsonate	−	+	−
R = carboxylate	−	±	−

Strength of binding is graded from negative (−) to very strong (+ + +). (From Landsteiner K, van der Scheer J: On cross reactions of immune sera to azoproteins. *J Exp Med* 1936; **63**:325.)

epitope, with the affinity of binding directly proportionate to the closeness of fit. The startling diversity of the antibody response is perhaps more comprehensible if antibody specificity is viewed as directed against a molecular shape rather than a particular chemical structure.

Immunodominance

Given a particular epitope, which may be the size of a tetrapeptide, the amino acid subunits of that epitope will contribute unequally to binding with antibody. The degree of the influence on reactivity is a measure of the immunodominance of the component.

Antibody specificity may be directed against conformational or sequential features of antigens. The former usually holds for globular proteins and helical structures. For example, polymers of the tripeptide L tyrosyl-L alanyl-L glutamic acid form an α-helix under physiologic conditions. The same tripeptide can be attached to a branched synthetic polypeptide (Fig 8–5). The tripeptide itself does not possess an ordered configuration. Antibodies to the 2 polymers do not cross-react, and the tripeptide binds antibodies produced against the branched polymer but not those made against the helical polymer. The immunodominant element of the helical polymer is its conformation. Antiserum against human hemoglobin A₁ combines better with the oxygenated form than with the reduced form, and this has been attributed to the difference in quaternary structure between the 2 forms. There are many examples of conformation-dependent antibody specificity.

Epitopes whose specificity is dictated by the sequence of subunits (amino acids or sugars) within the epitopes rather than by the macromolecular superstructure of the antigen molecule are designated **sequential epitopes.** In such cases, components of the epitope can act as haptens and bind with antibody, the reaction being demonstrable either directly, by such techniques as equilibrium dialysis or fluorescence quenching, or indirectly, by inhibition of the reaction between antigen and antibody. Sequential epitopes may be composed of terminal or internal sequences of macromolecules, or they may be artificially added to carriers, as in the case of the tripeptide Tyr-Ala-Glu. Characterization of the antigenic structure of several proteins has shown that sequential epitopes are always localized in hydrophilic regions of the molecule, where exposure to the aqueous environment is maximal.

When the epitope is a terminal sequence, the terminal residue of the sequence is almost invariably the immunodominant subunit. Again, many examples exist to illustrate this point, which was recognized by Landsteiner when he showed that the terminal amino acid of peptides coupled to a

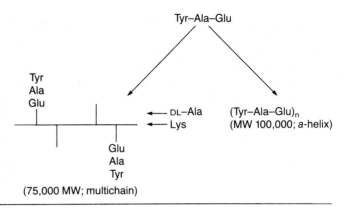

Figure 8-5. A synthetic branched polymer in which peptides of sequence Tyr-Ala-Glu are attached to the amino groups of side chains in multi-poly-DL-alanyl-poly-L-lysine *(left)* and a periodic polymer of the tripeptide Tyr-Ala-Glu *(right)*. (From Sela M: Antigenicity: Some molecular aspects. *Science* 1969;**166**:1365. Copyright© 1969 by the American Association for the Advancement of Science.)

protein carrier exerted a dominant effect on specificity. Goebel made the same observation with glycosides conjugated to protein carriers. In general, then, it may be concluded that all epitopes exhibit a gradient of immunodominance. When the epitope is composed of a terminal sequence, the gradient decreases from the most exposed portion inward.

In addition, epitopes may be continuous or discontinuous. If antibodies bind to a contiguous sequence of amino acids, the epitope is continuous. A discontinuous epitope, on the other hand, is composed of residues that are separated from one another in the sequence of the protein but are brought into proximity by tertiary folding. There are numerous examples of discontinuous epitopes in proteins. Conformational epitopes may be continuous or discontinuous, but sequential epitopes are always continuous.

IMMUNOGENIC DETERMINANTS

Immunogens are normally large molecules, and immunogenicity is, within limits, a function of molecular size and complexity. A characteristic of immunogens is their capacity to induce cellular immunity mediated by T lymphocytes (see Chapter 5), which haptens are unable to do. It is believed that an immunogen must possess at least 2 determinants to stimulate antibody formation, which is the function of another line of lymphocytes, B cells. At least one determinant must be capable of triggering a T cell response. Our concern here is with structural determinants of immunogens that interact with T and B lymphocytes. Early studies with small, well-defined immunogens supported the interpretation that specificities of the 2 cell types may be directed against different determinants of the antigen molecule. In recent years, more than 50 epitopes that activate T cells have been found on large proteins.

The pancreatic hormone glucagon consists of only 29 amino acids but is immunogenic. It has been functionally dissected into component determinants that interact with T cells (immunogenic determinants) and with antibody (haptenic determinants). Using isolated tryptic peptides of the hormone, it was found that antibodies recognized a determinant or determinants in the amino terminal part of the molecule, whereas T lymphocytes responded only to the carboxy-terminal fragment (Fig 8–6). The latter was therefore identified as the immunogenic or "carrier" portion of the molecule and the former as the haptenic region.

Several synthetic molecules about the size of a single antigenic determinant induce an almost purely cellular immune response, with little or no antibody production, but are capable of acting as carriers for conjugated haptens in much the same fashion as macromolecular immunogens are. One such unideterminant immunogen is the compound L-tyrosine-*p*-azobenzenearsonate (ABA-Tyr). Despite its molecular weight of only 409, ABA-Tyr

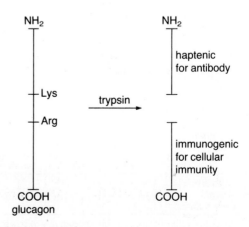

Figure 8-6. The functional dissection of glucagon into immunogenic and haptenic determinants.

induces cellular immunity with little or no antibody production in a variety of animal species. A hapten such as the dinitrophenyl group can be coupled to ABA-Tyr through a spacer group (6-aminocaproic acid) to produce a bideterminant or bifunctional immunogen (Fig 8–7). This antigen induces antibody specific for the dinitrophenyl haptenic determinant and cellular immunity directed against the ABA-Tyr immunogenic determinant. The concept of archetypal bifunctional immunogens has recently been applied to construction of synthetic peptide vaccines against infectious agents (see below).

Experiments with analogs of immunogenic determinants, designed along the lines of Landsteiner's classic studies on the specificity of antihapten antibodies, have shown that cellular (T cell) responses to antigens are as exquisitely specific as antigen-antibody reactions.

Recent findings indicate that in some instances different determinants on a protein antigen may activate different functional subpopulations of T cells (see Chapter 5). For example, different fragments of myelin basic protein induce suppression and immunity in rodents. Immunity is manifested as an autoimmune allergic encephalomyelitis. Animals presensitized with the suppressor-inducing fragment and subsequently challenged with the intact molecule did not develop encephalomyelitis. A determining factor in the selective activation of suppressor or helper T cells by particular determinants appears to be the genetic constitution of the animal. Thus, the same region (though perhaps not the identical determinant) of hen egg lysozyme induces suppression in strain B10 mice but helps in strain B10.A mice. Another example is the induction of suppression or help by a random synthetic copolymer of glutamic acid, alanine, and tyrosine in different inbred strains of mice.

The selective activation of help or suppression is being actively investigated, because it may eventually offer a rationale for manipulating the immune response in humans to such clinically important antigens as histocompatibility antigens, tumor antigens, and allergens.

THYMUS-INDEPENDENT ANTIGENS

eg. pure carbohydrates

A certain type of molecule may be immunogenic without the apparent participation of T lymphocytes. Such molecules appear to be able to directly trigger B lymphocytes (antibody-producing cells). Their characteristic feature is a structure that consists of repeating units. Bacterial polysaccharides and some polymerized proteins are thymus-independent antigens. However, not all repeating unit polymers behave this way. Poly-L-lysine, for example, is a thymus-dependent antigen in responder guinea pigs despite its simple, repetitive structure.

The mechanism by which thymus-independent antigens act is still unclear, but the immune response to such antigens differs from the response to more typical thymus-dependent antigens in that the antibody produced is largely or exclusively of the IgM class and little or no immunologic memory is engendered. Recent careful analysis of the responses to these antigens indicates that many, if not all, do require some degree of T cell help, although significantly less than that required by conventional thymus-dependent antigens. Therefore, it may be more accurate to consider them as thymus-efficient rather than as thymus-independent antigens.

SYNTHETIC VACCINES

Two promising new approaches to vaccine development have emerged in the modern era of biomedical technology. One is the cloning of genes coding for important surface proteins of infectious agents, with production of large quantities of the desired protein by microorganisms transfected with the gene. A recombinant vaccine containing the major surface protein of the hepatitis B virus has recently been approved and marketed.

The other approach is the chemical synthesis of short peptides from the known sequences of proteins from infectious organisms. The peptides

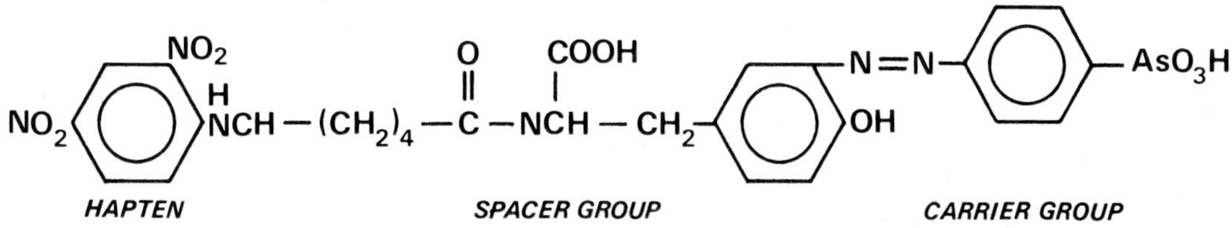

Figure 8–7. The bifunctional antigen dinitrophenyl-6-aminocaproyl-L-tyrosine-p-azobenzenearsonate.

may be linked to carriers, thereby becoming "synthetic antigens." This approach is predicated on the assumption that antibodies induced to short peptides of the order of 6–15 amino acids will react with the homologous sequences in the native proteins. Indeed, it has been shown that antibodies to many peptides representing sequences from the exposed surfaces of folded proteins, where they are accessible to antibody, do react with the native molecules, although the affinities of binding may be lower than with the peptides themselves. These findings offer promise for the manufacture of synthetic vaccines that are based on the hapten-carrier principle for use in human and animal prophylaxis. However, an important consideration is that immunologic memory in the response to hapten-carrier conjugates is directed primarily at the carrier, which bears the immunogenic determinants. Since the carriers are different in the synthetic vaccine and the native protein from which the peptide came, an encounter with the infectious agent following immunization with the synthetic vaccine should elicit little or no memory. Although sufficiently high antibody titers raised by the vaccine could provide substantial protection even without memory, this does represent a serious limitation for this type of vaccine.

An innovative way around the dilemma was taken in the design of a malaria vaccine based on the bifunctional immunogen concept discussed above. A helper T cell determinant on the circumsporozoite protein of *Plasmodium falciparum* was identified, synthesized, and covalently coupled to a second peptide representing the major haptenic determinant of the protein. The bifunctional conjugate elicited high-titer antibody responses in mice and induced anamnesis to the native protein. Although this vaccine technology is still in its infancy, it may signal the wave of the future.

SUMMARY

The immunologic properties of molecules include immunogenicity and antigenicity. Immunogenicity refers to the ability to induce an immune response, whereas antigenicity refers to the capacity to react with antibodies produced in an immune response. In general, immunogenicity is a function of foreignness of the immunogen to the individual being immunized, and increases with increasing molecular size and chemical complexity. However, peptides composed of only 8 or so amino acids can be immunogenic. The response to immunogens can be enhanced by adjuvants.

The subunit of an immunogen that actually binds with antibody is an antigenic determinant, or epitope. Large proteins possess many epitopes. The binding between antibody and antigen is exquisitely specific, but cross-reactions can occur between antibodies and other compounds bearing structurally related epitopes.

It is possible to raise antibodies to virtually any small compound (hapten) by coupling it to an immunogenic carrier and using the conjugate for immunization. The hapten is one of many epitopes of the complex conjugate and will react by itself with antibodies directed against it.

A number of immunogenic determinants or epitopes have been identified on immunogens. These structures are similar in size to antigenic determinants, but they trigger T cell responses and are responsible for immunogenicity. They may prove useful in the fabrication of relatively simple synthetic vaccines.

REFERENCES

Benjamin DC et al: The antigenic structure of proteins: A reappraisal. *Annu Rev Immunol* 1984;**2**:67.

Good MF et al: The T cell response to the malaria circumsporozoite protein: An immunological approach to vaccine development. *Annu Rev Immunol* 1988; **6**:663.

Goodman JW: Antigenic determinants and antibody combining sites. Page 127 in: *The Antigens*. Vol 3. Sela M (editor). Academic Press, 1975.

Goodman JW: Modelling determinants for recognition by B cells and T cells. *Prog Allergy* 1989;**56** (in press).

Goodman JW, Sercarz EE: The complexity of structures involved in T cell activation. *Annu Rev Immunol* 1983;**1**:465.

Goodman JW et al: Antigen structure and lymphocyte activation. *Immunol Rev* 1978;**39**:36.

Landsteiner K: *The Specificity of Serological Reactions*. Harvard Univ Press, 1945.

Lerner RA: Synthetic vaccines. *Sci Am* (Feb) 1983; **248**:66.

Livingston AM, Fathman CG: The structure of T cell epitopes. *Annu Rev Immunol* 1987;**5**:477.

Reichlin M: Amino acid substitution and the antigenicity of globular proteins. *Adv Immunol* 1975;**20**:71.

Sela M: Antigenicity: Some molecular aspects. *Science* 1969;**166**:1365.

Immunoglobulin Structure & Function

9

Joel W. Goodman, PhD

The immunoglobulins are proteins with antibody activity; ie, they combine specifically with the substance that elicited their formation (immunogen or antigen; see Chapter 8), and they make up the humoral arm of the immune response. With the possible exception of "natural" antibody, antibodies arise in response to foreign substances introduced into the body. They are therefore products of induced responses. The immunoglobulins, which circulate in body fluids, comprise a heterogeneous family of proteins, they account for approximately 20% of the total plasma proteins. In serum electrophoresis, the majority of immunoglobulins migrate as "gamma globulins," a historic but now archaic term.

The 2 hallmarks of immunoglobulins are the *specificity* of each for one particular antigenic structure and their *diversity* as a group, which meets the challenge of a vast array of antigenic structures in the environment. In addition to specifically binding antigens, the immunoglobulins express secondary biologic activities, which are important in defense against disease, eg, complement fixation, transplacental passage, and facilitation of phagocytosis. They are heterogeneous with respect to these activities, which are independent of the antigen-binding function of immunoglobulin molecules. This chapter explains how the structure of immunoglobulins accounts for their specificity, diversity, and secondary biologic activities.

BASIC STRUCTURE & TERMINOLOGY

Immunoglobulins are glycoproteins composed of 82–96% polypeptide and 4–18% carbohydrate. The polypeptide component possesses almost all of the biologic properties associated with antibody molecules. Antibodies are bifunctional molecules in that they bind specifically with antigen and also initiate a variety of secondary phenomena, such as complement fixation and histamine

release by mast cells, which are independent of their specificity for antigen. Antibody molecules are extremely heterogeneous, as might be expected in view of their enormous diversity with respect to antigen binding and their different biologic activities. This heterogeneity is easily demonstrated by serologic, electrophoretic, and amino acid sequence methods and severely hampered early structural studies.

Two major discoveries ushered in the period of detailed structural study of antibodies. The first was the finding that enzymes and reducing agents could be used to digest or dissociate immunoglobulin molecules into smaller components. The second was the realization that the electrophoretically homogeneous proteins found in serum and urine of patients with multiple myeloma were related to normal immunoglobulins. These myeloma proteins were found to be structurally homogeneous. They are also called monoclonal proteins, since they are synthesized by single clones of malignant plasma cells. A clone here refers collectively to the progeny of a single lymphoid cell.

Our present understanding of immunoglobulin structure is based collectively on studies of monoclonal and normal proteins. The discussion of the details of immunoglobulin structure is introduced with a list of definitions of the relevant terms used here and in Figs 9–1 and 9–2.

List of Definitions

Basic unit (monomer): Each immunoglobulin contains at least one basic unit or monomer comprising 4 polypeptide chains (Fig 9–1).

H and L chains: One pair of identical polypeptide chains contains approximately twice the number of amino acids, or is approximately twice the molecular weight, of the other pair of identical polypeptide chains. The chains of higher molecular weight are designated **heavy (H) chains** (Fig 9–1) and those of lower molecular weight **light (L) chains.**

V and C regions: Each polypeptide chain con-

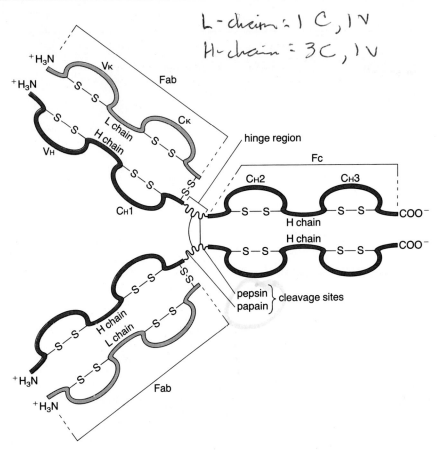

L-chain = 1 C, 1 V
H-chain = 3 C, 1 V

Figure 9-1. Simplified model for an IgG1 (κ) human antibody molecule showing the basic 4-chain structures and domains (V_H, C_H1, etc). V indicates the variable region; C indicates the constant region. Sites of enzyme cleavage by pepsin and papain are shown. Note portions of inter- and intrachain desulfide bonds.

tains an amino-terminal portion, the **variable (V) region;** and a carboxy-terminal portion, the **constant (C) region.** These terms denote the considerable heterogeneity or variability in the amino acid residues in the V region compared with the C region.

Domains: The polypeptide chains do not exist 3-dimensionally as linear sequences of amino acids but are folded by disulfide bonds into globular regions called domains. The domains in H chains are designated V_H and C_H1, C_H2, C_H3, and C_H4; and those in L chains are designated V_L and C_L.

Antigen-binding site: The part of the antibody molecule that binds antigen is formed by only small numbers of amino acids in the V regions of H and L chains. These amino acids are brought into close proximity by the folding of the V regions.

Fab and Fc fragments: Digestion of an immunoglobulin G (IgG) molecule by the enzyme pa-

pain produces 2 Fab (antigen-binding) fragments and one Fc (crystallizable) fragment.

Hinge region: The area of the H chains in the C region between the first and second C region domains (C_H1 and C_H2) is the hinge region. It is more flexible and is more exposed to enzymes and chemicals. Thus, papain acts here to produce Fab and Fc fragments.

F(ab)'₂ fragment: Digestion of an IgG molecule by the enzyme pepsin produces one F(ab)'₂ molecule and small peptides. The F(ab)'₂ molecule is composed of 2 Fab units and the hinge region, with intact inter-H chain disulfide bonds, since pepsin cleaves the IgG molecule on the carboxy-terminal side of the these bonds.

Disulfide bonds: Chemical disulfide (–S–S–) bonds between cysteine residues are essential for the normal 3-dimensional structure of immunoglobulins. These bonds can be interchain (H chain to H chain, H chain to L chain, L chain to L chain) or intrachain.

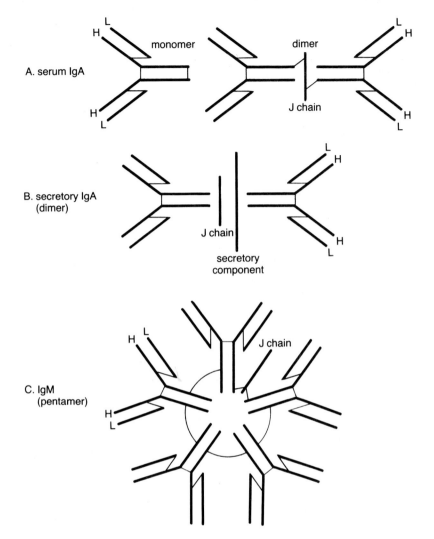

Figure 9-2. Highly schematic illustration of polymeric human immunoglobulins. Polypeptide chains are represented by thick lines; disulfide bonds linking different polypeptide chains are represented by thin lines.

Classes: There are 5 classes of immunoglobulins, designated IgG, IgA, IgM, IgD, and IgE (Table 9–1). They are defined by antigenic differences in the C regions of H chains. IgG, IgA, and IgM have been further subdivided into subclasses on the basis of relatively minor antigenic differences in C_H regions.

L chain types: L chains are divided into κ and λ types on the basis of antigenic determinants. Akin to the subclasses of H chains 4 subtypes of λ chains have been found.

Isotypes: These are the antigenic differences that characterize the class and subclass of H chains and the type and subtype of L chains. Each normal individual expresses all the isotypes characteristic of the species inasmuch as each isotype occupies a distinctive genetic locus in the genome.

Allotypes: These are polymorphic (allelic) forms of H and L chains that exhibit a mendelian pattern of inheritance. The antigenic determinants that characterize allotypes are usually localized to C regions. Thus, a particular isotype may have several alternative (allelic) structures.

Idiotypes: These are antigenic determinants that distinguish one V domain from all other V domains.

S value: The S value refers to the sedimentation coefficient of a protein, measured by the technique of Svedberg. S values of normal immunoglobulins range from 6S to 19S (Table 9–1). In general, the larger the S value of a protein, the higher its molecular weight.

Polymers: Immunoglobulins composed of more than a single basic monomeric unit are

Table 9-1. Properties of human immunoglobulin chains.

Designation	H Chains					L Chains		Secretory Component	J Chain
	γ IgG	α IgA	μ IgM	δ IgD	ε IgE	κ All classes	λ All classes	SC IgA	J IgA, IgM
Classes in which chains occur	IgG	IgA	IgM	IgD	IgE	All classes	All classes	IgA	IgA, IgM
Subclasses or subtypes	1,2,3,4	1,2	1,2	...	...	...	1,2,3,4	...	...
Allotypic variants	Gm(1)–(25)	A2m(1), (2)	...	...	...	Km(1)–(3)[2]	...	...	...
Molecular weight (approximate)	50,000[1]	55,000	70,000	62,000	70,000	23,000	23,000	70,000	15,000
V region subgroups	V_HI–V_HIV					$V_\kappa I$–$V_\kappa IV$	$V_\lambda I$–$V_\lambda VI$		
Carbohydrate (average percentage)	4	10	15	18	18	0	0	16	8
Number of oligosaccharides	1	2 or 3	5	?	5	0	0	?	1

[1]60,000 for γ3.
[2]Formerly Inv(1)–(3).

termed polymers. The main examples are IgA dimers (2 units) and trimers (3 units) and IgM pentamers (5 units).

J chain: This is a polypeptide chain that is normally found in polymeric immunoglobulins.

Secretory component: IgA molecules in secretions are most commonly composed of 2 IgA units, one J chain, and an additional polypeptide, the secretory component.

FOUR-CHAIN BASIC UNIT

Immunoglobulin molecules are composed of equal numbers of heavy and light polypeptide chains, which can be represented by the general formula $(H_2L_2)_n$. The chains are held together by noncovalent forces and usually by covalent interchain disulfide bridges to form a bilaterally symmetric structure (Fig 9–1). It has been shown that all normal immunoglobulins have this basic structure, although some, as we shall see, are composed of more than one 4-chain unit.

Each polypeptide chain is made up of a number of loops or domains of rather constant size (100–110 amino acid residues) formed by the intrachain disulfide bonds (Fig 9–1). The N-terminal domain of each chain shows much more variation in amino acid sequence than the others and is designated the variable region to distinguish it from the other relatively constant domains (collectively called the constant region in each chain). The zone where the variable and constant regions join is termed the "switch" region.

Immunoglobulins are rather insensitive to proteolytic digestion but are most easily cleaved about midway in the heavy chain in an area between the first and second constant region domains (C_H1 and C_H2) (Fg 9–1). The enzyme papain splits the molecule on the N-terminal side of the inter-heavy chain disulfide bonds into 3 fragments of similar size: 2 Fab fragments, which include an entire light chain and the V_H and C_H1 domains of a heavy chain; and one Fc fragment, composed of the C-terminal halves of the heavy chains. If pepsin is used, cleavage occurs on the C-terminal side of the inter-H chain disulfide bonds, yielding a large $F(ab)'_2$ fragment composed of about 2 Fab fragments. The Fc fragment is extensively degraded by pepsin. The region in the H chain susceptible to proteolytic attack is more flexible and exposed to the environment than the more compact, globular domains and is known as the "hinge" region. Antigen-binding activity is associated with the Fab fragments or, more specifically, with the V_H and V_l domains, while most of the secondary biologic activities of immunoglobulins (eg, complement fixation) are associated with the Fc fragment.

HETEROGENEITY OF IMMUNOGLOBULINS

As already noted, immunoglobulin molecules comprise a family of proteins with the same basic molecular architecture but with a vast array of antigen-binding specificities and different biologic activities. These different activities are, of course, reflections of structural differences dictated by the amino acid sequence of the polypeptide chains. This structural heterogeneity has been an obstacle for protein chemists, but plasmacytomas of human and murine origin provide homogeneous (monoclonal) immunoglobulins that have greatly facilitated the study of the amino acid sequence of antibody molecules. Furthermore, it is now possible to produce at will virtually unlimited quantities of monoclonal antibodies of prescribed antigen specificity by somatic cell fusion of plasmacytoma cells with normal antibody-producing cells from immunized animals. The monoclonal antibodies produced by such somatic cell hybrids, or "hybridomas," are being used on a vast scale as diagnostic reagents.

Light Chain Types

All L chains have a molecular weight of approximately 23,000 but can be classified into 2 types, kappa (κ) and lambda (λ), on the basis of multiple structural differences in the constant regions, which are reflected in antigenic differences (Table 9–1). The 2 types of L chains have been demonstrated in many mammalian species. Indeed, the amino acid sequence homologies between human and mouse κ chains are much greater than those between the κ and λ chains within each species, indicating that the 2 types separated during evolution prior to the divergence of mammalian species.

The proportion of κ to λ chains in immunoglobulin molecules varies from species to species, being about 2:1 in humans. A given immunoglobulin molecule always contains identical κ or λ chains, never a mixture of the two.

Heavy Chain Classes

Five classes of H chains have been found in humans, based again on structural differences in the constant regions detected by serologic and chemical methods. The different forms of H chain, designated γ, α, μ, δ and ϵ (Table 9–1), vary in molecular weight from 50,000 to 70,000, the μ and ϵ chains possessing 5 domains (one V and four C) rather than the 4 of γ and α chains. The δ chain has an intermediate molecular weight which is believed to be due to an extended hinge region. Likewise, the $\gamma3$ chain has an extended hinge region consisting of about 60 amino acid residues, including 14 cysteines, which account for the large number of inter-heavy chain disulfide bonds in IgG3 (Fig 9–3).

The class of the H chain determines the class of the immunoglobulin. Thus, there are 5 classes of immunoglobulins: IgG, IgA, IgM, IgD, and IgE. Two γ chains combined with either two κ or two λ L chains constitute an IgG molecule, the major class of immunoglobulins in serum. Similarly, two μ chains and two L chains form an IgM subunit; IgM molecules are macroglobulins which consist of 5 of these basic 4-chain subunits (Fig 9–2). IgA is polydisperse, comprising 1–5 such units. The other classes (IgD and IgE), like IgG, consist of a single 4-chain unit. The classification and properties of immunoglobulins and their component polypeptide chains are summarized in Tables 9–1 and 9–2.

Subclasses of Polypeptide Chains

Most of the H chain classes have been further subdivided into **subclasses** on the basis of serologic or physicochemical differences in the con-

stant regions. However, H chains representing the various subclasses within a class are much more closely related to each other than to the other classes. For example, there are 4 subclasses of γ chain in humans, γ1, γ2, γ3, and γ4 (Table 9–2), which yield IgG1, IgG2, IgG3, and IgG4 subclasses of immunoglobulin G molecules, respectively. The C regions of these γ chains are much more homologous to each other than to those of α, μ, δ, or ε chains. In some species, the charge spectra of the IgG subclasses differ sufficiently to permit their isolation by electrophoretic techniques. This is not true for human IgG subclasses, which have been recognized by serologic and chemical methods, facilitated by the existence of myeloma proteins and monoclonal antibodies.

A noteworthy aspect of the structural differences between the immunoglobulins subclasses is the number and arrangement of interchain disulfide bridges (Fig 9–3). In IgA2, the L chains are covalently linked to each other instead of to the H chains so that L–H binding is entirely by noncovalent forces. In other immunoglobulins, the

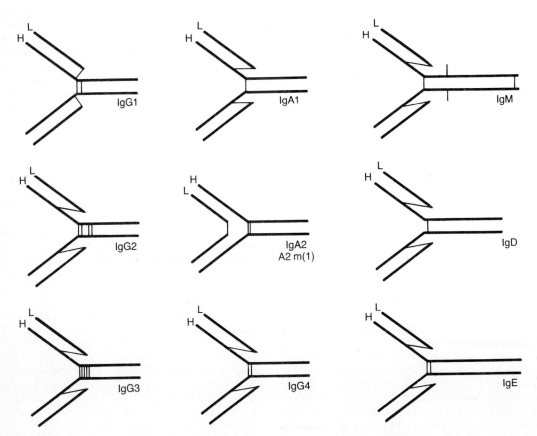

Figure 9–3. Distribution of interchain disulfide bonds in various human immunoglobulin classes and subclasses. H chains are represented by long thick lines and L chains by short thick lines. Disulfide bonds are represented by thin lines. The number of inter-heavy chain disulfide bonds in IgG3 may be as large as 14.

Table 9-2. Properties of human immunoglobulins.

	IgG	IgA	IgM	IgD	IgE
H chain class	γ	α	μ	δ	ϵ
H chain subclass	$\gamma 1, \gamma 2, \gamma 3, \gamma 4$	$\alpha 1, \alpha 2$	$\mu 1, \mu 2$		
L chain type	κ and λ	κ and λ	κ and λ	κ and λ	κ and λ
Molecular formula	$\gamma_2 L_2$	$\alpha_2 L_2$[1] or $(\alpha_2 L_2)_2 SC$[2]J[3]	$(\alpha_2 L_2)_5 J$[3]	$\delta_2 L_2$	$\epsilon_2 L_2$
Sedimentation coefficient (S)	6–7	7	19	7–8	8
Molecular weight (approximate)	150,000	160,000[1] 400,000[4]	900,000	180,000	190,000
Electrophoretic mobility (average)	γ	Fast γ to β	Fast γ to β	Fast γ	Fast γ
Complement fixation (classic)	+	0	+ + + +	0	0
Serum concentration (approximate; mg/dL)	1000	200	120	3	0.05
Serum half-life (days)	23	6	5	3	2
Placental transfer	+	0	0	0	0
Reaginic activity	?	0	0	0	+ + + +
Antibacterial lysis	+	+	+ + +	?	?
Antiviral activity	+	+ + +	+	?	?

[1] For monomeric serum IgA. [3] J chain.
[2] Secretory component. [4] For secretory IgA.

L–H bond may be formed close to the junction of the V_H and $C_H 1$ domains or, alternatively, near the junction between $C_H 1$ and $C_H 2$ in IgG1.

As for L chains, κ chains do not exhibit C region subclasses, but 4 distinct λ chain forms have been discerned in humans which have apparently arisen by tandem gene duplication. These are called subtypes to distinguish them from H chain subclasses, which determine the subclass of the intact molecule. Since all H chains may be combined with any of the L chains, the latter play no role in determining the class or subclass of immunoglobulin. Put another way, the complete repertoire of κ and λ chains is found in each immunoglobulin subclass.

Allotypic (Allelic) Forms of Heavy & Light Chains

Some H and L chain isotypes bear genetic markers that are inherited in typical mendelian fashion. These alternative forms at a given genetic locus are called **allotypes.** In humans, allelic forms have been found for γ and α H chains and κ L chains. The allotypes associated with γ chains are designated "Gm" (for gamma), those associated with α chains are termed "Am," and those associated with κ L chains are called "Inv" (abbreviation of a patient's name). Thus far, allotypic forms of λ L chains or the H chains of IgM, IgD, and IgE have not been found.

Allotypy has been detected by using homologous (same species) antisera that react with antigenic determinants foreign to the immunoglobulins of the host. For example, mothers may become immunized to paternal allotypic determinants on fetal immunoglobulins during the course of pregnancy. Alternatively, immunization may result from blood transfusions. Another source of detecting reagents has been the sera of some patients with rheumatoid arthritis, which contain "rheumatoid factors" reactive with IgG from some (not all) normal individuals. Such rheumatoid factors detect allotypic determinants. The structural differences that account for allotypic determinants usually involve only one or, at most, several amino acid substitutions in the constant regions of H and L chains.

SECRETORY COMPONENT & J CHAIN

Immunoglobulins are present not only in serum but also in various body secretions such as saliva, nasal secretions, sweat, breast milk, and colostrum. IgA is the predominant immunoglobulin class in the external secretions of most species. IgA usually exists in human serum as a 4-chain unit with a molecular weight of approximately 160,000 (7S). This unit may polymerize to give disulfide-bonded polymers with 8-chain, 12-chain, or larger structures. The IgA in secretions consists of two 4-chain units associated with one of each of 2 additional chain types, the secretory component and the J chain (Tables 9–1 and 9–2). The secretory component is associated only with IgA and is found almost exclusively in body secretions. The J chain is associated with all polymeric forms of immunoglobulins that contain 2 or more basic units. Fig 9–2 shows simplified models of secretory IgA and various polymeric serum immunoglobulins. Evidence suggests that binding of an

IgA to secretory component or J chain (or both) may promote the polymerization of additional monomeric 4-chain basic units. The secretory component may exist in free form or bound to IgA molecules by strong noncovalent interactions. The binding does not usually involve covalent bonding, although disulfide bonds have been implicated in a small fraction of human secretory IgA molecules. The secretory component is synthesized by nonmotile epithelial cells near the mucous membrane where secretion occurs. Its function may be to enable IgA antibodies to be transported across mucosal tissues into secretions.

The secretory component is a single polypeptide chain with a molecular weight of approximately 70,000. The carbohydrate content is high but not precisely known (Table 9–1). Its amino acid composition differs appreciably from that of every other immunoglobulin polypeptide chain, including J chain. No close structural relationship exists between the secretory component and any immunoglobulin polypeptide chain. Indeed, secretory component can be found free in secretions of individuals who lack mesurable IgA in their serum or secretions.

J chain is a small acidic polypeptide that is synthesized by cells which secrete polymeric immunoglobulins.

Quantitative mesurements indicate that there is a single J chain in each IgM pentamer or polymeric IgA molecule. J chain is covalently bonded to the penultimate cysteine residue of α and μ chains. Whether or not J chain is required for the proper polymerization of the IgA and IgM basic unit is controversial. Polymeric immunoglobulins of certain lower vertebrates such as nurse shark and paddlefish are apparently devoid of J chain. These observations indicate that J chain is not an absolute requirement for polymerization of the immunoglobulin basic units. Nevertheless, the presence of J chain does facilitate the polymerization of basic units of IgA and IgM molecules into their appropriate polymeric forms.

CARBOHYDRATE MOIETIES OF IMMUNOGLOBULINS

Significant amounts of carbohydrate are present in all immunoglobulins in the form of simple or complex side chains covalently bonded to amino acids in the polypeptide chains (Table 9–1).

The function of the carbohydrate moieties is poorly understood. They may play important roles in the secretion of immunoglobulins by plasma cells and in the biologic functions associated with the C regions of H chains.

The attachment in most cases is by means of an N-glycosidic linkage between an N-acetylglu-cosamine residue of the carbohydrate side chain and an asparagine residue of the polypeptide chain. However, other linkages have also been observed, including an O-glycosidic linkage between an amino sugar of an oligosaccharide side chain and a serine residue of the polypeptide chain. In general, carbohydrate is found in only the secretory component, the J chain, and the C regions of H chains; it is not found in L chains or the V regions of H chains. Exceptions to this rule have been found in a small number of myeloma proteins. The secretory component has more carbohydrate than either the α chain or the L chain; this accounts for the higher carbohydrate content in secretory IgA than in serum IgA. Studies on monoclonal immunoglobulins indicated that IgM and IgE generally have an average of 5 oligosaccharides each; IgG, one oligosaccharide; and IgA, 2 or 3 oligosaccharides. This agrees with the overall carbohydrate content of immunoglobulins, since IgM, IgD, and IgE have the largest amounts of carbohydrate, followed by IgA and then by IgG (Table 9–1). However, these studies were performed on a limited number of monotypic immunoglobulins. In view of the findings that (1) different myeloma proteins of the same class or subclass may differ from one another in carbohydrate content, (2) an individual myeloma protein occasionally exhibits microheterogeneity with respect to its carbohydrate content, and (3) V regions of a small number of immunoglobulin polypeptide chains contain carbohydrate, it is incorrect to assume that all immunoglobulins belonging to a given class or subclass have the same number of oligosaccharide side chains.

BIOLOGIC ACTIVITIES OF IMMUNOGLOBULIN MOLECULES

As already noted, immunoglobulins are bifunctional molecules that bind antigens and, in addition, initiate other biologic phenomena which are independent of antibody specificity. These 2 kinds of activity can each be localized to a particular part of the molecule; antigen binding to the combined action of the V regions of H and L chains, and the other activities to the C regions of H chains. These latter activities, some of which are listed in Table 9–2, will be considered in this section.

Immunoglobulin G (IgG)

In normal human adults, IgG constitutes approximately 75% of the total serum immunoglobulins. Within the IgG class, the relative concentrations of the 4 subclasses are approximately as follows: IgG1, 60–70%; IgG2, 14–20%; IgG3, 4–8%; and IgG4, 2–6%. These figures vary some-

CHO = Constant Heavy Only

what from individual to individual and correlate weakly with the presence of certain H chain C region allotypic markers. Thus, the capacity of a given individual to produce antibodies of one or another IgG subclass may be under genetic control.

IgG is the only class of immunoglobulin that can cross the placenta in humans, and it is responsible for protection of the newborn during the first months of life (see Chapter 17). The subclasses are not equally endowed with this property, IgG2 being transferred more slowly than the others. The adaptive or biologic value of this inequality, if any, is obscure.

IgG is also capable of fixing serum complement (see Chapter 14), and once again the subclasses function with unequal facility in the following order: IgG3 > IgG1 > IgG2 > IgG4. IgG4 is completely unable to fix complement by the classic pathway (binding of C1q) but may be active in the alternative pathway. The specific location of the C1q binding site on the IgG molecule appears to reside in the C_H2 domain.

Macrophages bear surface receptors that bind IgG1 and IgG3 and their Fc fragments. The passive binding of antibodies by such Fc receptors is responsible for "arming" macrophages, which can then function in a cytotoxic fashion (see Chapter 12). Fc receptors on macrophages also facilitate phagocytosis of particulate antigens, such as bacteria, which are coated with antibody, a phenomenon known as **opsonization** (Fig 9–4). The specific location of the Fc receptor binding site on IgG1 and IgG3 molecules seems to be in the C_H3 domain.

The major differences between the subclasses of human IgG are summarized in Table 9–3.

Immunoglobulin A (IgA)

IgA is the predominant immunoglobulin class in the mucosal immune system (see Chapter 15).

Each secretory IgA molecule consists of two 4-chain basic units and one molecule each of secretory component and J chain (Fig 9–2). The molecular weight of secretory IgA is approximately 400,000. Secretory IgA provides the primary defense mechanism against some local infections owing to its abundance in saliva, tears, bronchial secretions, the nasal mucosa, prostatic fluid, vaginal secretions, and mucous secretions of the small intestine. The predominance of secretory IgA in membrane secretions led to speculation that its principal function may not be to destroy antigen (eg, foreign microbial organisms or cells) but rather to prevent access of these foreign substances to the general immunologic system. However, secretory IgA has been shown to prevent viruses from entering and infecting host cells. Hence, it may be important in antiviral defense mechanisms.

IgA normally exists in serum in both monomeric and polymeric forms, constituting approximately 15% of the total serum immunoglobulins.

Immunoglobulin M (IgM)

IgM constitutes approximately 10% of normal immunoglobulins and normally exists as a pentamer with a molecular weight of approximately 900,000 (19S). IgM antibody is prominent in early immune responses to most antigens and predominates in certain antibody responses such as "natural" blood group antibodies. IgM (with IgD) is the major immunoglobulin expressed on the surface of B cells. IgM is also the most efficient complement-fixing immunoglobulin, a single molecule bound to antigen sufficing to initiate the complement cascade (see Chapter 14).

Immunoglobulin D (IgD)

The IgD molecule is a monomer, and its molecular weight of approximately 180,000 (7–8S) is slightly higher than that of IgG. This immuno-

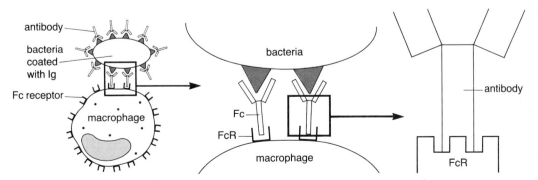

Figure 9–4. Schematic representation of phagocytosis of an antibody-coated bacterium. Note the Fc receptor (FcR) on the macrophage and its binding to the Fc portion of antibody and bound antigen (the bacterium).

Table 9-3. Properties of human IgG subclasses.

	IgG$_1$	IgG$_2$	IgG$_3$	IgG$_4$
Abundance (% of total IgG)	70	20	6	4
Half-life in serum (days)	23	23	7	23
Placental passage	+ + +	+	+ + +	+ + +
Complement fixation	+ +	+	+ + +	−
Binding to Fc receptors	+ + +	+	+ + +	−

globulin is normally present in serum in trace amounts (0.2% of total serum immunoglobulins). It is relatively labile to degradation by heat and proteolytic enzymes. There are isolated reports of IgD with antibody activity toward certain antigens, including insulin, penicillin, milk proteins, diphtheria toxoid, nuclear antigens, and thyroid antigens. However, the main function of IgD has not yet been determined. IgD (with IgM) is the predominant immunoglobulin on the surface of human B lymphocytes at certain stages of their development, and it has been suggested that IgD may be involved in the differentiation of these cells.

Immunoglobulin E (IgE)

The identification of IgE antibodies are reagins and the characterization of this immunoglobulin class marked a major breakthrough in the study of the mechanisms involved in allergic diseases. (see Chapter 11). IgE has a molecular weight of approximately 190,000 (8S). It constitutes only 0.004% of the total serum immunoglobulins but binds with very high affinity to mast cells via a site in the Fc region. Upon combination with certain specific antigens called allergens, IgE antibodies trigger the release from mast cells of pharmacologic mediators responsible for the characteristic wheal-and-flare skin reactions evoked by the exposure of the skin of allergic individuals to allergens. IgE antibodies provide a striking example of the bifunctional nature of antibody molecules. "Allergen" is an alternative term used by allergists for any antigen that stimulates IgE production. IgE antibodies bind allergens through the Fab portion, but the binding of IgE antibodies to tissue cells is a function of the Fc portion. Like IgG and IgD, IgE normally exists only in monomeric form. It may also be important in defense against parasitic infections.

THE VARIABLE REGION

The V regions, comprising the N-terminal 110 amino acids of the L and H chains, are quite heterogeneous. Indeed, no 2 human myeloma chains from different patients have been found to have identical sequences in the V region. However, distinct patterns are discernible, and V regions have been divided into 3 main groups based on degree of amino acid sequence homology. These are the V_H group for H chains, V_κ group for κ L chains, and V_λ group for λ L chains. These V region groups are associated with the appropriate C region subclasses or subtypes for that particular polypeptide only. For example, a V_H sequence will be found only on an H chain, never on a κ or λ L chain, and so forth. However, a particular V_H sequence may associate with any C_H class (γ, α, μ, δ, or ϵ). The genes coding for associated V and C regions are probably linked (see Chapter 10).

V Region Subgroups

When the sequences of the V regions of κ chains are compared, they can be further divided into 4 subgroups which have substantial homologies. The subgroups differ from one another principally in the length and position of amino acid insertions and deletions and bear much closer structural homology to each other than to λ or H chain V regions. Similar subdivisions have been made in H chain V regions and λ chain V regions.

Hypervariable Regions

The V regions are not uniformly variable across their spans but consist of relatively invariant positions, which define the type and subgroup to which the V region belongs, as well as highly variable zones or "hot spots." A plot of the known variations versus position in the sequence reveals 3 or 4 peaks, depending on the chain type. These peaks of extreme variability are known as **hypervariable regions** and have been shown to be intimately involved in the formation of the antigen-binding site. L chains appear to have 3 hypervariable regions, while H chains have 4, although only 3 of the 4 have been shown to contribute to the antigen-binding site (Fig 9-5). The approximate locations of the hypervariable regions in each chain are shown in Fig 9-6.

Idiotypes

The term "idiotype" denotes the unique V region sequences produced by each clone of antibody-forming cells. Idiotypic antigenic determinants of immunoglobulin molecules were identified by immunizing animals with specific antibodies raised

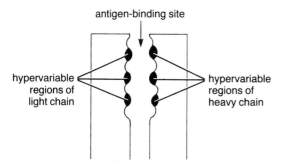

Figure 9-5. Schematic depiction of how the hypervariable regions in each heavy and light chain might form an antigen-binding site of an antibody molecule.

against a particular antigen in genetically similar animals. The only antigenic differences between the immunoglobulins of the donor and recipient were the unique V region sequences related to the specificity of the antibody. Thus, responses were restricted to such determinants. It is also possible to immunize across species lines to obtain anti-idiotype antisera, but in this case the antisera must be carefully absorbed with immunoglobulins from the donor species to render them specific for idiotypic markers.

In some cases, the reaction between anti-hapten antibody and anti-idiotypic antisera raised against that anti-hapten antibody can be inhibited by the hapten, indicating that the idiotypic antigenic determinants are close to or within the antigen-binding site of the antibody molecule. An antibody to idiotypic determinants is therefore regarded as an immunologic marker for the antibody combining

site. Although it is not yet formally proved, idiotypic determinants are believed to be associated with hypervariable regions, which determine antibody specificity.

It seems legitimate to extend the term "idiotype" to any combination of a particular L chain V region with a particular H chain V region. That is, any such combination will express a unique idiotypic specificity. Since any L chain may combine with any H chain and a common pool of V_H regions is shared by the 5 different classes of H chains, it follows that idiotypic determinants may be shared by different immunoglobulin classes. Idiotypic determinants are heritable, at least in some cases, as observed in certain inbred strains of mice.

THE THREE-DIMENSIONAL STRUCTURE OF IMMUNOGLOBULINS

Although the inference that the polypeptide chains of immunoglobulin molecules are folded into compact globular domains separated by short linear stretches was derived initially from amino acid sequence studies, confirmation of this structural model required examination of crystallized immunoglobulins or their component parts by x-ray diffraction analysis (Fig 9-7). This work has shown that all domains have a characteristic pattern of folding, regardless of their origin. Thus, V region and C region domains from L chains and H chains all have a very similar appearance. In addition, there is close physical approximation between corresponding domains, ie, V_H and V_L, C_H1 and C_L, and the identical H chain domains in the Fc portion. X-ray diffraction analysis of a crystallized myeloma protein complexed with hapten (see Chapter 8) revealed that the contact points between antigen and the antibody-combining site are located in the hypervariable regions of the H and L chains.

Other evidence in favor of the domain model has come from limited proteolysis of immunoglobulins, in which the major products appear to consist of one or more domains (as expected, based on the model, since the areas between the domains are more exposed and consequently more susceptible to enzymatic attack). It has also been found that some of the proteins present in patients with H chain disease have large deletions involving the entire C_H1 domain.

All domains, including those from the same polypeptide chain, different polypeptide chains, the same molecules, and different molecules, show a significant degree of amino acid homology. This led to the hypothesis that all immuno-

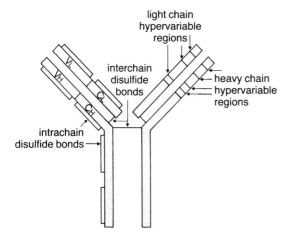

Figure 9-6. Schematic model of an IgG molecule showing approximate positions of the hypervariable regions in heavy and light chains.

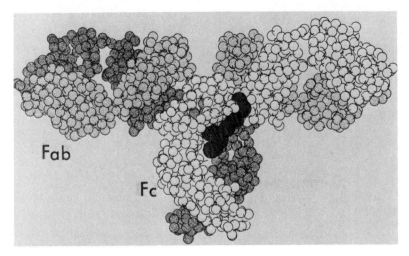

Figure 9-7. Three-dimensional structure of the immunoglobulin molecule. (Reproduced, with permission, from Silverton EW, Navia MA, Davies DR: Three-dimensional structure of an intact human immunoglobulin *Proc Natl Acad Sci USA* 1977;**74:**5140.)

globulin polypeptide chains evolved by a process of tandem gene duplication from a common ancestor that was equivalent to one domain.

CELL SURFACE IMMUNOGLOBULINS

Although, as noted earlier, IgM and IgD constitute the predominant membrane immunoglobulins, all classes of immunoglobulins have been found on the surfaces of B lymphocytes, where they function as antigen receptors. The membrane and secreted forms of μ, δ, and γ chains (and presumably α and ϵ chains as well) differ in structure. The membrane forms have an additional carboxy-terminal sequence of approximately 40 amino acid residues, which begins with a highly acidic sequence of 12–14 residues and terminates with a strikingly hydrophobic sequence of about 26 residues. The hydrophobic portion of the segment is believed to represent the transmembrane component anchoring the heavy chain in the cell membrane. It is similar in hydrophobicity and length to known transmembrane segments of other proteins, and it satisfies the requirements for the formation of a membrane-spanning alpha helix.

Whereas the acidic part of the membrane segment shows little amino acid sequence homology between heavy chain classes, the hydrophobic sequences of μ and γ chains show substantially greater homology than do the constant-region domains of those classes. This sequence conservation is puzzling, because transmembrane segments of other proteins seem to have little in common besides length and hydrophobicity.

SUMMARY

Immunoglobulins are glycoproteins and have a basic symmetric 4-chain structure composed of 2 identical heavy (H) and 2 identical light (L) chains, which are covalently joined by disulfide bonds. The chains are folded into domains consisting of about 100 amino acids, each of which is stabilized by an internal disulfide bond. The first domains of the H and L chains vary in structure (V domains) and make up the antigen-binding site. Thus, each immunoglobulin molecule has at least 2 identical binding sites (ie, it is bivalent). The structural variation between the V domains of different antibodies accounts for their specificity and diversity. The unique structure of each antibody V region is referred to as its idiotypic profile. The other domains make up the constant (C) regions of the 2 types of L chain (κ and λ) and the H chains. The 5 classes of immunoglobulins are distinguished by their H chain C (C_H) regions. Several classes are further divided into subclasses based on minor differences in the C_H regions. Allotypes are genetic markers within the C regions which can distinguish one individual from another.

The C_H regions are responsible for the biologic properties of each class of immunoglobulins, other than the function of binding antigen. IgG is the predominant class in serum and the only one that crosses the placenta and confers immunity on the fetus. It is also capable of fixing complement and promoting phagocytosis (opsonization). IgM exists in the pentameric form and fixes complement most efficiently. It is the earliest immunoglobulin to appear on the surface of developing B lymphocytes. IgA is the only class found in external secretions, where it is called secretory IgA and appears to be an efficient antiviral antibody. IgD is found on B lymphocytes at certain stages of their development and appears to be involved in their differentiation. IgE is responsible for many common allergies. It binds to receptors on mast cells and triggers degranulation of the cells upon contact with antigen. IgE may protect against parasitic infections.

REFERENCES

Alzari PM et al: Three-dimensional structure of antibodies. *Annu Rev Immunol* 1988;**6**:555.

Amos B (editor): *Progress in Immunology. I.* Academic Press, 1971.

Brent L, Holborow J (editors): *Progress in Immunology, II.* North-Holland, 1975.

Capra JD, Kehoe JM: Hypervariable regions, idiotypy, and the antibody-combining site. *Adv. Immunol* 1975:**20**:1.

Cunningham AJ (editor): *The Generation of Antibody Diversity: A New Look,* Academic Press, 1976.

Davie JM et al: Structural correlates of idiotypes. *Annu Rev Immunol* 1986;**4**:147.

Davies DR, Metzger H: Structural basis of antibody function. *Annu Rev Immunol* 1983;**1**:87.

Eisen HN: *Immunology.* Harper & Row, 1974.

Gergely J, Medgyesi GA (editors): *Antibody Structure and Molecular Immunology.* North-Holland, 1975.

Hilschmann N, Craig LC: Amino acid sequence studies with Bence Jones protein. *Proc Natl and Acad Sci USA* 1965;**53**:1403.

Hood L, Prahl JW: The immune system: A model for differentiation in higher organisms. *Adv Immunol* 1971;**14**:291.

Kehry M et al: The immunoglobulin μ chains of membrane-bound and secreted IgM molecules differ in their C-terminal segments. *Cell* 1980;**21**:393.

Koshland ME: The coming of age of the immunoglobulin J chain. *Annu Rev Immunol* 1985;**3**:425.

Mestecky J, Lawton AR (editors): *The Immunoglobulin A System.* Plenum Press, 1974.

Möller G (editor): Immunoglobulin D: Structure, synthesis, membrane representation and the function. *Immunol Rev* 1977; No. 37. [Entire issue.]

Natvig JB, Kunkel HG: Immunoglobulins: Classes, subclasses, genetic variants, and idiotypes. *Adv. Immunol* 1973;**16**:1.

Nisonoff A, Hopper JE, Spring SB: *The Antibody Molecule.* Academic Press, 1975.

Padian EA et al: Model-building studies of antigen-binding sites: The hapten-binding site of MOPC-315. *Cold Spring Harbor Symp Quant Biol* 1976;**41**:627.

Poljak RJ et al: Three-dimensional structure and diversity of immunoglobulins. *Cold Spring Harbor Symp Quant Biol* 1976;**41**:639.

Porter RR: Structural studies of immunoglobulins. *Science* 1973;**180**:713.

Spiegelberg HL: Biological activities of immunoglobulins of different classes and subclasses. *Adv Immunol* 1974;**19**:259.

Williams SF, Barclay AN: The immunoglobulin superfamily—domains for cell surface recognition. *Annu Rev Immunol* 1988;**6**:381.

Wu TT, Kabat EA: An analysis of the variable regions of Bence Jones proteins and myeloma light chains and their implications for antibody complementarity. *J Exp Med* 1970;**132**:211.

10

Immunoglobulin Genetics

Tristram G. Parslow, MD, PhD

To contend with the almost unlimited variety of antigens that it may encounter, the human immune system is able to produce an estimated 10^8 different antibody molecules, each with a unique specificity for antigen. How can so many different antibody proteins be encoded in the genes of every human being? The source of this diversity of antibodies lies in the structure of the immunoglobulin genes and in the remarkable ability of B cells to create and modify these genes by rearranging their own chromosomal DNA.

IMMUNOGLOBULIN GENES ARE FORMED THROUGH DNA REARRANGEMENT

The antigen specificity of an antibody is determined by amino acid sequences within its paired heavy (H) and light (L) chain variable (V) domains, which together form the antigen-binding site (see Chapter 9). To produce antibodies with many different specificities, the immune system must have the genetic capability to produce a very large number of different V domain sequences. The sequence of the constant (C) region, on the other hand, is generally the same for all H or L chains of a given immunoglobulin isotype and has no effect on antigen specificity. In fact, the entire family of immunoglobulin proteins consists of a relatively small number of different C region domains linked in various combinations with an almost unlimited assortment of V region sequences.

In 1965, Dreyer and Bennett first recognized that these interchangeable combinations of protein domains must be the result of an active reshuffling of gene fragments that takes place within the B cell chromosomes. This was a revolutionary insight, because it implied that a cell could efficiently manipulate its chromosomes to change the structure of genes that it had inherited. However, this proved to be only a part of the story: nearly a decade later, Tonegawa made the remarkable discovery that the inherited chromosomes contain no immunoglobulin genes at all, but only the building blocks from which these genes can

be assembled. Since that time, elegant molecular studies by Tonegawa and others have revealed in detail the extraordinary events that give rise to an immunoglobulin gene.

As with most human genes, the information that codes for an immunoglobulin protein is dispersed along the DNA strand in multiple coding segments **(exons)** that are separated by regions of noncoding DNA **(introns)**; after the gene is transcribed into RNA, the introns are removed from the transcript and the exons are joined by RNA splicing. Unlike nearly all other genes, however, the immunoglobulin DNA sequences that are found in germ cells or other nonlymphocyte cell types do not exist as intact, functional genes. This is because the exons that code for V domains are normally broken up along the chromosome into still smaller gene segments; these segments each lack some of the features needed for proper RNA splicing and so cannot function individually as exons. Before a developing B cell can begin to synthesize immunoglobulin, it must fuse 2 or 3 of these gene segments to assemble a complete V region exon. This fusion of gene segments is achieved through a highly specialized process that requires cutting, rearrangement, and rejoining of the chromosomal DNA strands. The enzymatic machinery that is needed to carry out this process of immunoglobulin gene rearrangement is found only in developing lymphocytes.

LIGHT CHAIN GENES

The kappa (κ) L chain genes are the simplest and will be considered first. All of the genetic information needed to produce κ chains lies within a single locus on chromosome 2 (Fig 10–1). The C domain of the protein (amino acid residues 109–214) is encoded by an exon called C_κ, and only one copy of this exon is found on the chromosome. The sequence encoding any given V domain, however, is contained in 2 separate gene segments called the variable (V_κ) and joining (J_κ) segments. The V_κ segment encodes approximately the first 95 amino acids of the V domain; the shorter J_κ

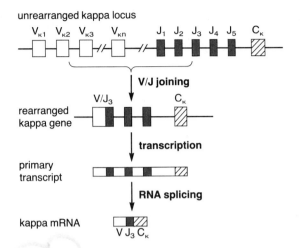

unrearranged kappa locus

Figure 10-1. The assembly and expression of the κ L chain locus. A DNA rearrangement event fuses one V segment (in this example, $V_{\kappa2}$) to one J segment ($J_{\kappa3}$) to form a single exon. The V/J exon is then transcribed together with the unique C_κ exon, and the transcript is spliced to form mature κ mRNA. Note that any unrearranged J segments on the primary transcript are removed as part of the intron during RNA splicing.

segment codes for the remaining 13 (amino acids 96–108). In contrast to the single C_κ exon, multiple V_κ and J_κ segments are present, each with a somewhat different DNA sequence. The 5 J_κ segments are clustered near the C_κ exon, whereas at least 100 different V_κ segments lie scattered over a region that spans more than 2 million base pairs of DNA (roughly 1% of the length of chromosome 2). This wide separation between the V_κ and J_κ segments is found in the DNA of all nonlymphoid cells. When an immature hematopoietic cell becomes committed to the B lymphocyte lineage, however, it selects one V_κ and one J_κ segment and fuses these to form a single continuous exon. In most cases, this process of "V/J joining" is

achieved by specific enzymatic deletion of the chromosomal DNA that normally separates the 2 segments. Transcription can then begin at one end of the V segment and pass through both the fused V_κ/J_κ exon and the nearby C_κ exon. When transcribed together, these 2 exons contain all of the information needed to synthesize a particular κ protein.

The organization of the κ genes thus accounts for the unusual properties of this L chain protein family. Because there is only one C_κ exon, for example, all κ proteins must have identical C region sequences. On the other hand, because the cell can choose from among many alternatives V_κ and J_κ segments and can join these together in various combinations, a large number of different V domain sequences can result. For example, 100 V_κ and 5 J_κ segments could give rise to 500 (100 × 5) different V domains. This reshuffling process, known as "combinatorial joining," is the most important source of light chain protein diversity.

Lambda L chains arise from a similar gene complex on chromosome 22. Joining of V_λ and J_λ segments occurs in a manner identical to that of the κ segments. A given chromosome 22, however, may contain 6–9 slightly different copies of the C_λ exon (corresponding to various subclasses of λ protein), each with a nearby J_λ segment. A V segment may fuse to any of these alternative J_λ segments, and the resulting V_λ/J_λ exon can then be transcribed together with the adjacent C_λ exon. The B cell selects only one of the available J_λ segments for V/J joining, and in so doing, it determines which C_λ subclass will be expressed (Fig 10-2).

HEAVY CHAIN GENES

All immunoglobulin H chains are derived from a single region on chromosome 14 (Fig 10-3). Each H chain C region is encoded by a cluster of several short exons. The μ C region, for example,

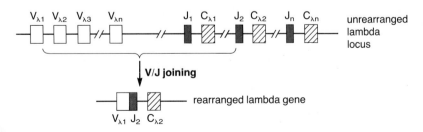

Figure 10-2. Assembly of a λ L chain gene. An individual λ locus contains 6–9 alternative C_λ exons, each with a nearby J_λ segment. In this example, DNA rearrangement fuses $V_{\lambda1}$ with $J_{\lambda2}$; the resulting gene will produce L chains that contain the λ2 C region.

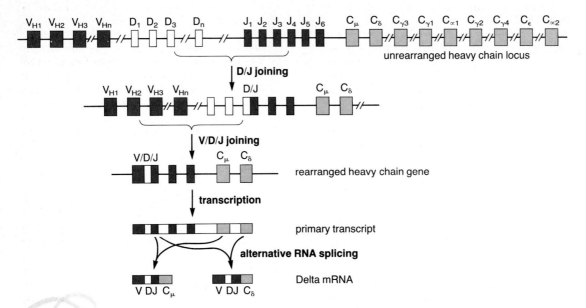

Figure 10-3. Rearrangement and expression of the H chain locus. Unlike the L chain genes, assembly of an H chain V region exon requires 2 sequential DNA rearrangement events involving 3 different types of gene segments. The D_H and J_H segments are joined first and are then fused to a V_H segment. Nine alternative C region sequences are present; of these, however, only the C_μ and C_δ sequences are initially transcribed. The primary transcript can be spliced in either of 2 ways to generate mRNAs that encode μ or δ H chains with identical V domains. This diagram is highly schematic: each C_H sequence is actually composed of multiple exons whose aggregate length is more than 3 times longer than that of the V/D/J exon.

is divided among 5 exons known collectively as the C_μ sequence. C region (C_H) sequences for each of the 9 heavy chain isotypes are arrayed in tandem along the chromosome in the following order: C_μ, C_δ, $C_{\gamma3}$, $C_{\gamma1}$, $C_{\alpha1}$, $C_{\gamma2}$, $C_{\gamma4}$, C_ϵ, $C_{\alpha2}$; only a single copy of each is present. The 6 J_H segments and a few hundred V_H segments (the exact number is unknown) are arranged in a manner analogous to those of the κ gene. In contrast to the L chain genes, however, a third type of gene segment, called the diversity (D_H) segment, must also be used in forming an H chain V region. At least 20 of these D_H segments, each coding for 2 or 3 amino acids, lie between the J_H and V_H segments on the unrearranged chromosome. In assembling the H chain gene, lymphocytes must complete 2 DNA rearrangement events, first bringing together one D_H and one J_H segment and subsequently linking these to a V_H segment (a sequence termed **V/D/J joining**).

Use of the D_H segment greatly increases the amount of H chain diversity that can be produced. For example, 200 V_H, 10 D_H, and 6 J_H segments could give rise to 12,000 (200 × 10 × 6) different H chain V domains, and these, when combined with 500 κ chain V domains, could form 6 million (500 × 12,000) different antigen-binding sites! Even using a relatively small number of gene

segments, then, the immune system can generate enormous antibody diversity through combinatorial joining.

THE MOLECULAR BASIS OF IMMUNOGLOBULIN GENE REARRANGEMENT

Active gene rearrangements of the type that produce V/J and V/D/J joining were first thought to be a unique property of the immunoglobulin genes. More recently, however, identical rearrangements have been found to give rise to genes that encode the antigen receptors of T lymphocytes, a diverse family of proteins which are functionally and genetically similar to immunoglobulins in many respects (see Chapter 6). There is evidence that rearrangement of both these gene families is carried out by the same molecular machinery: a presumably complex system of enzymes and other proteins known collectively as the **V/(D)/J recombinase.** This term must be used operationally because none of the enzymes involved in recognizing, cleaving, or religating the various gene segments has yet been purified and characterized.

V/(D)/J recombinase activity is found almost

exclusively in cells that are undergoing the early stages of B and T cell development. Potential sites for DNA rearrangement by the recombinase appear to be marked by the presence of a pair of short DNA sequences (7 and 9 base pairs, respectively) that are found adjacent to each unrearranged V, D, or J segment and are deleted in the course of rearrangement. The relative positions and orientations of these short sequences help to ensure that segments are joined in the proper order and alignment to produce a functional exon.

OTHER SOURCES OF ANTIBODY DIVERSITY

Additional diversity of V region sequences arises because the V/(D)/J rearrangement process is somewhat imprecise, so that the site at which one segment fuses with another can vary by a few nucleotides. As a result, the DNA coding sequence that remains at the junction between any 2 segments can also vary. Moreover, during assembly of a H chain gene, a few nucleotides of random sequence (called N regions) are often inserted at the points of joining between the V, D, and J segments; these insertions are thought to be produced by terminal deoxynucleotidyl transferase (TdT), an enzyme that is present in immature lymphocytes. The variations in gene sequence that result from imprecise joining or from the insertion of N regions contribute substantially to overall antibody diversity. At the same time, however, these processes greatly increase the risk that 2 segments may be joined in an improper translational reading frame, resulting in a nonfunctional gene. In practice, such unsuccessful rearrangements occur frequently and generally cannot be reversed or repaired; they represent a cost paid by the immune system in exchange for greater potential gene diversity.

Fully assembled V/J and V/D/J exons in lymphocytes have also been found to undergo point mutation at an unusually high rate, a phenomenon termed **somatic hypermutation**. Occasionally, such mutations alter the specificity or the affinity of the antibody molecule.

THE HEAVY CHAIN ISOTYPE SWITCH

occurs at DNA level

When first assembled, a V/D/J exon is transcribed together with the nearby C_μ exon to form μ H chain RNA. Exons corresponding to the other H chain isotypes lie farther downstream and are not transcribed. To express these other isotypes, the H chain gene must undergo a different type of DNA rearrangement known as isotype switching,

in which a new C_H sequence is placed adjacent to the original V/D/J exon. This is accomplished through a specific DNA deletion process that removes all of the intervening C_H sequences (Fig 10-4). Although isotype switching bears some resemblance to V/(D)/J joining, these 2 processes are thought to occur through different enzymatic pathways. In particular, switching takes place in cells that are no longer able to carry out V/(D)/J rearrangements (see below) and occurs at sites located several hundred bases away from the V/D/J and C_H exons themselves. Switching does not change the structure of the V/D/J exon and so does not affect antigen specificity.

Thus, V regions for all of the H chain classes are assembled from a single common pool of V_H, D_H, and J_H segments; once assembled, the V/D/J exon can then be linked to any one of the C region sequences through the process of isotype switching. By this means, the effector function of an antibody can be changed without altering its specificity for antigen. Because isotype switching occurs by deletion of one or more C_H regions, it is irreversible. The selection of a new C_H isotype may be influenced by lymphokines or other factors acting upon the B cell; for example, the microenvironment found in Peyer's patches of the gut appears to favor switching to $C_{\alpha1}$, resulting in the production of IgA.

In general, only the C_H region nearest the V/D/J exon can be expressed. One major exception to this rule is the C_δ sequence, which lies very near

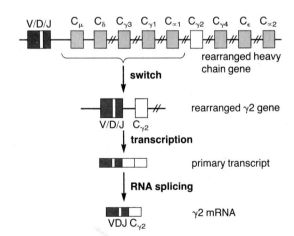

Figure 10-4. The H chain isotype switch. To express an isotype other than μ or δ, the fully assembled H chain locus undergoes an additional DNA rearrangement event that places a new C_H sequence adjacent to the V/D/J exon. This occurs by deletion of the intervening C_H exons and is carried out by an enzymatic pathway distinct from that of V/D/J rearrangement. In the example shown, the gene switches to the $C_{\gamma2}$ isotype.

the C_μ region and is often transcribed along with the V/D/J and C_μ exons. The resulting RNA can be spliced to yield either μ or δ mRNA, enabling the cell simultaneously to express IgM and IgD antibodies that have identical V domain sequences. Such coexpression of IgM and IgD on the surface membrane is a common phenotype among B lymphocytes.

IMMUNOGLOBULIN GENE REARRANGEMENTS & B CELL ONTOGENY

The DNA rearrangements that assemble immunoglobulin genes occur only at a very early stage in B cell development and follow a strict develop-

mental sequence (Fig 10–5). Joining of the D_H and J_H segments is one of the earliest events in the ontogeny of a B cell and occurs simultaneously on both copies of chromosome 14. The cell then attempts to join a V_H segment to the fused D_H/J_H segment on one chromosome. If this first attempt succeeds in producing a functional gene, the cell begins to synthesize μ (and perhaps also δ) H chains encoded by the rearranged gene. At this early stage of development (known as the pre-B stage), the H chains remain within the cytoplasm of the cell and are not displayed on the surface membrane. Through a mechanism that is not well understood, the expression of H chain protein is thought to inhibit any further rearrangement of H chain genes in the cell. If, however, the first rearrangement is not successful, a second attempt

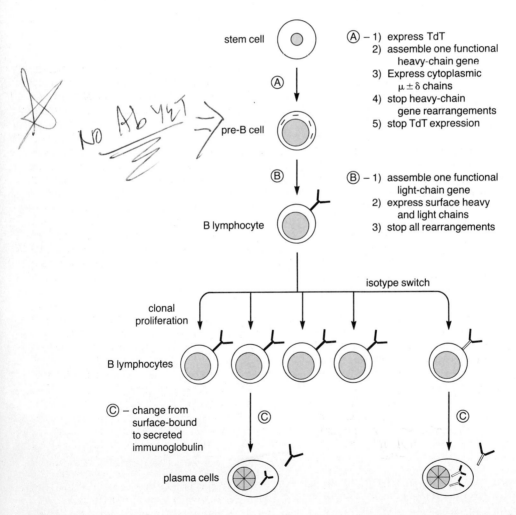

Figure 10–5. Major genetic events in B cell ontogeny. The sequence of events that marks the progression from each stage of development to the next is listed (A–C). Note that the ability to perform V/(D)/J rearrangements is lost by the time the cell becomes a mature B lymphocyte. Isotype switching does not change the antigen specificity of an immunoglobulin.

at V/D/J assembly can be made by using the other chromosome 14.

L chain gene rearrangements do not begin until the cell is actively producing cytoplasmic H chain protein (ie, after H chain V/D/J rearrangements have ceased). V/J joining is then attempted on each chromosome 2 or 22 in succession, until a functional κ or λ gene is produced. As soon as either type of L chain protein appears, the cell loses the ability to perform additional V/J rearrangements. The cell then enters the B lymphocyte stage of development, in which the H and L chain proteins are expressed together as disulfide-linked heterodimers on the cell surface membrane but are not secreted in appreciable quantities.

As mentioned above, successful assembly of a single H or L chain gene prevents all other genes of that type from undergoing rearrangement in the same cell. Consequently, only one H chain and one L chain gene can give rise to protein in any individual B lymphocyte, a phenomenon termed **allelic exclusion.** Moreover, when the lymphocyte divides, chromosomes bearing the active rearranged genes are passed on to its progeny, and the daughter cells continue to express these genes without performing further V/J or V/D/J rearrangements. For this reason, all of the immunoglobulin molecules produced by a given B lymphocyte and its progeny have identical antigen specificity and L chain isotype (κ or λ), a phenomenon known as **clonal restriction.** The diversity of antibody molecules produced by the immune system as a whole reflects cellular diversity, ie, the fact that innumerable B cell precursors each rearrange their genes independently and in different combinations, resulting in a large assortment of clones, each of which possesses a unique antigenic specificity.

The immunoglobulins on the surface membrane of a B lymphocyte serve as receptors for specific antigens. Mature lymphocytes tend to be quiescent cells and do not proliferate under ordinary circumstances. If, however, a B lymphocyte comes into contact with an antigen that can bind to its surface immunoglobulins, this binding stimulates the cell to undergo rapid clonal proliferation, producing daughter cells which bear identical surface-bound immunoglobulin. Many of these cells then undergo a final step in differentiation to become plasma cells, which secrete large amounts of this same immunoglobulin to form circulating antibodies. Such antigen-dependent proliferation and secretion form the essential basis of a humoral immune response. It is important to bear in mind that the specificity of this response depends upon the allelic exclusion and clonal restriction of immunoglobulin expression: each clone of lymphocytes can respond only to antigens that can bind to its unique pair of H and L chains,

and all of the antibodies secreted by the activated clone are directed against that particular antigen.

Although the H chain class also tends to be maintained during clonal B cell proliferation, isotype-switching rearrangements can still occur, occasionally giving rise to a daughter cell that expresses a different class of H chains and passes this new trait along to its progeny. More subtle changes in the H chain protein also determine whether an immunoglobulin will be membrane-bound or secreted. The final 2 exons of each C_H sequence encode a short hydrophobic tail, which serves to anchor the carboxyl terminus of the H chain onto the cell surface membrane. When a lymphocyte matures into a plasma cell, however, the H chain mRNA that it produces lacks these final exons; as a result, the immunoglobulins are secreted from the cell as soluble antibodies.

CLINICAL ASPECTS

Apart from their role in generating antibody diversity, immunoglobulin gene rearrangements are gaining increasing importance in clinical diagnosis and research. Rearrangement of these genes can be detected by using a technique known as **Southern blotting,** after its inventor, E. M. Southern (Fig 10–6). For this purpose, DNA is extracted from a population of cells contained, for example, in a tissue biopsy or sample of peripheral blood. The DNA is then digested with one or more restriction enzymes, a type of bacterial endonuclease that cleaves the long chromosomal DNA at defined sites to produce an array of shorter DNA fragments of various lengths. Next, these fragments are separated according to length by electrophoresis through an agarose gel and are treated with alkali to melt apart the complementary strands of the double helix in each fragment. A sheet of nylon or other suitable material is then pressed against the gel; the denatured DNA fragments bind tightly to the nylon and are drawn out of the gel. When the nylon is peeled away, it retains on its surface the immobilized DNA fragments, still arranged according to length, as they had been in the gel, but now exposed and accessible to further analysis. DNA fragments that contain a particular gene sequence can then be identified by their ability to bind specific DNA probes. Such probes simply consist of radioisotopically labeled single-stranded DNA molecules whose sequence is complementary to a portion of the gene in question and which are therefore capable of binding to the gene under appropriate conditions by base-pairing. Because the probe is radioactive, the fragments to which it binds can be identified by autoradiography, and the lengths of these frag-

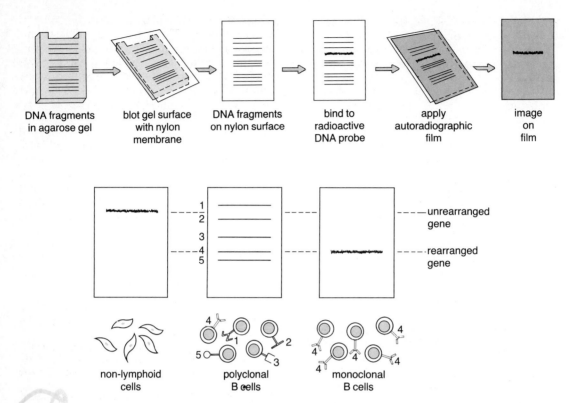

Figure 10-6. Detection of immunoglobulin gene rearrangements by the Southern blot technique. The blotting technique (**A**) is described in the text; it can be used to determine the size of DNA restriction fragments that encompass a specific gene. DNA rearrangement in lymphocytes alters the sizes of fragments bearing the immunoglobulin genes; the sizes of the immunoglobulin-specific fragments are characteristic of each B cell clone. This provides a means of detecting B cells and of assessing the clonal composition of B cell populations (**B**). DNA isolated from nonlymphoid cells contains only unrearranged immunoglobulin genes, whereas DNA from normal lymphocyte populations reveals many different rearranged genes—one from each of the many independent B cell clones. Detection of a only a single rearranged gene suggests that a lymphocyte population is monoclonal and therefore possibly malignant.

ments can be estimated by their positions along the agarose gel.

If all of the cells in a population contain DNA of identical sequence, the restriction enzyme should cleave at identical sites in the DNA of each cell. The fragment on which any particular gene resides will then have the same length for every cell and will appear as a single band on the autoradiogram. This is true of most cellular genes and of the unrearranged immunoglobulin loci found in nonlymphoid cells. Gene rearrangement in lymphocytes, however, dramatically changes the DNA sequences in and around an immunoglobulin locus and thus alters the size of the fragment that encompasses the locus (Fig 10–6). Because the size of the altered fragment varies according to the structure of the rearranged gene, its position on the Southern blot can serve as a distinctive "molecular fingerprint" that is unique to each B cell clone. By using the Southern blot to estimate the proportion of identically rearranged immuno-

globulin genes in DNA extracted from a population of lymphocytes, it is possible to determine whether any single B cell clone predominates—a possible indication of cancer. This technique also provides a sensitive means for detecting the recurrence of a malignant clone after treatment. Moreover, because immunoglobulin gene rearrangements occur almost exclusively among lymphoid cells, their presence can provide compelling evidence that an undifferentiated cancer is of lymphoid origin.

Just as importantly, errors in immunoglobulin gene rearrangement are now thought to contribute to the genesis of several major types of leukemia and lymphoma. For example, the cells of Burkitt's lymphoma, a B-lymphocytic cancer, usually contain a specific chromosomal abnormality called t(8,14), in which a portion of chromosome 8 has been translocated onto chromosome 14 (Fig 10–7). In this translocation, chromosome 14 breaks within the immunoglobulin H chain locus, while

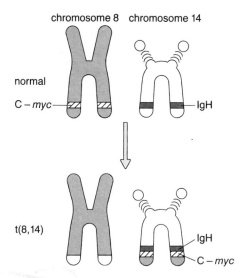

Figure 10-7. The t(8,14) chromosomal anomaly of Burkitt's lymphoma. A reciprocal exchange of genetic material occurs that involves the distal ends of the long arms of chromosomes 8 and 14. This transposes the c-*myc* proto-oncogene from chromosome 8 into the active immunoglobulin H chain locus on chromosome 14 and is thought to contribute to the development of a cancer.

the breakpoint on chromosome 8 coincides with a cellular proto-oncogene known as c-*myc*. As a result, the c-*myc* gene is moved to a position directly adjacent to the H chain gene. It is thought that this proximity to the active H chain locus alters the expression of the proto-oncogene and so contributes to malignant transformation. Less commonly, Burkitt's lymphoma may lack t(8,14) and instead exhibit a closely related anomaly in which the c-*myc* locus is translocated into the κ or λ L chain gene on chromosome 2 or 22. A different type of anomaly, called t(14,18), is observed in more than 85% of patients with follicular lymphoma, the most common human B cell cancer; here, the putative proto-oncogene *bcl-2* on chromosome 18 is translocated into the H chain locus on chromosome 14. In some of these translocations, chromosome breakage in the affected immunoglobulin locus occurs directly beside a J segment; this strongly implies that the translocation results in part from an error in immunoglobulin gene rearrangement.

SUMMARY

The remarkable properties of immunoglobulin genes provide a basis for understanding many as-

pects of B cell differentiation and of the humoral immune response. Through the active DNA rearrangements that assemble V/(D)/J exons or mediate isotype switching, the immune system is able to generate almost unlimited antibody diversity from a relatively small amount of chromosomal DNA. All of the immunoglobulin produced by an individual B lymphocyte, however, has identical antigen specificity. This specificity is determined by the structures of its V region exons and is established during the early stages of B cell ontogeny. Thereafter, V/(D)/J rearrangements cease, and the proliferative and secretory activity of each B cell clone depends upon the nature of antigens that it may subsequently encounter.

REFERENCES

**Immunoglobulin Gene Organization
& Rearrangements**
Dreyer WJ, Bennett JC: The molecular basis of antibody formations: A paradox. *Proc Natl Acad Sci USA* 1965;**54**:864.
Honjo T, Alt FW, Rabbitts TH (editors): *Immunoglobulin Genes.* Academic Press, 1989.
Leder P: The genetics of antibody diversity. *Sci Am* (May) 1982:102.
Tonegawa S: Somatic generation of antibody diversity. *Nature* 1983;**302**:575.

Mechanism & Ontogeny of Gene Rearrangements
Akira SJ, Okazaki K, Sakano H: Two pairs of recombination signals are sufficient to cause-immunoglobulin V-(D)-J joining. *Science* 1987; **238**:1134.
Lieber MR et al: Developmental stage specificity of the lymphoid V(D)J recombination activity. *Genes Dev* 1987;**1**:751.
Yancopoulos GD, Alt FW: Regulation of the assembly and expression of variable-region genes. *Annu Rev Immunol* 1986;**4**:339.

Other Sources of Antibody Diversity
French DL, Laskov R, Scharff MD: The role of somatic hypermutations in the generation of antibody diversity. *Science* 1989;**244**:1152.
Landau N et al: Increased frequency of N-region insertion in a murine pre-B-cell line infected with a terminal deoxynucleotidyl transferase retroviral expression vector. *Mol Cell Biol* 1987;**7**:3237.
Max EE et al: Variation in the crossover point of kappa immunoglobulin gene V-J recombination: Evidence from a cryptic gene. *Cell* 1980;**21**:793.

**Heavy Chain Isotype Switch
& Immunoglobulin Secretion**
Blattner FR, Tucker PW: The molecular biology of immunoglobulin D. *Nature* 1984;**307**:417.
Cebra JJ, Komisar JL, Schweitzer PA: CH isotype "switching" during normal B-lymphocyte development. *Annu Rev Immunol* 1984;**2**:493.
Early P et al: Two mRNAs can be produced from a

single immunoglobulin μ gene by alternative RNA processing pathways. *Cell* 1979;**20**:313.

Gene Rearrangements in Clinical Immunology

Arnold A et al: Immunoglobulin-gene rearrangements as unique clonal markers in human lymphoid neoplasms. *N Engl J Med* 1983;**309**:1593.

Bakhshi A et al: Lymphoid blast crises of chronic myelogenous leukemia represent stages in the development of B-cell precursors. *N Engl J Med* 1983;**309**:826.

Cleary ML, Warnke R, Sklar J: Monoclonality of lymphoproliferative lesions in cardiac-transplant recipients. *N Engl J Med* 1984;**310**:477.

Chromosomal Translocations & Oncogenesis

Croce CM, Nowell PC: Molecular basis of human B cell neoplasia. *Blood* 1985;**65**:1.

Tsujimoto Y et al: The t(14;18) chromosome translocations involved in B-cell neoplasms result from mistakes in VDJ joining. *Science* 1985;**229**:1390.

Mechanisms of Inflammation

11

Abba I. Terr, MD

The immune response generates a population of T lymphocytes and antibodies with specificity for recognizing an antigen on subsequent encounters. When the same antigen or a cross-reacting antigen containing the same antigenic epitope is subsequently encountered, several events may occur, known collectively as **effector mechanisms**. These are as follows.

Neutralization. The antibody blocks a toxic site on a microorganism or a chemical toxin, either by direct reaction with the toxic site or by steric hindrance, thereby preventing toxic damage to the host.

Cytotoxicity. The antibody lyses the cell containing the antigenic epitope through various mechanisms, such as complement-induced lysis or antibody-dependent cellular cytotoxicity (ADCC).

Cytostimulation. An autoantibody reacting with a host cell receptor stimulates metabolic processes within a cell by activating the receptor, thereby simulating a normal ligand, such as a hormone.

Inflammation. The reaction of specific T lymphocyte or antibody with antigen causes the recruitment of inflammatory cells and endogenous mediator chemicals. In some cases, the normal function of the organ or tissue is altered by an increase in vascular permeability and by contraction of visceral smooth muscle.

CLASSIFICATION

This chapter will describe the 3 principal classes of immunologically induced inflammation. The classification used here is based on the nature of the initiating immune response: (1) T cell-mediated generation of cytokines, (2) antigen-antibody complex-mediated generation of factors derived from the complement system, and (3) IgE antibody-mediated release of active chemicals from mast cells. A fourth type of inflammation, called cutaneous basophil hypersensitivity, will be mentioned only briefly, because its importance in human inflammation is not known. Although these mechanisms will be described separately, they can and often do operate simultaneously and synergistically in the in vivo immune response. Each class of inflammation is characterized by a particular histologic pattern with a cellular infiltration in the target tissue.

However, inflammation is a response that is not limited to just immunologic stimuli. The cells and chemical mediators of inflammation can be activated by nonimmunologic physical means, such as injury, trauma, heat, or environmental or endogenous tissue-damaging chemicals. Furthermore, inflammatory reactions that are induced immunologically may be accompanied by other immunologic effector responses, such as antigen neutralization and cytotoxicity.

PROTECTIVE & DELETERIOUS EFFECTS

Immunologically induced inflammation begins with the specific recognition of the antigen, but the events that ensue have no immunologic specificity. Although inflammation is an efficient means of protection against invading pathogenic microorganisms and recovery from infection, ie, protective immunity, the cells and chemical mediators participating in inflammation are also capable of damaging tissues and interfering with the functioning of organs within the host. The deleterious effects of inflammation are expressed as hypersensitivity (allergy) when immunologically induced inflammation is directed to a causative antigen that is not intrinsically harmful. Examples of antigens that can produce hypersensitivity include drugs, inhaled pollen grains or dust particles, ingested foods, and plant oils or chemicals in contact with the skin. In these cases, the tissues that are damaged and the organ functions that are disrupted are generally innocent bystanders with regard to the immune response directed at the foreign antigen. The harmful consequences of immunologically induced inflammation are also expressed in autoimmune diseases, wherein the effector mechanisms are misdirected to a host cell, possibly because of a defect in immune regulation.

METHODS OF STUDY

The accumulated knowledge about the mechanisms of human inflammation has been derived from many sources, including the analysis of tissue pathology, cytology, and biochemistry of mediators in tissues and body fluids during both naturally acquired and experimentally induced exposures to antigens. Historically, the first experimental model system of inflammation was the localized cutaneous reaction to an intradermal injection of antigen, ie, the skin test. This simple procedure, first used almost 100 years ago, continues to provide much essential information about the mechanisms of the various classes of inflammation (Table 11-1). Immunologic mechanisms have been determined by the technique of passive transfer skin testing, in which mixed populations of cells, purified lymphocyte preparations, serum, purified immunoglobulins, or immunoglobulin subclasses have been transferred from the sensitized (immunized) donor to a previously unimmunized recipient. The relevant mediators are analyzed by studying the effects of specific inhibitors of mediators on antigen-induced skin test reactions or by testing fluid obtained from suction-induced blisters of the skin test site.

This chapter will give a broad outline of the immunologic events that lead to inflammation. The inflammatory cells are discussed in more detail in Chapter 12, mediators of hypersensitivity in Chapter 13, cytokines that operate as mediators in cell-mediated immunity in Chapter 7, and the complement system in Chapter 14.

CELL-MEDIATED IMMUNITY

Cell-mediated immunity (CMI) is also known as delayed hypersensitivity or delayed-type hypersensitivity (DTH). These terms describe the same immunologic phenomenon, so the one used depends upon whether the effect on the host is protective or harmful. CMI and DTH refer to inflammation generated by the reaction of antigen with its corresponding antigen-specific T lymphocyte. In the previously immunized (sensitized) individual, the effector T cells that produce CMI and that can passively transfer that same antigen-specific immunity are known as TDH cells, a term which described the cell's activity and not a cell surface marker.

Mechanisms

The T lymphocyte responds on exposure to antigen only when the antigen is processed by an antigen-presenting cell (APC) (such as a macrophage) yielding peptide fragments and only in the context of the class II MHC molecule expressed on the surface of the APC along with the antigen peptide fragments (see Chapter 6). Exposure of the TDH cell to antigen for induction of CMI requires the same processing of antigen and genetically restricted presentation. Only in this way is the TDH cell activated. Activation of a small number of TDH cells results in the production and secretion of lymphokines. The action of these lymphokines on other cells both amplifies the size of the specific TDH cell population and recruits

Table 11-1. Classes of immunologically induced inflammation sharing the time course, cellular composition, relevant mediators, and immunologic mechanisms as reflected in the cutaneous response to skin testing.

Type of Inflammation	Skin Test Terminology	Time of Maximal Reaction (Hours)	Principal Inflammatory Cells	Primary Mediator	Immunologic Mechanisms of Inflammation
1. CMI, DTH	Delayed	36	Lymphocytes, macrophages (granuloma)	Lymphokines	TDH cell, cytokine, activated macrophage
2. Immune complex	Late	8	Polymorphonuclear neutrophils	Complement	Antigen-antibody complex, complement activation, neutrophil chemotaxis
3. IgE Immediate phase	Immediate	0.25	Eosinophils	Histamine, leukotrienes	Mast cell, fixed IgE, mediators
Late phase	Late	6	Eosinophils, neutrophils	PAF, other mediators	Chemotaxis from mast cell
4. Cutaneous basophil hypersensitivity	Delayed	36	Basophils	Unknown	Unknown

other immunologically nonspecific lymphocytes and other inflammatory cells. Although identification of the relevant lymphokines in this response is currently incomplete, certain functional activities can be described.

The cells attracted by lymphokine-induced chemotaxis include monocytes, granulocytes, B and T lymphocytes, and basophils. Activation of macrophages by lymphokines with macrophage-activating factor (MAF) not only causes these cells to express class II MHC molecules, but also enhances their phagocytic and bactericidal activities. Vasodilation occurs, effectively enhancing the availability of cells from the circulation. The coagulation-kinin system is activated, so that fibrin is formed and deposited. This material is probably important in a localization of the inflammatory reaction, and it gives the characteristic induration of the cutaneous DTH. These events are depicted in Figure 11-1.

Histopathology

The microscopic appearance of CMI is characteristic, and its occurrence in a number of clinical diseases suggests that this particular immunologic mechanism is involved in the pathogenesis. There

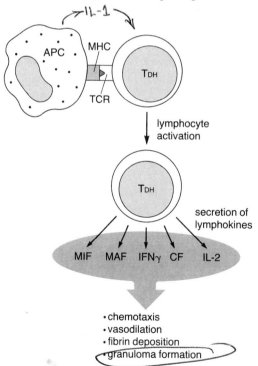

Figure 11-1. Schematic representation of the immunologic events in cell-mediated inflammation. Abbreviations: APC, antigen-presenting cell; MHC, major histocompatibility complex; TCR, T cell receptor; MIF, monocyte migration inhibitory factor; MAF, macrophage-activating factor; IFNα, alpha interferon; CF, complement fixation; IL-2, interleukin-2.

is a mononuclear cellular infiltration with monocytes and lymphocytes (often in a perivascular distribution) and granulocytes. In addition, fibrin deposition, edema, and tissue destruction occur. In advanced lesions there may be liquefaction of tissue, called caseation necrosis. A hallmark of CMI is the granuloma, a focal accumulation of monocytes, lymphocytes, neutrophils, plasma cells, and epithelioid giant cells that probably arises from coalescence of cells of the monocyte-macrophage series. The granuloma is considered to be the end result of CMI in which an antigen has persisted at the site because of low solubility and degradability, thereby causing persistent local antigenic stimulation. Granulomas occur in CMI from infections, in DTH to metals and organic particles, and in the disease sarcoidosis, in which the antigen is unknown.

Clinical Manifestations

A state of CMI/DTH is acquired naturally during the course of many infections, artificially by immunization, and through contact by many different sensitizing chemicals on the skin and mucous membranes.

Immunity to infection by obligate intracellular pathogenic organisms is mediated by CMI. The variety of organisms provoking this type of immunity is extensive and includes viruses, *Chlamydia,* fungi, bacteria, protozoa, and helminthic parasites. A major consequence of CMI in the primary infection is localization of the infection. However, as mentioned above, persistent antigenic stimulation in a granulomatous lesion may lead to tissue necrosis and systemic spread of organisms.

The primary disease in this category is allergic contact dermatitis. In this disease, the sensitizing antigens are usually haptens, which complex with skin protein carrier molecules before being processed by Langerhans cells in the skin. Examples of common contact sensitizers are pentadecyl catechol in the oil from poison ivy and nickel in jewelry.

Allograft rejection and the graft-versus-host reaction are complex immunologic phenomena that involve the class II MHC antigen as the target for rejection, but other antigenic cellular molecules and other immunologic effector mechanisms, especially cytotoxicity, are also involved. In a similar fashion, CMI participates along with other effector responses in tumor immunity and in autoimmune diseases.

Regulation

An active feedback inhibition regulating the extent of CMI is suggested by experimental evidence obtained with guinea pigs. The inhibitory effect appears to be antigenically nonspecific. A state of nonspecific depression of cellular immunity occurs in humans under certain circumstances and has been referred to as **anergy**. Anergy may accompany diseases with extensive granulomata, such as miliary tuberculosis, severe coccidioidomycosis, lepromatous leprosy, and sarcoidosis. It also occurs in Hodgkin's disease. A temporary loss of CMI occurs during the acute phase of certain viral infections such as measles. Anergy is usually defined as the absence of DTH skin tests to a panel of commonly encountered antigens or loss of a previously positive DTH skin test. Until the mechanism of anergy becomes known, the term should be considered an operational one without necessarily implying a mechanism.

IMMUNE COMPLEX-MEDIATED INFLAMMATION

Immune complex-mediated inflammation refers to the inflammatory cell response that occurs following a reaction of antigen and antibody and the subsequent activation of the complement system. Complement-generated inflammation functions both in immunity and in hypersensitivity. The 2 cardinal expressions of hypersensitivity in this case are the cutaneous Arthus reaction and systemic serum sickness. Both of these immunologic reactions were first recognized in the early 1900s, and since then the pathogenesis of immune-complex phenomena has been extensively studied by using rabbits. Rabbit models that apply to human diseases include the Arthus reaction on the skin, "one-shot" serum sickness, and chronic serum sickness produced by daily intravenous injections of antigen.

Mechanisms

The antigen may be either a high-molecular-weight protein, ie, a "complete antigen," or a hapten. However, the conditions necessary for complement activation require binding of the hapten to a host carrier protein. The chemical nature of the antigen is probably not as critical as its mode of exposure to the antibody. The reaction is antigen dose-related, especially in the serum sickness on first exposure to antigen, when the likelihood of this reaction increases with increasing dose of antigen. A prolonged period of antigen exposure also enhances the likelihood of serum sickness. An antigen with a net ionic charge could enhance the localization of the antigen-antibody complex to certain tissue sites bearing the opposite charge.

A. Complement-Activating Antibodies: The antibody must be capable of activating complement. IgM antibodies and IgG antibodies of all subclasses except for IgG4 activate the comple-

ment system through the classical pathway. IgM antibodies are more efficient than are IgG antibodies by virtue of their higher valence, permitting the development of large complexes with antigen. IgA antibodies activate complement through the alternative pathway. IgE antibodies have no effect on the complement system and therefore are not involved in this type of immune complex reaction, although it is possible that antigen-IgE antibody complexes have other pathogenic properties. IgD antibodies are not known to produce any form of inflammation.

B. Immune-Complex Formation: In the usual model of immune complex-mediated inflammation, antigen-antibody complexes cross-linked in a lattice fashion are formed in the circulation and secondarily deposited in tissues. In experimentally induced serum sickness with complexes formed at various points in the in vitro precipitin reaction (Fig 11-2), the complexes formed in moderate antigen excess are of the most effective size for activating complement and, furthermore, have the most prolonged residence in the circulation. Complexes formed in far antigen or antibody excess are small, because saturation of all antibody- or antigen-binding sites, respec-

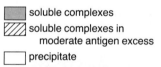

soluble complexes

soluble complexes in moderate antigen excess

precipitate

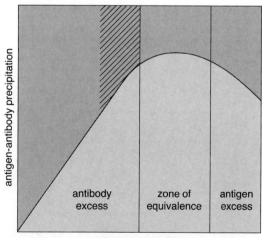

Figure 11-2. The precipitin reaction, showing the effect of increasing antigen concentration on the quantity of antigen-antibody precipitate formed in vitro. The concentration of antibody is constant. Soluble antigen-antibody complexes obtained from the supernatant in the region of moderate antigen excess are the most effective in activating complement.

tively, prevents multiple cross-linking required for lattice formation.

C. Immune-Complex Deposition: Soluble complexes of antigen and antibody formed in the circulation are deposited in various tissues. If the immune complexes are large enough, they become trapped, particularly on the basement membrane of the glomerulus and in blood vessels, where they deposit on the internal elastic lamina. The localization to these tissues may also depend on other secondary factors such as blood flow turbulence and the ionic charge of the immune complex. The size of the complex, however, appears to be the predominant factor in tissue localization. In the cutaneous Arthus reaction, a high concentration of immune complexes is generated locally because the antigen is injected directly into the skin, thereby creating focal deposits in blood vessels. In diseases in which antibody is formed to a cellular

autoantigen, the immune complex is formed by deposition of antibody on the cell-fixed antigen at that tissue site, rather than being deposited as an immune complex from the circulation.

D. Complement Activation: Complement activation can be initiated through either the classical or alternative pathway, depending on the immunoglobulin class of antibody within the immune complex (see Chapter 14). The principal inflammatory factor derived from the complement cascade appears to be C5a, which is chemotactic for neutrophils from the circulation and from surrounding tissues. The resulting vasculitis is made up of several elements (Fig 11–3). Neutrophils release lysosomal enzymes and generate toxic oxidants in the process of phagocytizing the immune complex, thereby causing destruction of the internal elastic lamina of the blood vessel wall. Blood vessel endothelial cells swell and prolifer-

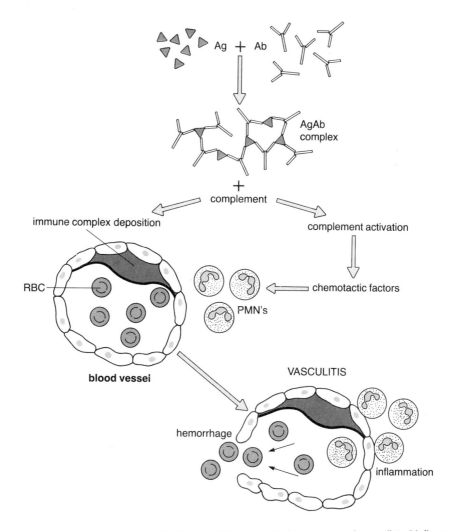

Figure 11–3. Schematic representation of the immunologic events in immune complex-mediated inflammation.

ate, and there is aggregation of platelets. Later, mononuclear cells infiltrate the area, but the mechanism of their attraction is unknown.

E. Control Mechanism: Recently a possible control mechanism has been described which could limit the extent of immune-complex inflammation. It has been shown that immune complexes are solubilized by C3 convertase. This enzyme is formed by activation of C3 by factor B of the alternative complement pathway. When C3 convertase is bound to immune complexes at equivalence, C3 fragments dissociate antigen-antibody binding, thereby breaking up the immune complex.

F. Normal Immune-Complex Formation: Small quantities of immune complexes are formed normally in the absence of disease. The antigens responsible for these normal antigen-antibody complexes are not all known, although at least some are antigens from ingested foods. Other environmental antigens and possibly autoantigens could be responsible for these normal circulating complexes. Nevertheless, they are promptly eliminated through phagocytosis by cells of the mononuclear phagocyte system (formerly called the reticuloendothelial system), which contain receptors for the Fc portion of IgG and for C3. Immune-complex disease therefore requires (1) large amounts of antigen; (2) generation of immune complexes large enough to activate complement; and (3) in some cases, impaired function of the mononuclear phagocyte system, possibly because of an abnormality of the Fc receptor.

Clinical Manifestations

In immunity, immune-complex inflammation is accompanied by other complement-mediated phenomena such as opsonization, immune adherence, and ADCC of bacteria and other microorganisms by antibodies to surface antigens on these pathogens. In certain hypersensitivity states, on the other hand, immune complex inflammation is recognized as an important isolated pathogenic mechanism.

A. Arthus Reaction: The Arthus reaction as described for rabbit skin occurs in humans as a frequent consequence of immunotherapy for allergy; it is present in a very mild form, consisting of edema and tissue inflammation but with little or no significant vasculitis. It appears occasionally as a response to insect bites or injected medications.

A single injection of a large quantity of foreign protein antigen into a rabbit produces a characteristic acute "one-shot" serum sickness. The associated immunologic events are depicted in Figure 11-4. During an initial equilibration phase lasting 12–24 hours, the injected antigen load reaches equilibrium between the circulation and extravas-

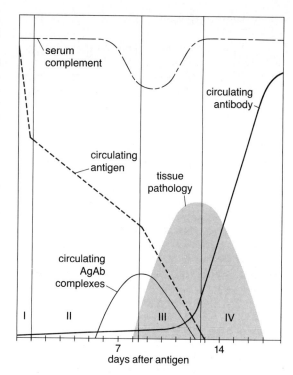

Figure 11-4. Immunologic events in experimental "one-shot" serum sickness in rabbits. The pathogenesis of human serum sickness is similar. A single high dose of antigen is given intravenously on day 0. Phase I: Equilibration of antigen between blood and tissues. Phase II: Primary antibody response. Near the end of this phase, antibody combines with antigen, forming circulating immune complexes. Phase III: Tissue pathology and progression of clinical disease. Circulating complexes activate complement and deposit in tissues. The serum complement level falls transiently, and residual antigen is rapidly cleared from the blood. Phase IV: Remission. Antigen is no longer available, and the level of circulating antibody rises. No further immune complexes form, complement levels return to normal, pathologic lesions repair, and symptoms subside.

cular space as the immune response begins. Over the next 5–7 days, as the primary antibody response takes place, residual antigen is slowly degraded. This is followed by the immune elimination phase, in which circulating antigen is rapidly cleared because newly generated antibody enters the circulation, combines with antigen, and forms circulating antigen-antibody complexes. During this brief phase of several days, circulating immune complexes can be detected in the serum, and this is reflected by a transient drop in the level of serum complement. It is during this phase that immune complexes are deposited in tissues, complement activation occurs, and the pathologic events described above ensue.

B. Serum Sickness: The clinical symptoms of serum sickness, include fever, lymphadenopathy, arthralgias, and dermatitis. The final phase begins when free antigen is no longer available, immune complexes no longer form, the serum complement level returns to normal, and free antibody appears in the circulation. No new pathologic lesions develop, and healing with gradual subsidence of symptoms takes place. Serum sickness was once a common reaction to the administration of large quantities of foreign hyperimmune serum used to treat a variety of infectious and toxic diseases prior to the era of antibiotic therapy. Today, heterologous serum is no longer used to treat infections, but it is used in transplantation as a source of anti-lymphocyte or anti-thymocyte antibodies and experimentally as a source of antibodies to specific lymphocyte antigens, such as CD3 for therapeutic immunomodulation. Serum sickness also occurs as an allergic reaction to penicillin and during the prodromal phase of some viral infections, most notably viral hepatitis.

C. Autoimmune Diseases: In 2 autoimmune diseases, thyroiditis and Goodpasture's syndrome, a localized form of immune-complex inflammation results from the action of antithyroglobulin antibodies and anti-glomerular basement membrane antibodies, respectively.

An experimental chronic serum sickness can be induced in rabbits by daily intravenous infusions of a quantity of antigen calculated to maintain a prolonged state of moderate antigen excess, based on quantitative antibody determinations. In animals requiring small doses of antigen because of a relatively weak antibody response, this disease model produces membranous glomerulonephritis; in animals requiring large daily doses of antigen because of a brisk antibody response, the predominant lesion is an immune alveolitis in the lungs. These experiments have been used as a model for the pathogenesis of systemic lupus erythematosus, rheumatoid arthritis, polyarteritis nodosa, and other diseases of unknown etiology that are characterized by the presence of circulating immune complexes and vasculitis. The serum sickness model cannot be used to explain all of the pathology and clinical manifestations of these diseases, and the antigen responsible for vasculitis in these conditions is unknown. Solubilization of immune complexes by C3 convertase, discussed above, could explain the frequent occurrence of systemic lupus erythematosus in patients with inherited complement deficiencies.

IgE-MEDIATED INFLAMMATION

IgE-mediated inflammation refers to the inflammatory response mediated by the reaction of antigen with IgE antibodies that occupy receptor sites on mast cells. The interaction of antigen with these cell-fixed antibodies causes the mast cell to degranulate, release certain preformed mediators, and generate other mediators de novo. The result is a 2-phase response, with an initial immediate effect on blood vessels, smooth muscle, and secretory glands, followed by a later cellular inflammatory response. This type of inflammatory response is commonly known as immediate hypersensitivity.

Mechanisms

IgE-mediated inflammation is common. Antigens include a variety of environmental inhaled and ingested allergens; drugs given by injection, inhalation, or orally; and certain microorganisms, especially helminths. The antigen may be complete or haptenic, and its physicochemical nature is probably not important, because known antigens include proteins, carbohydrates, low-molecular-weight organic compounds, and metals. The dose of antigen, however, is important. In contrast to immune complex-mediated inflammation, IgE antibodies are typically formed to very small doses of antigen, and once these antibodies are formed, extremely small quantities of antigen are sufficient to evoke a response.

A. IgE Antibody: The unique feature of IgE antibodies is a structural component of the ϵ heavy chains that binds specifically to a high-affinity receptor (FcϵRI) on the mast cell surface membrane. There is no similar structure on other immunoglobulin heavy chains that can either stimulate the mast cell receptor or block the occupation of the receptor by IgE antibodies. The chemistry of this reactive portion of the IgE antibody is currently unknown, but it involves the normal conformation of the intact molecule and is destroyed by heating at 56°C for 4 hours.

B. Mast Cells and Basophils: The mast cells and basophils both bear the surface FcϵRI at high density. The average number of receptors has been calculated at 270,000 per basophil, but the number on mast cells has not been determined. The high affinity of this receptor for IgE is reflected by an equilibrium constant (K_a) of 2.8 $\times$ 10^{-9} mol/L. Binding is reversible, but the dissociation constant is low. This explains the very small quantities of IgE antibody required for response and the persistence of that response. Despite the high affinity, the binding of IgE antibody to its receptor is noncovalent. IgE antibodies in circulation are in equilibrium with antibodies on mast cells and basophils. Recently it has been shown that both human and rodent IgE antibodies can react with the human mast cell receptor, but it is not known whether human IgE antibody can occupy the rodent mast cell receptor.

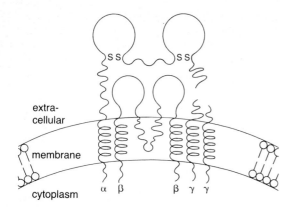

Figure 11-5. The high-affinity mast cell receptor for IgE (FcεRII).

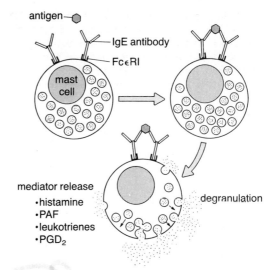

Figure 11-6. Schematic representation of the immunologic events in IgE-mediated inflammation.

The high-affinity mast cell receptor for IgE is composed of 4 polypeptide chains (Fig 11-5). The α chain (MW 50,000) contains the binding site for IgE and is exposed on the cell surface. It contains 2 domains and has 30% carbohydrate. The β chain (MW 30,000) is located entirely within the cell membrane. There are 2 identical disulfide-linked γ chains on the cytoplasmic aspect of the cell surface membrane. A different low-affinity (K_a 10^{-5} mol/L) receptor (FcεRII) is present on eosinophils, monocyte-macrophages, lymphocytes, and platelets. This receptor is expressed when those cells are activated, and it plays no known role in the release of mediators of inflammation.

Cellular events of IgE-mediated inflammation are depicted in Figure 11-6. A multivalent antigen (or hapten-carrier complex) reacts with 2 or more IgE antibodies occupying FcεRI receptors; this results in physical bridging of the receptors owing to receptor motion in the plane of the cell membrane, which is in a relatively fluid state. Receptors bound to antigen in this way migrate and form a cap on one pole of the cell. Receptor motion is believed to be the initial signal for mast cell activation.

C. Mediators: Once the cell is activated, generation and release of mediators are accompanied by a rapid series of intracellular biochemical events. The first of these is activation of membrane-associated enzymes serine oxidase, phospholipase C, and adenylate cyclase. This is followed by the same methyltransferase reaction that accompanies ligand-receptor activation in many other cell systems. The critical action of phospholipase C on inositol phospholipids and methylation of membrane phospholipids precedes the influx of extracellular calcium ion into the cell. The initial enzyme reactions are maximal within 15 seconds after the antigen-IgE antibody union has taken place, and calcium uptake is maximal within 2–3 minutes.

Other intracellular reactions include mobilization of protein kinase C from the cytosol to the cell membrane, where it is activated, and an increase in intracellular cyclic AMP (cAMP). The effect of these intracellular enzyme reactions is the fusion of membranes of the cytoplasmic granules with each other and with the mast cell membrane; this is reflected microscopically as degranulation. Preformed mediators, such as histamine, are present within these granules prior to exposure of the cell to antigen and are therefore released from the cell. Active membrane-associated mediators, such as the products of arachidonic acid (prostaglandins and leukotrienes), are then generated.

The variety of mediators that are described in more detail below have different effects on different end organs (blood vessels, smooth muscles, afferent nerve endings, and secretory glands). However, the release of mediators from mast cells follows a clear biphasic course of an immediate response that is maximal at 15–30 minutes and a later response that is maximal at 6 hours.

D. Immediate and Late Phases: The immediate response is mediated principally by the effects of histamine and leukotrienes from the mast cell. The late response requires a number of mediators, of which platelet-activating factor (PAF) is probably the most important, although the arachidonic acid metabolites (leukotrienes and prostaglandins) are probably also important. The late response is characterized by recruitment of inflammatory cells, especially neutrophils and eosinophils. Eosinophils release major basic protein, whereas neutrophils, eosinophils, and mast cells release lysosomal enzymes.

Pathology

pruritus = itching

The immediate response consists grossly of erythema, localized edema in the form of a wheal, and pruritus, all of which can be explained by the actions of histamine. The microscopic pathology consists of vasodilation and edema with a mild cellular infiltrate initially of granulocytes followed by eosinophils. The late response appears grossly as erythema, induration, heat, burning, and itching. Microscopically, neutrophils predominate, along with edema, degranulated mast cells, and a perivascular distribution of eosinophils. There are some mononuclear cells and free eosinophilic granules in the later stages. Fibrin deposition probably occurs transiently. There are no signs of immunoglobulin or complement deposition.

Clinical Manifestations

IgE-mediated inflammation is responsible for atopic allergy (hay fever, asthma, and atopic dermatitis), systemic anaphylaxis, and allergic urticaria. It is at least in part responsible for immunity to infestation by helminths. It may play a facilitative role as a "gatekeeper" in immune complex–mediated immunity and CMI because of its ability to provide rapid vasodilation, resulting in the formation of a portal of entry into tissues for circulating soluble factors and cells.

CUTANEOUS BASOPHIL HYPERSENSITIVITY

Cutaneous basophil hypersensitivity, formerly known as Jones-Mote hypersensitivity, is a form of inflammation that at present has uncertain significance. It is elicited by protein antigens, which, when injected into the skin, cause a localized area of swelling which is softer than that of DTH, and it is pruritic. It generally follows the same time course as DTH, but it differs histologically from DTH, since there is prominent infiltration with basophils, but no granulomas or other characteristics of DTH. It can be transferred passively with serum or B cells, indicating that it is an antibody-mediated phenomenon and not CMI, although T cells might be required for its expression. Its clinical significance is unknown. The presence of basophils in renal allografts suggests that it may be involved as one component of the transplant rejection phenomenon.

SUMMARY

The inflammatory response is the primary means by which the immune system functions in immunity. Inflammation is also responsible for hypersensitivity reactions and for many of the clinical effects of autoimmunity.

There are 3 principal pathways of immunologically induced inflammation. CMI/DTH involves the interaction of antigen with the effector T lymphocyte, causing the generation of lymphokines that give rise to a mononuclear cellular inflammation and the formation of granulomas. Immune complex–mediated inflammation involves the interaction of antigen with antibody of certain immunoglobulin isotypes that activate the complement cascade. This generates a variety of chemotactic factors that induce neutrophilic inflammation and vasculitis. IgE-mediated inflammation involves the interaction of antigen with IgE antibodies occupying mast cell receptors. Activation of the mast cell releases mediators with effects on blood vessels, smooth muscles, and secretory glands, causing changes in vascular permeability and the functioning of visceral organs.

The inflammation in infectious, allergic, and autoimmune diseases may involve one or more of these immunologically induced inflammatory pathways.

REFERENCES

Barnett EV: Circulating immune complexes: Their biologic and clinical significance. *J Allergy Clin Immunol* 1986;**78:**1089.

Bielory L et al: Human serum sickness: A prospective analysis of 35 patients treated with equine anti-thymocyte globulin for bone marrow failure. *Medicine* 1988;**67:**40.

Boros DL, Yoshida T (editors): *Basic and Clinical Aspects of Granulomatous Diseases.* North Holland Publishing Co, 1980.

Buhner D, Grant JA: Serum sickness. *Dermatol Clin* 1985;**3:**107.

Dvorak HF, Galli SJ, Dvorak AM: Expression of cell-mediated hypersensitivity in vivo: Recent advances. *Int Rev Exp Pathol* 1980;**21:**119.

Erffmeyer JE: Serum sickness. *Ann Allergy* 1986;**56:**105.

Galli SJ, Askenase PW: Cutaneous basophil hypersensitivity. Pages 321–369 in: *The Reticuloendothelial*

System. Philips SM, Escobar MR (editors). Plenum, 1986.

Ishizaka T, Ishizaka K: Activation of mast cells for mediator release through IgE receptors. *Prog Allergy* 1984;**34**:188.

Metzger H et al: The receptor with high affinity for immunoglobulin E. *Annu Rev Immunol* 1986;**4**:419.

Naguwa SM, Nebon BL: Human serum sickness. *Clin Rev Allergy* 1985;**3**:117.

Serafin WE, Austen KF: Current concepts: Mediation of immediate hypersensitivity reactions. *N Engl J Med* 1987;**317**:30.

Van Es LA: Factors affecting the deposition of immune complexes. *Clin Immunol Allergy* 1981;**1**:281.

Inflammatory Cells: Structure & Function

12

David H. Broide, MB, ChB

The inflammatory response, like the immune response, can be generated both from cells (neutrophils, eosinophils, basophils, macrophages, mast cells, platelets, and endothelium) and from circulating proteins (components of the complement, coagulation, fibrinolysis, and kinin pathways) (see Chapter 13). The cellular inflammatory response is the mechanism by which the body defends against infection and repairs tissue damage. However, persistent inflammation can result in disease states and thus be detrimental to the host. The clinical expression depends on the site (lung, joint, or blood vessel) and cellular nature (neutrophil or eosinophil) of the inflammatory response. To rapidly activate the cellular inflammatory response and to protect the body from the potent cellular inflammatory mediators, these mediators are stored either preformed in cytoplasmic granules or as phospholipids available to be newly generated in the cell surface membrane. Furthermore, there is both a mobile (circulating) and a stationary (noncirculating) cellular inflammatory capacity. Thus, in the inflammatory response, a distinction can be made between short-lived circulating inflammatory cells (neutrophils, eosinophils, and basophils) and cells that preexist in the tissue as long-lived resident noncirculating inflammatory cells (mast cells and macrophages) (Table 12–1). For some inflammatory cells (neutrophils and

macrophages) the primary function is phagocytosis, and for others (mast cells and basophils) it is the secretion of inflammatory mediators. The phagocytic cells, by eliminating particles or organisms that have gained access to the host, act as a protective barrier between the environment and the host. In contrast, the secretory cells contain both inflammatory mediators, which increase vascular permeability, and chemotactic factors, which recruit other inflammatory cells, thus contributing to host defense either by amplifying the effects of the phagocytic cells or by having a direct effect on target cells.

This chapter will describe the ultrastructure and identification of each of the inflammatory cells, as well as their subtypes, receptors, and cellular changes during inflammation (activation, degranulation, and metabolism).

NEUTROPHILS

Polymorphonuclear neutrophils are the predominant leukocytes in the circulation, where they have a brief existence between their formation in the bone marrow and their subsequent phagocytic and microbicidal activity in the tissue sites of inflammation. They are primarily responsible for maintaining normal host defenses against invading microorganisms, being the major cellular elements in most forms of acute inflammation, particularly during the earlier stage of the inflammatory response. Their cytoplasmic granules contain a potent array of digestive enzymes, which may either remove tissue debris or act intracellularly or extracellularly to kill and degrade microorganisms. To perform their function in tissues, neutrophils are equipped to adhere to vascular endothelium, diapedese through the walls of small blood vessels, and migrate toward particles to be ingested (**chemotaxis**). In a coordinated, sequential series of steps, they can recognize, attach to, and engulf particles (**phagocytosis**); discharge cytoplasmic granule contents into phagocytic

Table 12-1. Inflammatory Cells.[1]

Circulating	Tissue Resident
Neutrophils	Mast cells
Eosinophils	Macrophages
Basophils	Endothelium
Platelets	

[1]The cells participating in the inflammatory response can be categorized into (1) circulating and (2) noncirculating, tissue-resident inflammatory cells. Another useful way to classify inflammatory cells, as either primary phagocytic cells (macrophages, neutrophils) or primary secretory cells (mast cells, basophils), has the potential disadvantage of ignoring the secretory capacity of primary phagocytic cells such as macrophages.

vacuoles (**degranulation**); and generate a burst of oxidative metabolism. Phagocytosed microorganisms, coated with complement and specific antibody (**opsonization**), are killed by a combination of neutrophil-generated toxic oxygen radicals and cytotoxic cytoplasmic granule-derived proteins.

Origin & Tissue Distribution

Neutrophils are bone marrow-derived members of the granulocyte series, which arise from pluripotential stem cells in the bone marrow. Stromal cells in the bone marrow produce specific glycoprotein colony-stimulating factors termed granulocyte colony-stimulating factor (G-CSF), granulocyte-macrophage colony-stimulating factor (GM-CSF), and interleukin 3 (IL-3) (see Chapter 7). These factors stimulate neutrophil progenitor cells in the bone marrow to proliferate and differentiate into mature neutrophils. The mature cells remain in the marrow storage compartment for approximately 5 days and then circulate for about 10 hours before entering the tissues at sites of inflammation. It has been estimated that more than 100 billion neutrophils enter and leave the circulation of a 70 kg person daily under normal conditions. This enormous turnover can be increased up to 10-fold during an acute infection.

Ultrastructure & Identification

The neutrophil has a characteristic segmented, multilobe (2–5 lobes) nucleus, which contains densely clumped chromatin and no nucleoli. The neutrophil cytoplasm contains fine granules that stain pink with Wright's stain. In contrast, Wright-stained eosinophil and basophil cytoplasmic granules are larger and stain bright orange (eosinophils) or purplish-black (basophils). The mature neutrophil is conspicuously deficient in rough endoplasmic reticulum, which indicates that the synthesis of new protein is not an important function.

Enzymes associated with neutrophil cytoplasmic granules are capable of hydrolyzing a wide variety of both natural and synthetic substrates, including simple and complex polysaccharides, proteins, and lipids. These enzymes are important in maintaining normal host defenses and in mediating inflammation. Two major types of neutrophil cytoplasmic granules are distinguishable by their morphology, staining characteristics, enzyme content, and order of synthesis during myeloid development. Primary granules are also known as **azurophil granules** because of their blue appearance on Wright's stain. They contain myeloperoxidase and other lysosomal hydrolases, and they appear in the cytoplasm of neutrophils during the promyelocyte stage of development, arising from the concave surface of the Golgi com-

plex. Secondary granules, also known as **specific granules,** are formed from the convex surface of the Golgi complex during the myelocyte stage of development and contain predominantly lysozyme and iron-binding lactoferrin. Azurophil granules, which are more dense and generally larger than the peroxidase-negative specific granules, contain all the neutrophil myeloperoxidase, β-glucuronidase, elastase, and cathepsin G, whereas specific granules contain all the neutrophil lactoferrin. Specific granules outnumber azurophil granules 3:1. The neutrophil ultrastructure is shown in Fig 12–1.

Receptors

A. Immunoglobulin Fc Receptors: Approximately 75–90% of peripheral blood neutrophils have cell surface receptors for the Fc portion of IgG (FcγR) (Table 12–2). There are 3 distinct FcγR's, 2 of which are present on neutrophils. They have apparent molecular weights of 42,000 and 50,000–70,000. The heavier one preferentially binds to antigen-IgG antibody complexes or IgG-coated particles. Binding of immune complexes to this neutrophil FcγR exceeds the binding by the corresponding monomeric IgG. It has been hypothesized that either IgG antibodies in immune complexes have more binding sites available to attach to neutrophil FcγR's or the complexes produce allosteric changes in the conformation of immunoglobulin molecules, thereby

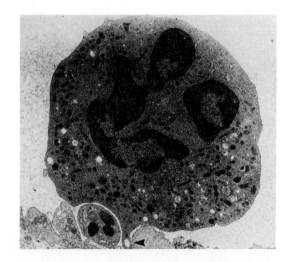

Figure 12–1. Electron micrograph of a neutrophil depicting its characteristic morphology. The nucleus is hypersegmented with abundant heterochromatin and no nucleoli. The cytoplasm contains cytoplasmic granules of heterogeneous size and electron density. The neutrophil is in the process of diapedesing between endothelial cells (arrow). (Courtesy of Henry C Powell, University of California, San Diego.)

Table 12-2. Inflammatory-cell immunoglobulin Fc receptors.

Receptor	Present on:					
	Neutrophils	Monocytes	Mast Cells	Basophils	Eosinophils	Platelets
IgM	−	−	−	−	−	−
IgG						
IgG1	+	+	−	?	+	+
IgG2	+	+	−	−	?	+
IgG3	+	+	−	−	?	+
IgG4	+	+	−	−	?	+
IgA	+	+	−	−	?	−
IgD	−	−	−	−	+	−
IgE	−	+	+	+	+	+
FcεRI	−	−	+	+	−	−
FcεRII	−	+	?	?	+	+

[1]Symbols: +, receptor present; −, receptor absent; ?, presence unknown.

altering the tertiary structure of immunoglobulin and exposing sites capable of interacting with the neutrophil FcγR. Both types of neutrophil FcγR bind to multivalent forms of IgG, but exhibit weak or undetectable binding to monomeric IgG. In addition to IgG receptors, neutrophils have Fc receptors for IgA but appear to lack Fc receptors for IgE and IgD. Studies attempting to demonstrate binding of IgM to human neutrophils have generally not been successful.

B. Complement Receptors: Activation of either the classic complement pathway by antigen-antibody reactions or the alternative complement pathway by certain bacterial products generate complement fragments, which are able to amplify the inflammatory response by attracting and activating neutrophils. Complement fragment C3b mediates these effects through neutrophil cell surface complement receptors, which are described in Chapter 14.

In addition to receptors for IgG and C3b, neutrophils contain receptors for f-Met-Leu-Phe (FMLP), leukotriene B4 (LTB4), hematopoietic growth factors (GM-CSF and G-CSF), and complement fragments C5a and C3a.

Adherence & Chemotaxis

Peripheral blood contains 2 exchangeable pools of neutrophils, a central circulating axial pool and a marginal pool moving slowly along the vascular endothelium. One of the earliest events in acute inflammation is an increase in the adherence of circulating neutrophils to vascular endothelium. In response to IL-1 and other inflammatory mediators, endothelial cells become adhesive for neutrophils. Although the molecular nature of the endothelium-neutrophil adherence is at present incompletely understood, it is known that adherence of neutrophils to cells and surfaces is mediated partly by a related group of cell suface glycoproteins that include the CR3 receptor (C3bi), lymphocyte function antigen-1 (LFA-1), and p150,95. In

addition, neutrophils possess receptors for the extracellular matrix components laminin and fibronectin, which could facilitate the attachment of neutrophils to host tissue or microbial surfaces.

There are a large number of chemotactic factors that can recruit neutrophils to sites of tissue inflammation. The best-characterized of these are FMLP, LTB4, and C5a. They are derived from cellular as well as circulating plasma sources, including proteins (C5a and C567 derived from the complement pathway, fibrin fragments, and collagen fragments), enzymes (plasma kallikrein and C3bBb derived from the alternative complement pathway), lipids (LTB4, platelet-activating factor [PAF]), synthetic N-formyl methionyl peptides (derived from bacterial protein and mitochondrial protein breakdown). Cellular sources of factors chemotactic for neutrophils include bacteria, macrophages, lymphocytes, platelets, and mast cells. At nanomolar concentrations of chemotactic factors, neutrophils respond by an increase in adhesiveness, an increase in chemotactic factor receptor number, and the release of specific cytoplasmic granule contents, and they are primed for the oxidative burst.

In contrast to tissue eosinophils, which are present in normal tissues at epithelial surfaces in contact with the environment, the neutrophil is not normally found in tissues unless recruited from the circulation to sites of tissue inflammation.

Phagocytosis

The internalization of extracellular substances by invagination of the plasma membrane (**endocytosis**) can be further defined as **phagocytosis** (the ingestion of particulate material) or **pinocytosis** (the internalization of fluids and solutes) (Fig 12-2). Attachment of a neutrophil to a suitable small particle results in the formation at the site of attachment of pseudopodia, which surround the particle and ultimately fuse at its distal pole. The neutrophil cell surface then completely

1. neutrophil maintains viability

(a) 'regurgitation during feeding'

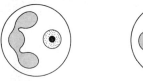

normal phagosome   incompletely sealed
                          phagosome

(b) reverse endocytosis

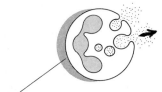

immune complexes or aggregated immunoglobulins deposited on solid surfaces

2. neutrophil cell death

(a) cell death

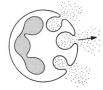

(b) perforation from within

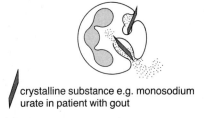

crystalline substance e.g. monosodium
urate in patient with gout

Figure 12-2. Neutrophil events during phagocytosis and degranulation. See the text for a description.

surrounds the engulfed particle, forming a phagocytic vesicle or **phagosome,** which moves into the cell and fuses with intracellular cytoplasmic granules. This provides a local environment in which the opportunity for particle degradation by cytoplasmic granule enzymes in the phagosome is enhanced. Phagocytosis requires metabolic energy and an active cytoplasmic contractile protein system. Although neutrophils are capable of phagocytosing particles in the absence of IgG antibody or complement, phagocytosis is stimulated by the presence of both C3b and IgG antibody, which have separate but synergistic roles in phagocytosis. Activation of the neutrophil C3b receptor primarily promotes recognition and attachment of bound or adherent particles, whereas occupation of the neutrophil IgG receptor by antibody appears necessary for optimal phagocytosis.

Degranulation

Neutrophil cytoplasmic granules (modified lysosomes) contain a potent array of destructive enzymes, which may act either inside or outside the neutrophil. Since mature neutrophils are deficient in their ability to synthesize new protein molecules, the cytoplasmic granules cannot be regenerated once they have been lost. Intracellular degranulation, the "internal digestive system" of the neutrophil, is not a uniform process, as neutrophil azurophil and specific cytoplasmic granules discharge their contents at different rates during phagocytosis. During phagocytosis, neutrophil cytoplasmic granule membranes fuse with the membranes of the phagocytic vacuole. The process of neutrophil degranulation involves discharge of the neutrophil cytoplasmic granule contents into the newly formed **phagolysosome.** The formation of phagolysosomes is crucial to host defense, as the ingested microorganisms are killed and digested within phagolysosomes. Although the contents of neutrophil cytoplasmic granules most often are discharged intracellularly into phagosomes, in certain circumstances they can be released extracellularly. The extracellular degranulation of neutrophils could contribute significantly to inflammation, as neutrophils are richly endowed with a variety of neutral and acidic proteases that are collectively capable of activating complement, of generating kinins, of enhancing vascular permeability, and of degrading elastin, collagen, and a variety of other proteins. The mechanisms of neutrophil extracellular degranulation include neutrophil cell death as well as the extrusion of neutrophil cytoplasmic granule contents from incompletely sealed neutrophil phagosomes, open at their external borders to the extracellular space (Fig 12–2).

Neutrophils can also degranulate in the absence of phagocytosis when stimulated by immune complexes or aggregated immunoglobulins deposited on solid surfaces. This process is termed "reverse endocytosis," during which the merger of neutrophil cytoplasmic granules with the plasma membrane results in the discharge of granule constituents directly to the outside of the cell. This mechanism of cytoplasmic granule release from neutrophils could be pertinent to the pathogenesis of tissue injury in several diseases in which immune complexes are deposited upon cell surfaces or extracellular structures such as vascular basement membrane.

Oxidative Metabolism

Oxygen-derived free radicals generated by the neutrophil play an important role as microbicidal oxidants as well as mediators of inflammation and tissue injury (Table 12–3). The bulk of oxygen consumed by stimulated neutrophils is converted directly to superoxide anion radicals (O_2^-) by the enzyme NADPH oxidase. The superoxide is rapidly converted to hydrogen peroxide and hydroxyl radicals, which provide most of the microbicidal activity within the phagosome and extracellular environment. Additional oxidants such as hypochlorous acid and free chlorine are formed in the presence of hydrogen peroxide, halide, and neutrophil cytoplasmic granule–derived myeloperoxidase. The neutrophil is able to protect itself from the injurious effects of toxic oxygen radicals by the presence in the neutrophil cytosol of potent protective enzymes and scavengers such as superoxide dismutase, catalase, and the glutathione peroxidase-reductase cycle.

The generation of toxic oxidants in neutrophils is stimulated immunologically by a variety of microorganisms coated with the appropriate antibody (opsonin). Other stimuli include concanavalin A, FMPL, NaF, phorbol myristate acetate, C5a, the calcium ionophore A23187, serum-acti-

Table 12–3. Generation of toxic oxygen products by the respiratory oxidant burst in leukocyte phagolysosomes.[1]

I. Electron transfer by oxygen burst

$$\text{Glucose } + \text{ NADP}^+ \xrightarrow{\text{hexose monophosphate pathway}}$$

$$\text{Pentose } PO_4 + \text{NADPH}$$

$$\text{NADPH } + O_2 \xrightarrow{\text{NADPH oxidase}} \text{NADP}^+ + \boxed{O_2^-}$$

II. Spontaneous generation of toxic oxygen products

$$2O_2^- + 2H^+ \longrightarrow H_2O_2 + \boxed{^1O_2}$$

$$O_2^- + H_2O_2 \longrightarrow \boxed{\cdot OH} + OH^- + \boxed{^1O_2}$$

III. Peroxidase generation of halogenating compounds

$$H_2O_2 + Cl^- \xrightarrow{\text{peroxidase}} \boxed{OCl^-} + H_2O$$

$$OCl^- + H_2O \longrightarrow {}^1O_2 + Cl^- + H_2O$$

[1]The toxic products that kill bacteria during phagocytosis are shown in outline. O_2^-, superoxide anion; $^1O_2$, singlet oxygen; $\cdot OH$, hydroxyl free radical; OCl^-, hypochlorous anion. The leukocyte contains protective enzymes superoxide dismutase and catalase (equations not shown).

vated zymosan particles, latex beads, and various microorganisms coated with appropriate opsonins. As is the case with degranulation, enhanced oxidative metabolism by neutrophils can be stimulated in the absence of phagocytosis. The neutrophil respiratory oxidant burst is associated with increased oxygen consumption, superoxide generation, the emission of light (chemiluminescence), and increased glucose oxidation via the hexose monophosphate pathway.

Heterogeneity

Morphologically indistinguishable circulating neutrophils are heterogeneous in density, cell surface antigens, Fc receptor expression, and functional properties (eg, surface adherence, response to chemoattractants, aggregation, and phagocytosis). The origin and significance of this neutrophil heterogeneity are at present unknown. Whether the evidence for neutrophil heterogeneity reflects distinct stem cells or represents functional maturational differences within a common cell line awaits further study.

MAST CELLS

Mast cells are tissue cells with a prominent role in IgE-mediated inflammation. They are especially abundant in tissues at host-environment interfaces in organs such as the skin (10^4 mast cells/mm^3), lungs (10^6 mast cells/g, gastrointestinal tract, and nasal mucous membrane. They are thus strategically positioned to interact rapidly with inhaled or ingested antigens and to secrete a potent array of proinflammatory preformed and newly generated mediators, which produce increased vascular permeability, smooth muscle contraction, and mucus secretion. In addition, mast cell-derived factors are chemotactic for other inflammatory cells including eosinophils, neutrophils, and mononuclear cells (see Chapter 13).

Ultrastructure & Receptors

Mast cells are characterized by the presence of the high-affinity cell surface IgE receptor (FcεRI) and histamine-containing cytoplasmic granules (50–200 per cell) (Table 12–2). Mast cells are relatively large (10–15 μm in diameter). They possess a single round or oval, eccentrically located nucleus and membrane-bound cytoplasmic granules (0.1–0.4 μm in diameter) that are smaller than the cytoplasmic granules of basophils (1.0–1.2 μm in diameter). Although mast cells and basophils both have histamine-containing cytoplasmic granules and high-affinity cell surface IgE receptors, mast cells differ from basophils in morphology, mediator content, and sensitivity to pharmacologic modulation. In tissues, human mast cells are vari-

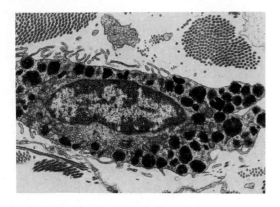

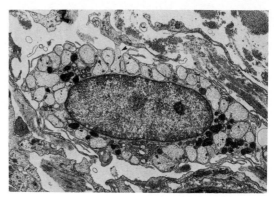

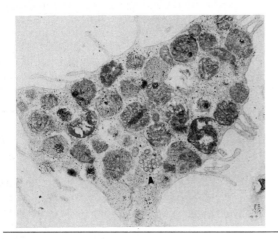

Figure 12-3. A: Electron micrograph of a resting skin mast cell. (Courtesy of Marc M Friedman, Georgetown University, Washington, DC.) **B:** Electron micrograph of a stimulated skin mast cell (ragweed antigen, 5 minutes) with swollen, lucent secretory granules. The arrowhead indicates extrusion of flocculent granule matrix material through a surface pore into the extracellular connective tissue. (Courtesy of Marc M Friedman.) **C:** Some of the electron-dense mast cell cytoplasmic granules have a crystalline substructure of scrolls, whorls (arrowhead), and multiwalled rectangles. (Courtesy of Karen Oetkon, University of California, San Diego.)

able in shape, appearing as round, oval, or spindle-shaped cells. Electron-microscopic analysis of human mast cells (Fig 12–3) reveals cytoplasmic granules that are heterogeneous in substructural pattern and exhibit scroll-like configurations, amorphous electron-dense granular zones, and highly ordered crystalline arrays. Individual cytoplasmic granules are frequently characterized by more than one of these patterns in sharp juxtaposition. During IgE-mediated mast cell activation, the crystalline structure of human skin and lung mast cell cytoplasmic granules is lost. The mast cell plasma membrane possesses numerous cell surface projections. The identification of mast cells by light microscopy is assisted by their characteristic staining properties. Mast cell cytoplasmic granules contain preformed mediators, including anionic proteoglycans. When stained with toluidine blue, the proteoglycans give the mast cell granule a metachromatic red or violet color.

IgE-mediated mast cell degranulation (described in Chapter 11) is characterized by a series of events, including enlargement of cytoplasmic granules, granule solubilization (disorganization and electron lucency of granules), and membrane fusion of adjacent cytoplasmic granules and the cell surface membrane. The conduits formed between the cytoplasmic granules and the outer cell membrane permit communication of the solubilized cytoplasmic granules with the extracellular space. Mast cell cytoplasmic granules contain much larger amounts of histamine ($5 \ \mu g/10^6$ cells) than do basophils ($1 \ \mu g/10^6$ cells).

Subtypes

The concept of mast cell heterogeneity was initially defined for the rat small intestine by the identification of a population of mucosal type mast cells differing in their staining and fixation properties from those of the rat connective tissue mast cell. Mucosal mast cells have subsequently been shown to differ from connective tissue mast cells in their T cell dependence, preformed cytoplasmic granule mediators (proteoglycan, protease), mediators generated from arachidonic acid, and functional responses to secretagogues (neuropeptides, compound 48/80) and antiallergic compounds.

Evidence for human mast cell heterogeneity is less conclusive. However, histochemical and biochemical analysis of mast cells derived from skin, lungs, nose, and intestines shows that there are 2 types of mast cells, which differ in content of the 2 cytoplasmic granule neutral proteases, tryptase and chymase. T mast cells contain tryptase and are the predominant type of mast cells in the lungs and gastrointestinal mucosa, whereas TC mast cells contain both tryptase and chymase and are the predominant mast cell type in the skin and gastrointestinal submucosa. The T lymphocyte dependence of T but not TC mast cells is suggested from studies of patients with congenital or acquired T lymphocyte defects (ie, patients with combined immunodeficiency or AIDS) in whom there is a deficiency of T mast cells in the gastrointestinal mucosa.

BASOPHILS

Basophils are circulating neutrophils with many of the functional properties of tissue mast cells. Mature basophils (5–7 μm in diameter) are the smallest cells in the granulocyte series. Basophils share with mast cells high-affinity IgE receptors and cytoplasmic granules containing histamine, but differ from mast cells in that they differentiate and mature in the bone marrow, circulate in the blood, and are not normally found in connective tissue (Table 12–4). The morphology of basophils also distinguishes them from mast cells. Basophils possess lobular bilobed or multilobed nuclei, peripherally condensed nuclear chromatin, and electron-dense aggregates of cytoplasmic glycogen (Fig 12–4). In contrast, mast cells have a single eccentric nucleus and uniformly distributed cell surface membrane processes, and they lack both the peripherally condensed nuclear chromatin and the electron-dense aggregates of cytoplasmic glycogen that are present in basophils. Another distinguishing feature between mast cells and basophils is the presence of 2 surface membrane proteins, Charcot-Leyden crystal protein and major basic protein, in the cell surface membrane of basophils but not mast cells. The basophil cell surface membrane is smooth, has occasional, irregularly distributed, short, blunt folds or uropods, and contains an average of 270,000 high-affinity receptors for IgE (Table 12–2). Basophils contain

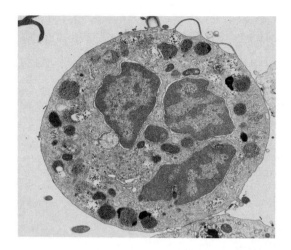

Figure 12–4. Electron micrograph of a peripheral blood basophil. The basophil has a multilobed nucleus and a smooth cell surface with occasional irregularly distributed short blunt folds or uropods. (Courtesy of Marc M Friedman.)

fewer cytoplasmic granules than mast cells and make up 0.2–1% of nucleated cells in bone marrow and peripheral blood.

Small to moderate numbers of basophils are found in a variety of inflammatory conditions involving the skin (late phase skin reaction to allergen, cutaneous basophil hypersensitivity reactions, lesions of bullous pemphigoid), small intestine (Crohn's disease), kidneys (allergic interstitial nephritis, renal allograft rejection), nose (allergic rhinitis), and eyes (allergic conjunctivitis). Although mast cells have an established role in IgE-mediated inflammation, the importance of basophils in immunity and hypersensitivity has yet to be determined.

EOSINOPHILS

Eosinophils are found in the tissues in many diseases, but predominantly in 2 forms of inflamma-

Table 12–4. Structural characteristics distinguishing basophils from mast cells[1]

Characteristic	Basophils	Mast Cells
Size	5–7 μm	10–15 μm
Nucleus	Lobular bilobed or multilobed nucleus with peripherally condensed nuclear chromatin	Single nucleus
Cytoplasm	Contains electron-dense aggregates of cytoplasmic glycogen not present in mast cells ALSO HAVE HISTAMINE GRANULES	Electron-dense, histamine-containing, membrane-bound secretory granules are smaller than cytoplasmic granules of basophils
Cell surface	Smooth with occasional irregularly distributed short blunt folds or uropods	Numerous cell surface projections
Distribution	Primarily circulating in blood	Tissue resident

[1]Mast cells and basophils are the only inflammatory cells with histamine-containing cytoplasmic granules and high-affinity cell surface IgE receptors

tion: allergy and parasitic infection. Eosinophils, like basophils and neutrophils, are bone-marrow-derived granulocytes, which can be distinguished from the other 2 members of the granulocyte series on the basis of morphology, staining properties, mediator content, and association with differing disease states. Although the eosinophil stem cell is not morphologically identifiable, the eosinophil promyelocyte is clearly distinguishable from the promyelocyte of neutrophils and the basophils by its characteristic cytoplasmic granules. The life span of an eosinophil is relatively short; it has a bone marrow maturation time of 2–6 days, a circulating half-life of 6–12 hours, and a connective tissue residence time of several days. The number of circulating blood eosinophils, which make up about 1–3% of circulating leukocytes, is a very small portion of the total body eosinophil count. It is estimated that for every circulating eosinophil, there are approximately 200 mature eosinophils in the bone marrow and 500 eosinophils in connective tissue. Although a precise model of human eosinophil proliferation and differentiation in vivo is not possible at present, in vitro studies suggest that hematopoietic growth factors such as GM-CSF, IL-3, and IL-5 (eosinophil-differentiating factor) are important factors in regulating eosinophilopoiesis.

Ultrastructure

The eosinophil nucleus is bilobed and lacks a nucleolus (Fig 12–5). The most distinctive feature of eosinophils is their specific or secondary cytoplasmic granules, which contain an electron-dense crystalloid core surrounded by a less dense matrix. Human eosinophils have approximately

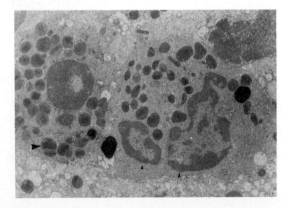

Figure 12–5. Electron micrograph of 2 tissue eosinophils depicting their distinct bilobed nuclei (small arrowheads) lacking nucleoli. The cytoplasm contains characteristic specific or secondary granules with a central electron-dense crystalline core running parallel to the long axis of the cytoplasmic granules (large arrowhead). The electron-dense core of the cytoplasmic granules is surrounded by a less electron-dense matrix.

200 secondary cytoplasmic granules per cell, one-tenth the number present in neutrophils. Eosinophils also have primary cytoplasmic granules, which are round, uniformly electron-dense, and characteristically seen in promyelocytes. Human eosinophils are slightly larger than neutrophils, being approximately 12–17 μm in diameter. The cytoplasmic granules are often spherical or ovoid and are 0.5 μm in diameter. The high content of a biochemically distinct peroxidase and the presence of at least 3 other basic proteins are the distinguishing features of the eosinophil cytoplasmic granules. One of these, the major basic protein, has a strong affinity for acidic dyes such as eosin, resulting in the characteristic intense red staining of the eosinophil cytoplasmic granules.

Receptors

A. Immunoglobulin Fc Receptors: A low-affinity IgE receptor (FcϵRII) identified on human eosinophils has a 100-fold-lower affinity to IgE than does the high-affinity IgE receptor (FcϵRI) present on mast cells and basophils, but its affinity for IgE is comparable to the affinity of FcγR for IgG (Table 12–2). Unlike other Fc receptors sequenced to date, FcϵRII is not a member of the immunoglobulin gene superfamily, but belongs to a primitive superfamily of vertebrate and invertebrate lectins (including CD23, the transferin receptor, the invariant chain of class II MHC antigens, influenza virus neuraminidase, and β-galactosidase 2,6-sialyltransferase). A common feature of this family of molecules is their unusual membrane orientation, with a cytoplasmic amino terminus and an extracellular carboxy terminus.

Approximately 10–30% of eosinophils from normal individuals have IgG receptors. Activation of the eosinophil IgG receptor with IgG-coated schistosomula or Sepharose-coated beads induces degranulation and the release of the newly generated mediator LTC$_4$. The generation of the eosinophil-derived LTC$_4$, in response to IgG activation, is increased up to 10-fold in "activated" hypodense eosinophils compared with normodense eosinophils (see below).

B. Complement Receptors: In normal individuals approximately 40–50% of eosinophils compared with 90% of neutrophils display complement receptors. The percentage of eosinophils bearing complement receptors is increased in the hypereosinophilic syndrome, helminth infections, and atopy. This suggests that activation of eosinophil complement receptors in these disorders may play a role in the inflammatory response of the eosinophil. The eosinophil CR3 receptor (which binds C3bi) appears to be more important than the CR1 receptor in mediating adherence and parasite cytotoxicity to antibody-schistosomula targets.

Activated Eosinophils

When peripheral blood eosinophils are separated on a density gradient, a subpopulation of low-density or "hypodense" eosinophils can be separated from normal or "normodense" eosinophils. Evidence that the hypodense eosinophils are cells that have been activated and degranulated in vivo includes (1) an altered expression of cell surface antigenic determinants, (2) an increased expression of IgG and IgE Fc receptors, (3) altered oxidative metabolism, (4) increased generation of LTC_4 after incubation with IgG-coated particles, and (5) an increased capacity to kill schistosomula of the parasite *Schistosoma mansoni* in vitro. Peripheral blood "activated" hypodense eosinophils have been found in patients with atopy, asthma, chronic helminthic infections, the idiopathic hypereosinophilic syndrome, and neoplasms. Eosinophils can be activated by vascular endothelium, T cell-derived cytokines (GM-CSF, IL-3, and IL-5), and monocyte-macrophage-derived cytokines (IL-1 and tumor necrosis factor [TNF]).

Effector Function

Helminthic (metazoan) parasites, especially those with tissue-dwelling phases, are associated with a prominent blood and/or tissue eosinophilia. This does not occur in protozoan infections. Eosinophil chemotactic and activating factors derived from mast cells, monocytes, and T lymphocytes appear to regulate eosinophil effector function in killing parasites. In vitro a number of parasites, including *Trichinella*, schistosomes, and *Fasciola*, can be killed or damaged by eosinophils. As the parasite represents a large, noningestible microorganism to the eosinophil, eosinophil cytotoxicity requires direct eosinophil-parasite cell contact. In vivo studies have shown that eosinophils accumulate around parasites in tissues and deposit toxic cytoplasmic granule contents on tissue parasites. The eosinophil, with its cationic secondary cytoplasmic granules and potent generated oxidants, is well equipped to destroy these multicellular organisms.

The role of eosinophilic inflammation in allergy has been studied most thoroughly in the pathogenesis of the airway inflammatory response in asthma. The hexagonal, bipyramidal Charcot-Leyden crystals, first found in 1872 in the sputum of patients with asthma, are "footprints" of the eosinophil inflammatory response in the airway. The Charcot-Leyden crystal is a protein with lysophospholipase activity derived from the eosinophil cell surface membrane. Major basic protein liberated from eosinophil cytoplasmic granules has been shown to be toxic to respiratory epithelium, and its levels are elevated in the sputum and bronchoalveolar lavage fluid of asthmatic patients.

Although eosinophils are able to function as phagocytes, they are less efficient than neutrophils both in the rate of phagocytosis and in the quantity of material ingested. Eosinophils are able to ingest bacteria, fungi, mycoplasmas, inert particles, and antigen-antibody complexes in vitro, but conclusive evidence for a functional role as phagocytic cells in vivo is still awaited.

MACROPHAGES

Macrophages share with neutrophils a central role in host defense against infection, which includes ingesting and killing invading organisms and releasing a number of factors involved in host defense and inflammation. They also function as antigen-presenting cells (APC) during the development of specific immunity (see Chapter 5). They are similar to neutrophils in their phagocytic capacity and in their potent array of cytoplasmic granule-derived hydrolytic enzymes and production of toxic oxygen metabolites. In contrast to neutrophils, macrophages have long life spans, can differentiate in situ, respond to external stimuli with a relatively slow and sustained time course, and usually become prominent in inflammatory lesions after the first 8–12 hours. Macrophages and neutrophils differ in their distribution of cytoplasmic granuloenzymes, reuse phagolysosomes to reconstruct their plasma membranes, and secrete nonlysosomal proteins.

Monocyte-Macrophage Formation

The cells in the mononuclear phagocyte system (previously termed the reticuloendothelial system) include promonocytes and their precursors in the bone marrow, monocytes in the circulation, and tissue macrophages. In the bone marrow, over a period of approximately 6 days, a committed progenitor cell termed "colony-forming unit granulocyte macrophage" (CFU-GM) differentiates under the influence of locally produced colony-stimulating factors (CSF) into a monoblast. The monoblast differentiates into a promonocyte and subsequently is released into the circulation as a monocyte. Monocytes are large cells with an oval, indented, or "folded" nucleus possessing lacy to strandlike chromatin and plentiful, gray-blue cytoplasm containing fine azurophilic granules. Human monocytes, circulating in the bloodstream, have a half-life of about 1–3 days. Migration of monocytes into the different tissues appears to be a random phenomenon in the absence of localized inflammation. Compared with neutrophils, monocytes have a much smaller bone marrow reserve, a longer intravascular half-life, and a larger extravascular tissue compartment. The tissue macrophage arises either by immigration of monocytes from the blood (probably the predominant mechanism) or by proliferation of precursors in local sites. Macrophages differ from monocytes in their relative enzymatic activities, their phagocytic capacities, and their cell surface membrane characteristics. The macrophage cell surface membrane has more immunoglobulin and complement receptors than the precursor monocyte does. During differentiation of monocytes to macrophages, azurophilic peroxidase-containing cytoplasmic granules are lost and lysosymes containing hydrolytic enzymes become prominent. Monocytes are richly endowed with myeloperoxidase, whereas tissue macrophages are not.

In the presence of helper T cells, macrophages may become actively endocytic cells organized into structures (granulomas) that are the hallmark of delayed hypersensitivity reactions. Macrophages that have accumulated at a site of chronic inflammation often differentiate further to form epithelioid cells, or they may fuse to form multinucleated giant cells.

Ultrastructure & Receptors

The ultrastructure of the macrophage is shown in Fig 12–6. The macrophages of the liver (Kupffer cells), lungs (alveolar macrophages), connective tissue (histiocytes), bone (osteoclasts), skin (Langerhans cells), central nervous system (microglial cells), and serous cavities (pleural and peritoneal macrophages) all belong to the mononuclear phagocyte series. Characteristic features of macrophages include the ability to adhere to glass, phagocytose, ruffle their membranes, display immunoglobulin Fc receptors, and stain positively for nonspecific esterase and peroxidase. The macrophage samples and senses its environment through specific cell surface membrane receptors, which include receptors for immunoglobulin and complement (IgG, IgE, C3b, C5a), hematopoietic growth factors (M-CSF, GM-CSF), lipoproteins, peptides, and polysaccharides (Table 12–2). Binding of agonists to these receptors is the initial step in the series of actions that eventuate in macrophage proliferation, chemotaxis, phagocytosis, secretion, or oxygen consumption. Occupancy of these receptors can activate the macrophage to secrete soluble products (including IL-1, hydrolytic enzymes, and products of oxidative metabolism) that endow the macrophage with the capacity to exert pro- or anti-inflammatory effects on the function of other cell types.

Activation

Activated macrophages exhibit morphologic, metabolic, and functional differences from resting macrophages. In its most commonly accepted sense, an "activated" macrophage is one that has an enhanced capacity to kill facultative intracellular microorganisms or tumor cells. During an infection, specific effector T lymphocytes, sensitized to antigens from the infecting organism, release soluble factors, such as gamma interferon and GM-CSF, that can activate macrophages. In this manner the induction of macrophage activation is immunologically specific (T cell-microbial antigen interaction), whereas its expression (macrophage activation) is nonspecific and consists, in essence, of an enhanced antimicrobial capacity. Macrophages are attracted to sites of inflammation by chemotactic factors derived from serum (C5a), lymphocytes, neutrophils, and fibroblasts. As with the neutrophil, phagocytosis is influenced by the presence of opsonins for the invading microorganism (IgG, complement, and perhaps fibronectin) as well as by the inherent surface properties of the microorganism. Macrophage activation is evident from morphologic changes (larger size, ruffling of the plasma membrane, increased formation of pseudopods, increased number of pinocytic vesicles), metabolic changes (increased glucose metabolism and respiratory oxidant burst), and functional changes (more vigorous migration in response to chemotactic factors, increased microbicidal activity) exhibited by the activated macrophage.

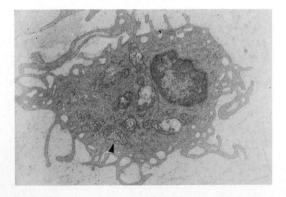

Figure 12–6. Electron micrograph of a macrophage revealing a cell with a single nucleus and cytoplasm containing modest numbers of mitochondria (arrowhead). The numerous cell surface projections (filopodia) are consistent with the motile nature of this phagocytic cell. (Courtesy of Henry C Powell.)

Phagocytosis & Secretion

Macrophages are able to internalize material external to the cell (endocytosis) by means of phagocytosis (the ingestion of particulate material) or pinocytosis (the ingestion of soluble materials). The generation of pinocytic vesicles is a constitutive event, which proceeds without known exogenous stimuli in an energy-dependent manner. In this way large amounts of the plasma membrane are continually recycled, allowing a constant re-utilization of the plasma membrane and its receptors, as well as allowing a constant flow of solutes into the cell. Particle ingestion by macrophages is usually accompanied by a respiratory oxidant burst similar to that in neutrophils and eosinophils. Macrophage phagocytosis requires the expenditure of metabolic energy in the form of high-energy phosphate. The source of high-energy phosphate is creatine phosphate in the macrophage, compared with ATP in the neutrophil.

In addition to their role as phagocytic cells, macrophages are secretory and regulatory cells. The macrophage is an extraordinarily active secretory cell, having the capacity to produce approximately 100 different substances affecting the inflammatory response. Some of the macrophage products are secreted constitutively (lysosome, lipoprotein lipase), whereas others follow ligand-receptor interaction. Some ligands, such as immune complexes, trigger secretion in seconds to minutes after macrophage stimulation, whereas others, including lymphocyte mediators, require days after the stimulus for macrophage secretion.

In general, the antimicrobial spectrum of macrophages exceeds that of neutrophils, although neutrophils kill many organisms more rapidly than do macrophages. In addition to antimicrobial activity, macrophages subserve a number of important effector functions including antitumor function, immunoregulatory function, wound healing, and selective removal of autologous cells (senescent cells, cells targeted by autoimmune reactions, and metabolically defective cells). Macrophages can also play an important role in the resolution of acute inflammation. In addition to secreting extracellular proteases, which help liquefy the residual inflammatory exudate, macrophages phagocytose cellular debris, inflammatory exudate, and senescent neutrophils.

PLATELETS

Platelets, which arise in the bone marrow from megakaryocyte cytoplasm and thus lack a nucleus, are the smallest circulating cells (2 μm in diameter). Unstimulated platelets, which contain 3 types of cytoplasmic granules (dense bodies, α granules, and lysosomal granules), circulate as flattened disks remaining within the intravascular space during their 10-day life span. Platelet activation is characterized by a change in platelet morphology, platelet aggregation, generation of arachidonic acid metabolites (prostaglandins G_2 and H_2, thromboxane A_2), and secretion of plate-

let cytoplasmic granule contents. Although the content of preformed cytoplasmic granule mediators in platelets resembles that in other secretory inflammatory cells, the confinement of platelets to the intravascular compartment (intact platelets are rarely found extravascularly at inflammatory sites) suggests that platelets have a more limited role than the other cells in inflammation. This does not exclude the possibility that intravascularly activated platelets generate inflammatory mediators which might exert their effects at extravascular sites of tissue inflammation.

The role of platelets in inflammatory reactions is therefore not as well defined as that of the neutrophil, eosinophil, macrophage, or mast cell. However, activated platelets may contribute to inflammatory responses by releasing clotting and growth factors, amines, and lipids with vasoactivity, as well as neutral and acid hydrolases. Activated platelets may also aggregate and serve as foci that trap responding leukocytes and help produce vascular occlusion. Platelets are able to interact with the immune system through platelet cell surface $Fc\gamma R$ and $Fc\epsilon RII$. The interaction of platelets with components of the immune system includes platelet binding of IgG and generation of platelet-derived proinflammatory mediators in response to IgG-immune complex platelet activation. Platelets also express 6×10^4 $Fc\epsilon RII$ per cell (Table 12–2). Activation of $Fc\epsilon RII$ on the platelet induces the formation of a factor cytotoxic to parasites (probably hydrogen peroxide or oxygen metabolites), but it does not lead to the release of the contents of the platelet cytoplasmic granules, nor to platelet aggregation. Activation of the platelet $Fc\epsilon RII$ also induces production of PAF, a potent inflammatory mediator. The platelet therefore may play a role in cellular inflammation, in addition to its role in hemostasis and thrombosis.

ENDOTHELIUM

Recent evidence has led to the appreciation that endothelial cells are not merely conduit cells lining blood vessels and thus passive bystanders in the inflammatory response, but, rather, are actively involved in modulating the inflammatory response of the circulating inflammatory cells. Endothelial cells "activated" by various inflammatory cytokines (IL-1, TNF) exhibit increased adhesivity for many circulating inflammatory cells (monocytes, neutrophils). This increased endothelial adhesivity is probably important in recruiting circulating inflammatory cells to sites of tissue inflammation. Endothelial cells are also capable of secreting the cytokines IL-1 and GM-CSF, which are important modulators of the inflammatory response (see Chapter 7).

SUMMARY

Although the inflammatory cells differ in morphology, mediator content, stimuli for cell activation, and time course for mediator release, they do have many features in common. These common cellular features include common receptors (immunoglobulin and complement), cytoplasmic granules containing potent hydrolytic enzymes, the generation of arachidonic acid metabolites, and the ability to phagocytose or secrete. As tissue inflammation may be mediated by serum proteins or inflammatory cells, the control of the interrelated feedback systems is important to host defense. Cellular inflammation is a double-edged sword, being a crucial form of host defense but having serious deleterious effects if it is either inadequately or excessively activated.

In attempting to define the precise roles played by the different cell types in inflammation, important advances have been made in characterizing the structure and function of purified populations of the various inflammatory cells. However, the local environment in inflamed tissues represents a complex milieu in which many different inflammatory cells and serum proteins are present, raising the possibility of important modulating effects, which will not be recognized when only pure cell populations are studied. Despite the complexity of the inflammatory responses, it seems likely that there is considerable coordination and cooperation between the different cell types, which is mediated through inflammatory mediators and shared common receptors (ie, immunoglobulin and complement). Further characterization of the various inflammatory cells and their subtypes will assist in improving our understanding of the complex cellular interactions involved in cellular inflammation.

REFERENCES

Neutrophils

Cohen AM, et al: In vivo stimulation of granulopoieses by recombinant human granulocyte colony-stimulating factor. *Proc Natl Acad Sci USA* 1987;**84**:2484.

Goetzl EJ, Goldstein IM: Granulocytes. Chap 19, pp 322–345, in: *Textbook of Rheumatology,* 3rd ed. Kelley WN et al (editors). Saunders, 1989.

Lehrer RI et al: Neutrophils and host defense. *Ann Intern Med* 1988;**109**:127.

Malech HL, Gallin JI: Neutrophils in human diseases. *N Engl J Med* 1987;**317**:687.

Metcalf D: The molecular biology and functions of the granulocyte-macrophage colony-stimulating factors. *Blood* 1986;**67**:257.

Sklar LA: Ligand-receptor dynamics and signal amplification in the neutrophil. *Adv Immunol* 1986;**39**:95.

Macrophages

Adams DO: Molecular interactions in macrophage activation. *Immunol. Today* 1989;**10**:33.

Clark SC, Kamen R: The human hematopoietic colony-stimulating factors. *Science* 1987;**236**:1229.

Henson PM et al: Phagocytic cells: Degranulation and secretion. Chap 22, pp 363–390, in: *Inflammation: Basic Principles and Clinical Correlates.* Gallin JI et al (editors). Raven Press, 1988.

Johnston RB Jr: Current concepts in immunology: Monoctyes and macrophages. *N Engl J Med* 1988;**318**:747.

Roska AK, Lipsky PE: Monocytes and macrophages. Chap 20, pp 346–366, in: *Textbook of Rheumatology,* 3rd ed. Kelley WN et al (editors). Saunders, 1989.

Stossel TP: The molecular biology of phagocytes and the molecular basis of non-neoplastic phagocyte disorders. Chap 14, pp 499–533, in: *The Molecular Basis of Blood Diseases.* Stamatoyannopoulos G. et al (editors). Saunders, 1987.

Unanue ER, Allen PM: The basis for the immunoregulatory role of macrophages and other accessory cells. *Science* 1987;**236**:551.

Mast Cells & Basophils

Charlesworth EN et al: Cutaneous late phase response to allergen. Mediator release and inflammatory cell infiltration. *J Clin Invest* 1989;**83**:1519.

Helm B et al: The mast cell binding site on human immunoglobulin E. *Nature* 1988;**331**:180.

Irani AA et al: Two types of human mast cells that have distinct neutral protease compositions. *Proc Natl Acad Sci USA* 1986;**83**:4464.

Lemanske RF Jr, Kaliner M: Late-phase IgE-mediated reactions. *J Clin Immunol* 1988;**8**:1.

Schwartz LB et al: Tryptase levels as an indicator of mast cell activation in systemic anaphylaxis and mastocytosis. *N Engl J Med* 1987;**316**:1622.

Serafin WE, Austen KF: Mediators of immediate hypersensitivity reactions. *N Engl J Med* 1987; **317**:31.

Stevens RL, Austen KF: Recent advances in the cellular and molecular biology of mast cells. *Immunol Today* 1989;**10**:381.

Stevens RL et al: Biochemical characteristics distinguish subclasses of mammalian mast cells. Pages 183–203, in: *Mast Cell Differentiation and Heterogeneity.* Befus AD, Bienenstock J, Denburg JA (editors). Raven Press, 1986.

Eosinophils

Campbell HD et al: Molecular cloning, nucleotide sequence, and expression of the gene encoding human eosinophil differentiation factor (interleukin 5). *Proc Natl Acad Sci USA* 1987;**84**:6629.

Gleich GJ: Current understanding of eosinophil function. *Hosp Pract* 1988;**23**:137.

Gleich GJ, Adolphson CR: The eosinophil leukocyte: Structure and function. *Adv Immunol* 1986;**39**:177.

Rothenberg ME et al: Eosinophils co-cultured with endothelial cells have increased survival and functional properties. *Science* 1987;**237**:645.

Wardlaw AJ, Kay AB: The role of the eosinophil in the pathogenesis of asthma. *Allergy* 1987;**42**:321.

Platelets

Ginsberg MH: Role of platelets in inflammation and rheumatic disease. *Adv Inflamm Res* 1986;**2**:53.

Kunicki TJ, George JN (editors): *Platelet Immunobiology: Molecular and Clinical Aspects.* Lippincott, 1989.

Endothelium

Jaffe EA: Cell biology of endothelial cells. *Hum Pathol* 1987;**18**:234.

13

Mediators of Inflammation

Stephen I. Wasserman, MD

The various inflammatory cells discussed in Chapter 12 mediate their responses by releasing or generating chemical compounds or by recruiting other cells to release or activate additional chemical mediators. Our current knowledge of the chemistry, sources, actions, and mechanisms of generation of inflammatory mediators comes largely from studies of allergic diseases, especially IgE-mediated hypersensitivity.

Mediators of inflammation therefore are endogenous chemicals arising from the activation of inflammatory cells by an immune reaction. They are also released or generated from direct stimulation of the cells by cytokines or releasing factors or by exogenous drugs or chemicals. Mediators may be classified by function: (1) those with vasoactive and smooth-muscle-constricting properties, (2) those that attract other cells and are termed chemotactic factors, (3) enzymes, (4) proteoglycans, and (5) reactive molecules generated from the metabolism of oxygen (Table 13–1).

VASOACTIVE & SMOOTH-MUSCLE-CONSTRICTING MEDIATORS

Histamine

Histamine is a vasoactive and smooth-muscle-constricting mediator that is found preformed in the granules of mast cells and basophils (Fig 13–1). Other mediators with these properties are generated from inactive precursors following cell activation. Histamine is generated in this site by the action of histidine decarboxylase upon the amino acid histidine. Mast cells and basophils store approximately 5 and 1 μg of histamine/10^6 cells, respectively. Histamine may make up as much as 10% of the weight of the granule of these cells. It is bound through ionic linkages to proteoglycans and proteins within the mast cell and basophil granule and is particularly tightly bound to mast cell heparin. It is displaced from its binding sites in the granule by exposure to an increased ionic concentration. Levels of histamine in the blood are highest in the morning and lowest in the late afternoon; they approximate 0.3 ng/mL. A small proportion of histamine, approximating 12–16 μg/24 h, is excreted unchanged in the urine, and the remainder is excreted as metabolic products of the action of histamine methyltransferase and diamine oxidase.

Histamine is found almost exclusively throughout the organism in mast cells and basophils, and therefore tissue levels are particularly high in the intestine, lungs, and skin. Histamine is released from its cellular stores when the cells are activated immunologically by the action of antigen on cell-bound IgE antibodies or when they are activated by nonimmunologic mechanisms, as described in Chapter 11. Increased amounts occur in the circulation of patients with mastocytosis, and the levels are further elevated during attacks of this disorder. Elevated blood levels may also be detected during anaphylaxis, asthma, and a variety of physical urticarias. Increases in local concentrations of histamine have been identified in bronchoalveolar lavage fluid of patients experiencing allergic reactions during allergen provocation or during experimental provocation of asthma and in blister fluids of patients with experimentally induced urticaria.

Histamine exerts its physiologic action by interacting with one of 3 separate target cell receptors, termed H1, H2, and H3 (Table 13–2). The primary H1 functions of histamine, identified by the inhibitory effects of the classic antihistamines, are (1) contraction of smooth muscle of bronchi, intestine, and uterus, and (2) augmentation of vascular permeability between post-capillary venular endothelial cells. Other H1 actions of histamine include pulmonary vasoconstriction, elevation of intracellular levels of cyclic GMP, augmentation of nasal mucus production, enhanced leukocyte chemokinesis, and production of prostaglandins from lung tissue. Stimulation of the H2 receptor augments gastric acid secretion, stimulates airway mucus production, augments intracellular levels of cyclic AMP, inhibits leukocyte chemokinesis,

Table 13-1. Mediators.

Vasoactive and smooth-muscle-constricting mediators
  Preformed
    Histamine
  Generated
    Arachidonic acid metabolites (PGD$_2$, LTC$_4$)
    PAF
    Adenosine
Chemotactic mediators
  Eosinophil-directed
    ECF-A
    ECF oligopeptides
    PAF
  Neutrophil-directed
    HMW-NCF
    LTB$_4$
    PAF
  Monocyte-directed
    Uncharacterized
  Basophil-directed
    Uncharacterized
  Lymphocyte-directed
    Uncharacterized
Enzymatic mediators
  Neutral proteases
    Tryptase—all mast cells
    Chymase—connective-tissue mast cells
  Lysosomal hydrolases
    Arylsulfatase
    β-Glucuronidase
    β-Hexosaminidase
  Other Enzymes
    Superoxide dismutase
    Peroxidase

Table 13-2. Histamine receptors.

Receptor	Histamine Actions
H1	Increased post-capillary venular permeability Smooth muscle contraction Pulmonary vasoconstriction Increased cGMP levels in cells Enhanced mucus secretion Leukocyte chemokinesis Prostaglandin production in lungs
H2	Enhanced gastric acid secretion Enhanced mucus secretion Increased cAMP levels in cells Leukocyte chemokinesis Activation of suppressor T cells
H3	Histamine release inhibition Histamine synthesis inhibition

and stimulates suppressor T lymphocytes. Stimulation of the H3 receptor has been best studied in central nervous tissue, where it inhibits the release and blunts the synthesis of histamine. Co-stimulation of H1 and H2 receptors causes maximal vasodilatation, cardiac irritability, and pruritus.

The clinical consequences of the release of histamine or its instillation into tissue include wheal-and-flare reactions in the skin associated with pruritus and flushing, bronchoconstriction and mucus secretion in the airways, intestinal cramping, gastric acid and enzyme release, intestinal mucus production, hypotension, and cardiac dysrhythmias. H1 actions of histamine can be blunted through the use of any of the large number of H1-directed antihistamines; H2 actions can

be prevented by a number of compounds (eg, cimetidine and ranitidine); and H3 actions can be blocked by certain investigational compounds not available as drugs.

Metabolites of Arachidonic Acid

Prostaglandins and leukotrienes, products of the enzymatic cyclo-oxygenation and lipoxygenation, respectively, of arachidonic acid derived from cell membrane phospholipid, are two major families of inflammatory mediators (Fig 13-2). Their actions are broad, varying with the target tissue, and encompass vasoactive, smooth-muscle-active, and chemotactic properties.

Arachidonic acid, a 20-carbon, 4-double-bond fatty acid, is liberated from membrane phospholipids either through the sequential action of phospholipase C and diacylglycerol lipase or by the direct action of phospholipase A$_2$ upon membrane phospholipid. Once liberated, arachidonic acid is

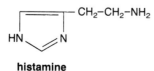

histamine

Figure 13-1. Chemical structure of histamine.

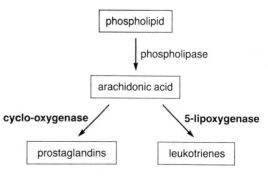

Figure 13-2. Derivation of prostaglandins and leukotrienes from arachidonic acid by the enzymes cyclo-oxygenase and 5-lipoxygenase, respectively.

reesterified or metabolized by either the cyclo-oxygenase or lipoxygenase pathways.

A. Cyclo-oxygenase Products: The product of cyclooxygenase action upon arachidonic acid in mast cells is prostaglandin D_2 (PGD$_2$) (Fig 13-3). Basophils, on the other hand, do not generate cyclo-oxygenase products of arachidonic acid. Connective tissue-type mast cells, when activated, appear to preferentially generate PGD$_2$ from liberated arachidonic acid. As is true of other prostaglandins, PGD$_2$ production is inhibited by nonsteroidal anti-inflammatory drugs, which, however, do not alter the release of other mast cell mediators. PGD$_2$ induces more prolonged erythema and wheal-and-flare vasopermeability responses in skin than histamine does.

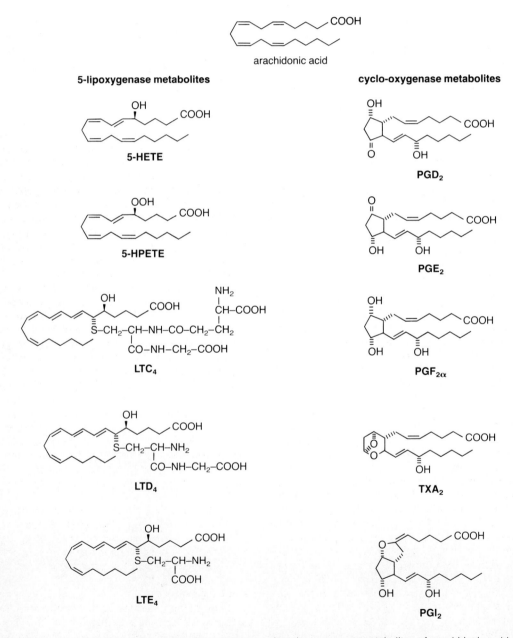

Figure 13-3. Chemical structures of the 5-lipoxygenase and cyclo-oxygenase metabolites of arachidonic acid. The compounds depicted in the figure are physiologically active mediators of inflammation.

It also mediates a neutrophil infiltrate into skin and augments chemotaxis and chemokinesis of leukocytes in vitro. The systemic flushing and hypotensive episodes in patients with systemic mastocytosis have been attributed to this arachidonic acid product.

B. Lipoxygenase Products: When arachidonic acid is metabolized via the lipoxygenase pathway, a family of compounds is generated that contains 4 principal biologically active compounds, termed leukotrienes: leukotriene B_4 (LTB_4), LTC_4, LTD_4, and LTE_4 (Fig. 13–3). These are the predominant products of mucosal mast cells. LTB_4 is a dihydroxylated product with chemotactic potency (see below). LTC_4 is generated from lipoxygenase-modified arachidonic acid following the addition of the tripeptide glutathione; it forms one of the moieties of what was once termed "slow-reacting substance of anaphylaxis." The sequential modification of the terminal amino acids on the Cys-Gly-Glu tripeptide leads to the production of LTD_4 and LTE_4. This modification occurs through the action of γ-glutamyltranspeptidase and a variety of other peptidases found in biologic materials. These modified lipoxygenase products, known as the sulfidopeptide leukotrienes, are potent inducers of smooth muscle contractility, bronchoconstriction and mucus secretion in the airway, and the wheal-and-flare reaction in the skin. When injected intravenously, they may cause hypotension and cardiac dysrhythmias. The leukotrienes are several-hundredfold more potent on a molar basis than is histamine and are therefore believed to have an important role in the genesis of allergic disorders. At present, there are no inhibitors of leukotrienes that are sufficiently selective for clinical use.

Platelet-Activating Factor

Platelet-activating factor (PAF) is generated from a complex lipid that is stored in the precursor state in cell membranes. This lipid has a glycerol backbone modified in 3 ways: (1) on the first carbon of the glycerol backbone is located a long-chain alcohol molecule, usually of 16–18 carbons; (2) the second position in the storage form is generally arachidonic acid; and (3) on the third carbon is a phosphorocholine moiety (Fig 13–4). The activation of cells leads to the liberation of the arachidonic acid from the 2-position, and the addition at this site of an acetate group leads to the generation of fully active PAF. This molecule was originally named because it activates rabbit platelets. More recently, it has been determined that it has a number of other biologic effects, but the original descriptive name has been retained.

The biologic activity requires a long-chain alcohol of 16–18 carbons in the 1-position, the acetate group in the 2-position, and the phosphorocnoline

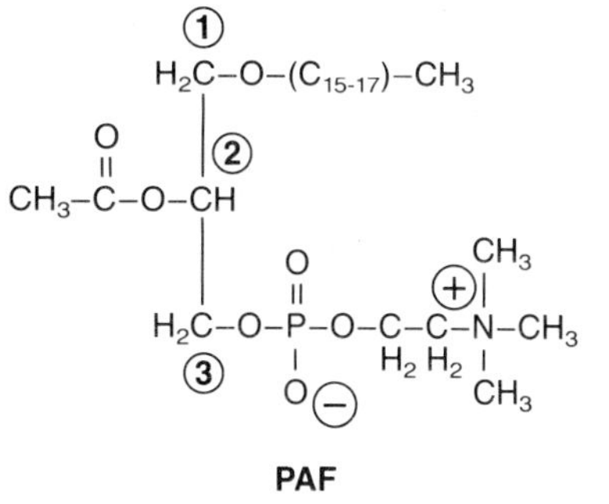

Figure 13-4. Chemical structure of platelet-activating factor (PAF). The biologically active moieties 1, 2, and 3 are discussed in the text.

moiety. PAF activates a variety of cell types, including platelets, whose mechanism of activation involves induction of aggregation and release of platelet granule constituents. It also activates neutrophils and eosinophils, causing the release of granular constituents, and is the most potent eosinophil chemoattractant yet described. When it is injected intravenously, its effects on those target cells are evidenced by transient neutropenia, thrombocytopenia, and basopenia. In addition, intravenous injection is associated with marked hypotension. When injected in the skin, PAF causes a wheal-and-flare reaction and leukocyte infiltration. When inhaled, it causes bronchoconstriction, an eosinophil infiltrate, and a state of nonspecific bronchial hyperreactivity that may persist for days to weeks following a single administration. Many of the actions of PAF are platelet-dependent, so that abrogation of platelets in animal models diminishes the ability of PAF to alter pulmonary resistance and compliance, although without affecting its ability to attract leukocytes or to induce hypotension or cardiac depression. In vivo, PAF is rapidly degraded by an acid-labile acetylhydrolase enzyme found in plasma, and it can also be degraded by a variety of phospholipases present in cells and tissues throughout the body.

Inhibitors of PAF action have been identified in biologic extracts from the Gingko tree, and a variety of other compounds are currently being studied for inhibition of this interesting molecule, but none are yet available for clinical use.

Adenosine

Adenosine is a nucleoside that is liberated from mast cells following the utilization of ATP during the degranulation process (Fig 13–5). It may be degraded by adenosine deaminase or may be taken up again by the cell and phosphorylated into

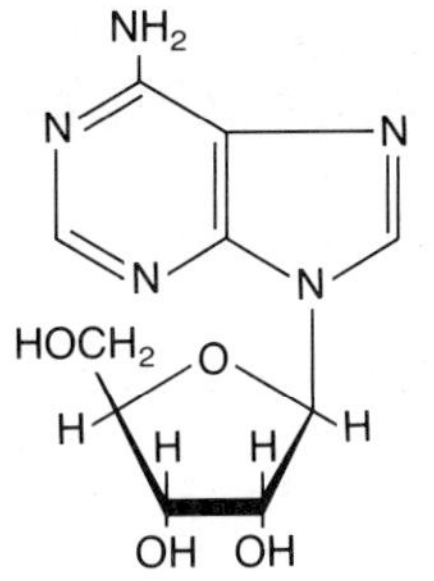

Figure 13-5. Chemical structure of adenosine.

AMP. The blood levels of adenosine approximate 0.3 μmol/L, a concentration at which this molecule is minimally biologically active. These levels increase during hypoxia and antigen bronchoprovocation challenge of patients with asthma. Adenosine interacts with 2 receptors, termed A1 and A2, on cell surfaces. The A2 receptor is linked to elevations in intracellular levels of cyclic AMP and is blocked by methylxanthine drugs, further supporting a role for adenosine in asthma. When inhaled, adenosine causes bronchoconstriction, which can be inhibited by antihistamine. In vitro, adenosine does not cause mast cell mediator release, but it potentiates IgE-induced mast cell mediator release through an action on mast cell adenosine A2 receptors. This potentiation is believed to occur through a protein phosphorylation step, whose exact properties remain to be elucidated. Adenosine is also capable of inducing fluid and electrolyte secretion from intestinal epithelia.

CHEMOTACTIC MEDIATORS

Mast cells and basophils generate and release compounds that are capable of interacting with other leukocytes in augmenting their nonspecific or directed migration and are therefore termed **chemotactic mediators.** Some of these mediators are cell-specific, whereas others are directed at a variety of lymphocyte populations.

Eosinophil Chemotactic Mediators

It has long been known that immediate hypersensitivity reactions are associated with peripheral blood and tissue eosinophilia. For this reason, eosinophil chemotactic factors were the first to be investigated and identified. Two low-molecular-weight tetrapeptides of the sequence Val-Gly-Ser-Glu and Ala-Gly-Ser-Glu were isolated and termed collectively the eosinophil chemotactic factor of anaphylaxis (ECF-A). These molecules are very weak chemoattractant substances for eosinophils and are capable of augmenting eosinophil expression of complement receptors and of PAF synthesis. Molecules of similar molecular weight and charge have been identified in the blood of patients undergoing experimental bronchoprovocation challenge and patients with physical urticaria. Another family of chemotactic mediators of molecular weight between 1500 and 3000, which are presumed to be peptides, have also been identified in experimental model systems of asthma and urticaria. They are also capable of attracting eosinophils in vitro, but their other biologic potencies have yet to be investigated. The most potent eosinophil chemoattractant factor yet identified is PAF (see above). This molecule, although capable of attracting a variety of leukocytes, demonstrates at concentrations of 10^{-6}–10^{-11} mol/L a dose-dependent chemoattractant effect for eosinophils, far more potent than any other mediator yet identified.

Neutrophil-Directed Chemoattractant Factors

Three main molecular species capable of modulating neutrophil chemokinesis and chemotaxis are generated during mast cell mediated reactions. A protein of MW 660,000, termed high-molecular-weight neutrophil chemotactic factor (HMW-NCF), is the most unusual of these. It has been identified during experimental induction of physical urticaria and allergen-mediated bronchoconstriction. The molecule appears in the circulation very shortly after experimental challenge and during the late phase of IgE-mediated reactions. Its release is inhibited by pretreatment of allergic subjects with cromolyn, but its exact cell source and biologic role remain to be identified. It causes a transient neutrophilic leukocytosis and an increased expression of complement receptors upon neutrophils. Two low-molecular-weight mediators capable of modulating neutrophil chemotaxis are also generated by mast cells: (1) LTB$_4$, the dihydroxy product of the action of the lipoxygenase pathway upon arachidonic acid, and (2) PAF. These molecules are active at 10^{-6}–10^{-10} mol/L, similar in potency to C5a and much greater than any other neutrophil chemoattractant molecules. The exact role of these molecules in activating neutrophils during inflammation remains to be identified. However, as the chemotactic activation of neutrophils is associated with the production of toxic oxygen species (see below), their relevance to allergic inflammation may be more pertinent than previously assumed.

ENZYMATIC MEDIATORS

A variety of enzymes are present in mast cell and basophil granules and are released upon activation of these cells. Two major categories have been identified: (1) neutral proteases and (2) lysosomal hydrolases.

Neutral Proteases

Human and animal mast cells contain several neutral proteases, which not only are useful in characterizing the cells and identifying them in tissue, but also are believed to have important biologic properties. The first to be identified is a tryptic protease present in all mucosal and connective-tissue mast cells. This is a 4-chain heterodimer of MW 144,000, with trypsin-like potency. This enzyme makes up 25–50% of the granular protein in mast cell granules and is resistant to the action of circulating antiproteases. It is stabilized by its binding to granular heparin, and its biologic activity rapidly decays when this binding is broken. Although tryptase possesses some tryptic specificity, it differs from trypsin in the molecules that it cleaves, and therefore one cannot predict which substrates are susceptible to its action. It is known to cleave C3, to generate C3a, and to alter many of the blood-clotting proteins, but it is inactive on C5. A number of protease effects have been identified within supernatants of challenged human mast cells, including activation of kallikrein and cleavage of kininogen.

A second neutral protease with the specificity of chymotrypsin has also been identified and localized to human connective tissue but not mucosal mast cells. It is also abundant in the mast cell granule and may make up 10–20% of the granule protein in connective tissue mast cells. It may be distinguished from the tryptic protease by its lower molecular weight (26,000–30,000) and by its specificity for peptide substrates. One of its substrates appears to be angiotensinogen, but its natural substrate remains to be clearly elucidated, and its role in allergic pathophysiology is uncertain. Another mast-cell-neutral protease, carboxypeptidase A, has also been identified, and it, too, is richly present in mast cell granules.

Acid Hydrolases

A number of acid hydrolases, which are broadly distributed in primary lysosomes of a number of cells, are also found in mast cells. These hydrolases include β-hexosaminidase, which has been used as a marker of mast cell activation in vitro, β-glucuronidase, and arylsulfatase. Superoxide dismutase and peroxidase have been found in mast cell granules. It is speculated that these enzymes are capable of degrading ground substances such as chondroitin sulfates, but their specific functions are unknown.

PROTEOGLYCANS

The structural matrix of mast cell and basophil cytoplasmic granules contains chemical compounds known as **proteoglycans,** which are important in the storage and release of mediators from these cells. The major granular proteoglycan found in human mast cells is heparin. This proteoglycan (MW 60,000) is found at levels of approximately 5 μg/10^6 cells; it is an anticoagulant, and is also capable of modulating tryptase action. It is believed to act as a structural matrix for granular protein and amine binding. In addition to heparin, a highly sulfated granular proteoglycan, chondroitin sulfate E, is present in mast cells, whereas basophils contain chondroitin sulfates A and C. These compounds appear not only to act as structural molecules, but also to provide binding sites for the other mediators present within the mast cell granule.

TOXIC OXYGEN MOLECULES

Toxic oxygen molecules are liberated by activation of neutrophils, eosinophils, and probably also mast cells. Furthermore, mast cell chemoattractant molecules permit these cells to interact with neutrophils and eosinophils. As described in Chapter 12 (Table 12–3), NADPH oxidase donates an electron to oxygen to generate superoxide anion, which itself can interact with hydrogen ion to form hydrogen peroxide. Although the superoxide anion is short-lived, hydrogen peroxide is a rather stable molecule that can further mediate extracellular events, possibly leading to the generation of the hydroxyl radical, particularly in the presence of iron or other metal catalysts. In the presence of peroxidase, either myeloperoxidase from the neutrophil or the unique eosinophil peroxidase, hydrogen peroxide and a halide ion can generate a variety of hypohalous acids of the structure HOX. These molecules are capable of adding their halide ion, such as chloride, to a variety of biologic substrates, and they are believed to be important in biologic reactions in killing microorganisms. Other biologic reactions may be a consequence of the generation of hypohalous acids, for example, the generation of chloramines, which are relatively strong oxidants. Thus, the activation of the neutrophil, the eosinophil, or, presumably, the mast cell can lead to the sequential generation of superoxide anion, hydrogen peroxide, hydroxyl radical, hypohalous acid, and chloramines through the intercession of enzymes including NADPH oxidase and myeloperoxidase in the presence of a variety of metal ions as catalysts.

MEDIATOR INTERACTIONS

The panoply of mediators generated in allergic reactions and their overlapping biologic effects suggest that they may well interact in a synergistic or additive fashion. Known interactions include the interaction of histamine and leukotrienes, the interaction of heparin and tryptase, and, in cascade fashion, the induction of prostaglandins by histamine. Undoubtedly, other interactions remain to be discovered.

THE BIOLOGIC ROLE OF MEDIATORS

The best evidence for the role of mediators in allergic disease has come from studies of patients who are known to be sensitive to specific antigens and who are challenged by bronchoprovocation with aerosolized allergen. This causes acute bronchoconstriction within a few minutes of inhalation of antigen and spontaneous recovery within 30–60 minutes. In at least half of the subjects, a second, late-phase, IgE-mediated response occurs, which may begin within 2–4 hours and may persist for 4–18 hours (see Chapter 12).

In the early (immediate)-phase reaction, there is bronchial mucosal edema, erythema, mucous secretion, and bronchoconstriction. This reaction is accompanied by the release of histamine and a variety of neutrophil and eosinophil chemoattractants into the blood and the release of histamine, leukocyte chemoattractants, PGD_2, and sulfidopeptide leukotrienes in the bronchoalveolar lavage fluid. The late bronchial inflammatory reaction is accompanied in the blood by chemoattractant factors for neutrophils and eosinophils and by the evidence of neutrophil and particularly eosinophil infiltration into the airways. It appears, therefore, that the early reaction is dependent on vasoactive and bronchospastic mediators, particularly histamine, PGD_2, PAF, sulfidopeptide leukotrienes, and adenosine. Since potent H1 antihistamines and nonsteroidal anti-inflammatory drugs blunt this early-phase response, it is likely that PGD_2 and histamine play a role in its expression. Although there are no specific inhibitors of the late-phase reaction, leukocyte infiltration is an important component, so PAF and other leukocyte chemoattractants probably play a major role in its expression.

More recent work has indicated that the mast cell growth and differentiation promoting cytokines, IL-3, IL-4, and GM-CSF, as well as other cytokines such as histamine-releasing factor generated from macrophages and lymphocytes, may activate mast cells to generate mediators. Therefore, the role of mast cells in inflammation may not be restricted to antigen-IgE antibody systems, but they may also interact with inflammatory systems dependent upon macrophages and lymphocytes. Although the participation of each of the mediators discussed above in the inflammatory responses in immunity and hypersensitivity has been well documented, the role, if any, of these mediators in normal physiologic functioning and homeostasis of the organism is unknown.

SUMMARY

The mediators of immediate hypersensitivity possess a sufficiently broad biologic spectrum of activity and potency to play a major role in human disease. Asthma, allergic rhinitis, and urticaria clearly owe their signs, symptoms, and chronicity to these mediators. Many other inflammatory disorders such as rheumatoid arthritis, vasculitis, and inflammatory bowel disease have, at least in the past, had manifestations due to these mediators. Important roles for these compounds in wound repair, angiogenesis, osteoporosis, and neural functioning have been suggested by well-controlled investigations. Clearly, the next decade holds extraordinary promise in expanding and elucidating the role for mediators of immediate hypersensitivity in health and disease.

REFERENCES

Wasserman SI: Mast cell mediators in the blood of patients with asthma. *Chest* 1985;**87**:13S.

Wasserman SI: Mediators of immediate hypersensitivity. *J Allergy Clin Immunol* 1983;**72**:101.

Wasserman SI: Platelet activating factor as a mediator of bronchial asthma. *Hosp Pract* 1988;**23**:49.

Weiss SJ: Toxic effects of neutrophils. *N Engl J Med* 1989;**320**:365.

Complement & Kinin

14

Michael M. Frank, MD

Complement activation, kinin generation, blood coagulation, and fibrinolysis are physiologic processes that occur through sequential cascadelike activation of enzymes normally present in their inactive forms in plasma. Although they are 4 distinct systems and perform different functions, they interact with each other and with various cell membrane proteins. The first two—complement and kinin—are the subjects of this chapter because of their involvement in immunologic effector responses.

THE COMPLEMENT SYSTEM

Complement is a collective term used to designate a group of plasma and cell membrane proteins that play a key role in the host defense process. Table 14–1 lists the major proteins, their molecular weights, and their serum concentrations.

FUNCTIONS OF COMPLEMENT

This complex system, which now numbers more than 25 proteins, acts in at least 3 major ways. The first and best-known function of the system is to cause lysis of cells, bacteria, and enveloped viruses. The second is to mediate the process of opsonization, in which foreign cells, bacteria, viruses, fungi, etc, are prepared for phagocytosis. This process involves the coating of the foreign particle with specific complement protein fragments that can be recognized by receptors for these fragments on phagocytic cells. Interaction with these receptors leads to binding of the particle to the cell membrane of the phagocyte, the first step in the phagocytic process.

The third function of the complement proteins is the generation of peptide fragments that regulate features of the inflammatory and immune response. These proteins play a role in vasodilatation at the site of inflammation, in adherence of the phagocytes to blood vessel endothelium and egress of the phagocyte from the vessel, in directed migration of phagocytic cells into areas of inflammation, and, ultimately, in clearing infectious agents from the body. Most of the early-acting proteins of this system are present in the circulation in an inactive form. The proteins undergo sequential activation to ultimately cause their biologic effects.

PATHWAYS OF COMPLEMENT ACTIVATION

Two major pathways of complement activation operate in plasma. A general scheme of the system is shown in Fig 14–1. The first complement activation pathway to be discovered is termed the **classic complement pathway.** Under normal physiologic conditions, activation of this pathway is initiated by antigen-antibody complexes. The second pathway, known as the **alternative complement pathway,** was discovered more recently, although phylogenetically it probably is the older activation pathway. It does not have an absolute requirement for antibody for activation. Both pathways function through the interaction of proteins termed components. Both proceed by means of sequential activation and assembly of a series of proteins, leading to the formation of a complex enzyme capable of binding and cleaving a key protein, C3, which is common to both pathways. Thereafter, the 2 pathways proceed together through binding of the terminal components to form a membrane attack complex, which ultimately causes cell lysis.

NOMENCLATURE

The proteins of the classic pathway and the terminal components are designated by numbers fol-

Table 14-1. Molecular weights and serum concentrations of complement components.

Classic Pathway Component	Molecular Weight	Serum Concentration (μg/mL)
C1q	410,000	70
C1r	85,000	34
C1s	85,000	31
C2	95,000	25
C3	195,000	1,200
C4	206,000	600
C5	180,000	85
C6	128,000	60
C7	120,000	55
C8	150,000	55
C9	79,000	60
Alternative pathway component		
Properdin	153,000	25
Factor B	100,000	225
Factor D	25,000	1
Inhibitors		
C1 Inhibitor	105,000	275
Factor I	105,000	34
Regulatory proteins		
C4-binding protein	560,000	8
Factor H	150,000	500

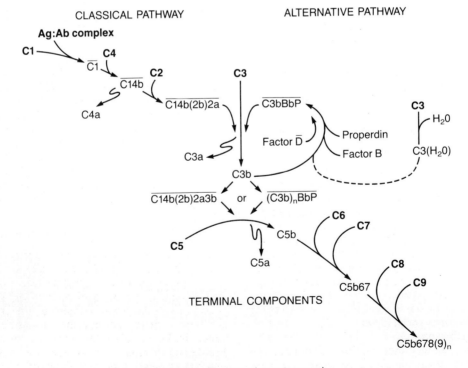

Figure 14-1. The complement cascade.

lowing the letter C. Proteins of the alternative pathway are generally given letter designations, as are other proteins that have major regulatory effects on the system. Under certain circumstances, which will be discussed briefly below, the pathways can be activated by nonimmunologic mechanisms, leading to the generation of biologically active products.

The proteins of each pathway interact in a precise sequence. When a protein is missing, as occurs in some of the genetic deficiencies, the sequence is interrupted at that point. The early steps in the activation process are associated with the assembly of complement cleavage fragments to form enzymes that bind the next proteins in the sequence to continue the reaction cascade. These enzymes are designated with a bar placed over the symbol of the component to indicate active enzymatic activity.

THE CLASSIC COMPLEMENT PATHWAY

The Function of Antibody & C1

In most cases, the classic pathway is initiated by the binding of antibody to an antigen. A single molecule of IgM antibody on an antigenic surface or 2 side-by-side molecules of IgG of the appropriate subclasses bind and activate C1, a macromolecular complex composed of 3 proteins—C1q, C1r, and C1s—held together in the presence of calcium ion. Binding to the antibody occurs via the C1q portion of the molecule. If the antibody-binding sites (epitopes) on a target antigen are too low in density for proper arrangement of antibody molecules, C1 binding may not occur. This is seen with erythrocytes coated with anti-Rh_0 (D) antibody. Although complement-activating subclasses of IgG are formed in response to this antigen, complement is not usually activated and has no role in the destruction of erythrocytes coated with anti-Rh_0 (D) antibody, because the proper complement-binding antibody doublets are not formed. The ability of antigen-antibody complex to interact with the C1q subcomponents of C1 serves as the basis for a group of assays used to detect immune complexes in serum samples: the C1q-binding assays. C1q is bound by IgM, IgG1, IgG2, and IgG3. It is not bound by IgG4, IgE, IgA, or IgD, so these antibody isotypes do not activate the classic pathway.

Nonimmunologic Classic Pathway Activators

It is of interest that a number of nonimmunologic activators of the classic pathway exist. Certain bacteria (eg, certain *Escherichia coli* and *Sal-*

monella strains of low virulence) and viruses (eg, parainfluenza virus) interact with C1q directly, causing C1 activation and, in turn, classic pathway activation in the absence of antibody. Such an interaction obviously would aid the host natural defense process. Other structures, eg, the surface of urate crystals, myelin basic protein, denatured DNA, bacterial endotoxin, and polyanions such as heparin, also may activate the classic pathway directly. Such activation by urate crystals is thought to contribute to the inflammation and pain associated with gout.

For simplicity, a series of block diagrams showing the interaction of the components is depicted in Figure 14-2. C1q is shown as a molecule with a central core and 6 radiating arms, each of which ends in a podlike structure. Each C1q molecule is composed of 18 separate polypeptide chains, divided into 3 chain types with 6 chains of each type. The amino-terminal segments of these chains closely resemble collagen and have a triple-helix, collagenlike structure. Thus, the arms of C1q are highly flexible. The globular heads contain the carboxy-terminal ends of the polypeptide chains and bind to the C_H2 domain of the appropriate immunoglobulin. The enzymatic potential of C1 resides in the C1r and C1s chains, which are associated with the collagenlike portion of the molecule. Each chain has a molecular weight of about 85,000 and is a proenzymatic form of a serine protease. There are one C1q, 2 C1r, and 2 C1s chains making up each C1 macromolecular complex.

Mechanism of C1 Activation

Binding of C1 to antibody is followed by activation of C1r and, in turn, C1s. This activation is associated with cleavage of the 2 identical C1r chains and of the 2 C1s chains. Each chain is cleaved into long and short fragments, with the appearance of an enzymatic site on the short fragment. It is believed that the function of the activated C1r enzyme, $\overline{C1r}$, is to cleave C1s, which then develops enzymatic activity. $\overline{C1s}$ cleaves the next portion in the sequence, C4 (Figs 14-1 and 14-2).

C4 & C2

C4 is a 3-chain molecule. The largest of the 3 chains, the α chain, is cleaved at a single site by $\overline{C1s}$, with the release of a small peptide, C4a. The larger peptide, consisting of most of the α chain together with the β and γ chains of C4, binds to the target cell to continue the complement cascade. Binding involves the formation of a covalent amide or ester bond between the target cell and the α chain of C4 (see the discussion of chemistry under C3 below). In the presence of magne-

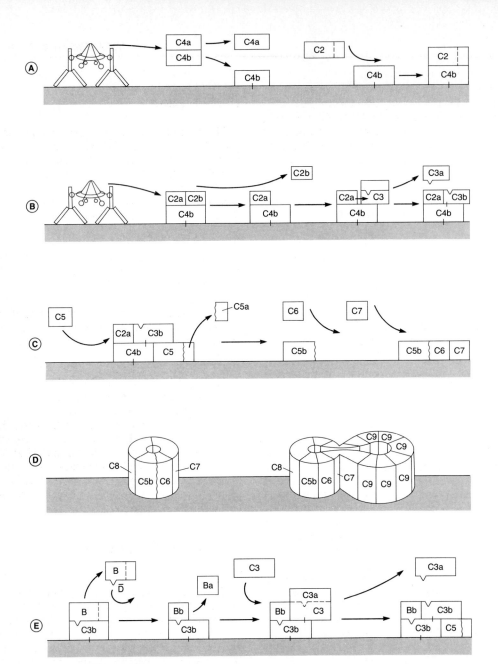

Figure 14–2. Diagram of the complement cascade. **A:** The classic complement pathway. A doublet of IgG antibody molecules on a surface can bind and activate C1, a 3-part molecule composed of C1q, C1r, and C1s. C1q has a core and 6 radiating arms, each of which ends in a pod. The pod recognizes and binds to the Fc fragment of the IgG. Upon activation the C1 binds and cleaves C4. The small fragment, C4a, is released. The large fragment binds to the target to continue the cascade. In the presence of magnesium ion, C2 recognizes and binds to C4b. **B:** Once C2 is bound to C4b, it can be cleaved by C1. A small fragment, C2b, is released, and the large fragment, C2a, remains bound to the C4b. This newly formed complex of 2 protein fragments can now bind and cleave C3. This molecule is, in turn, cleaved into 2 fragments, C3a and C3b. The small fragment, C3a, is released, and the large fragment, C3b, can bind covalently to a suitable acceptor. C3b molecules that bind directly to the C4b continue the cascade. **C:** The complex formed of C2a, C4b, and C3b can bind and cleave C5. A small fragment of C5, C5a, is released. The large fragment, C5b, does not bind covalently. It is stabilized by binding to C6. When C7 binds the complex of C5b, C6 and C7 becomes hydrophobic. It is partially lipid-soluble and can insert into the lipid of the cell membrane bilayer. **D:** When the C5b67 binds C8, a small channel is formed in the cell membrane. Multiple molecules of C9 can bind and markedly enlarge the channel. The channel has a hydrophobic outer surface and a hydrophilic central channel that allows passage of water and ions. **E:** The alternative complement pathway. In the presence of magnesium ion, C3b on a surface can bind factor B, just as C4b can bind C2. Factor D, a fluid-phase factor, can cleave bound factor B into 2 fragments, Ba and Bb. Ba is released. The C3bBb complex can now bind an additional molecule of C3 and cleave it, just as C4b2a can bind and cleave C3. C3a is released, and the new complex of C3bBbC3b, usually written (C3b)2Bb, can bind C5 to continue the cascade.

sium ion, C4b on a target cell is capable of interacting with and binding the next component in the series, a single-chain molecule of MW 95,000, termed C2. C2 binds to C4b and, in the presence of C̄1̄s̄, is cleaved. The larger cleavage fragment of C2 (C2a), which contains the enzymatic site, remains in complex with C4b to continue the complement cascade. The complex of C4b and C2a develops a new capacity: the ability to bind and cleave the next component in the series, C3. For this reason it is termed the classic pathway C3 convertase. The peptide complex C̄4̄b̄2̄ā is unstable and decays with loss of the C2 peptide from C4b as an enzymatically inactive fragment from its binding site on the C4b. Target-bound C4b can accept another C2 and, in the presence of active C1, will regenerate a convertase capable of continuing the complement cascade. These early steps in the classic pathway are under tight regulation, as discussed below.

C3

The C3 convertase of the classic pathway as described above binds and activates C3, a glycoprotein (MW 195,000) present at a concentration of 1.2 mg/ mL of plasma. The molecule has 2 disulfide-linked chains, termed α and β (MW 120,000 and 75,000, respectively). Like C4, C3 contains an internal thiolester bond buried in a hydrophobic pocket that links 2 amino acids in the α chain, twisting the α chain into a strained configuration. On cleavage of the thiolester, the molecule undergoes a major conformational change, which alters its biochemical properties. When C3 is activated by the C̄4̄b̄2̄ā convertase, a peptide, C3a (MW 9,000), is cleaved from the α chain. The internal thiolester is exposed to the surrounding medium and is immediately cleaved. The half-life of the intact but reactive thiolester is in the range of 30–60 microseconds. It will interact with any suitable acceptor in the environment. Suitable acceptors include molecules that have reactive hydroxyl or amino groups on their surface. If the thiolester does not form a covalent bond with an acceptor, the reactive group interacts with water, is hydrolyzed, and can no longer form a covalent bond with the target. A particle coated with C3b is opsonized and may interact with cells with C3b receptors (see the section on receptors below). To continue the complement cascade sequence, it appears that C3b must interact directly with target C4b, forming a covalently bound complex. C3b also has a strong tendency to interact with IgG present in the area of activation. The dimer formed from C3b and the IgG molecule is a more potent opsonin than is C3b alone (see the section on opsonization below).

THE CLASSIC PATHWAY C5 CONVERTASE

The complex on a target surface consisting of C4b, C2a, and C3b (C̄4̄b̄2̄ā3̄b̄) has a newly expressed enzymatic activity: it can coordinate with and cleave C5. Again, 2 fragments, C5a and C5b, are formed, with C5a being the smaller. In this case the larger fragment does not have an internal thiolester linkage and cannot form a covalent bond with the target. It remains associated with the C̄4̄b̄2̄ā3̄b̄ complex and is available to interact with later components. It is C5b that initiates that segment of the complement cascade that leads to membrane attack.

In summary, the early steps of the complement cascade lead to the generation of a series of enzymatically active peptides and peptide complexes. As each complex is formed, it has a different specificity from the preceding complex, interacting with the next protein in the complement cascade. Each enzyme will interact with multiple molecules of the next substrate protein in the cascade of reactions either until it decays, as occurs with C̄4̄b̄2̄ā and C̄4̄b̄2̄ā3̄b̄, which interact with C3 and C5, respectively, or until it is inhibited by regulatory proteins present on cells or in plasma. Thus, there is a potential for considerable biologic amplification; a limited number of antigen-antibody complexes will lead to the activation of large numbers of complement molecules.

THE ALTERNATIVE COMPLEMENT PATHWAY

C3 not only acts as a centrally important component of the classic pathway but also is the key component in the functioning of the alternative pathway. As described above, C3 can have 2 molecular forms: a native form that circulates in plasma with an intact thiolester, and a conformationally altered form, C3(H₂O), in which the thiolester bond has been hydrolyzed. Once the conformational change has occurred, C3(H₂O) in the presence of magnesium ion can interact with another circulating protein, factor B of the alternative pathway—a protein analogous to C2. Factor B has similar thermostability properties to C2 and requires magnesium ion to interact with its ligand, conformationally altered C3. The genes for factor B and C2 are located side by side on chromosome 6. It is reasonable to believe that C2 arises from a gene duplication of factor B. In the presence of factor D, a C1-like serine protease, the factor B bound to C3(H₂O), is cleaved. Thus, in many respects the alternative pathway is like the classic pathway. Conformationally altered C3(H₂O) resembles C4b; factor D resembles C1 in its function, although it has no binding site for the target and therefore is much less efficient in function. Factor B, acting much like C2, binds to altered C3 and is cleaved. Together, these proteins form an alternative pathway C3 convertase that can bind and activate C3, much as the classic pathway convertase binds and activates C3. As in the classic pathway, the activated C3 is cleaved into C3a and C3b. C3b with a cleaved thiolester has the same general conformation as $C3(H_2O)$. C3b binds factor B, and in the presence of factor D, it continues alternative pathway activation.

Thus, whereas the classic pathway proceeds in a fashion that is strictly sequential (C1 being required before C4, before C2, etc.), the alternative pathway activation is in many ways circular. C3 in the circulation is slowly hydrolyzed to $C3(H_2O)$. In the altered conformation it interacts with factors B and D of the alternative pathway to form a C3-cleaving enzyme that will bind fresh C3 and form C3a and C3b. The newly formed C3b can, of course, bind to suitable acceptors on targets and can itself continue alternative pathway activation. Thus, the slow cleavage of C3 in the circulation acts as a nidus to initiate alternative pathway activation. Once again, control proteins under normal circumstances prevent this nidus, which appears to form physiologically at all times, from inducing massive alternative pathway activation.

Alternative Pathway Amplification

The ability of hydrolyzed C3 to interact with alternative pathway components to form C3a and C3b and continue alternative pathway activation is termed the "feedback amplification system." The alternative pathway convertase (C3bBb) is extremely unstable and decays rapidly under normal physiologic conditions. Such rapid decay would markedly reduce its effectiveness. Properdin, a protein in plasma, binds to the alternative pathway convertase and stabilizes it, thus slowing its decay and allowing it to continue the complement cascade.

Cobra Venom Factor

It is interesting that for years investigators have used a protein derived from cobra venom (cobra venom factor) to activate complement. Recent investigation has shown that this protein is a fragment of cobra C3 and is a physiologic analogue of C3b in this reptile. This protein, when added to human plasma, activates complement just as C3b, derived physiologically, activates the alternative pathway. C3b generated by complement activation in normal serum is under tight regulatory control by plasma proteins, as mentioned below. However, cobra venom factor is not inhibited by these regulators and therefore can induce massive complement activation.

THE LATE COMPONENTS C5-9 & THE MEMBRANE ATTACK COMPLEX

As described above, C5 is bound and then cleaved by either the alternative or classic pathway convertase into C5a and C5b. C5a is released. Its biologic activity is described in a later section. C5b continues the lytic sequence; however, it does not form a covalent bond with the surface of its target. C5b is rapidly inactivated unless it is stabilized by binding to the next component in the cascade, C6. The C5b6 complex now can bind C7, the third protein involved in membrane attack. The C5b67 complex becomes increasingly hydrophobic and will interact with nearby membrane lipids. It is capable of inserting into the lipid bilayer of cell membranes. In that location, one C5b67 complex can accept one molecule of C8 and multiple molecules of C9, ultimately forming a cylinderlike structure, $C5b678(9)n$, which has been termed the **membrane attack complex (MAC)** (Fig 14-3). This structure has a hydrophobic outer surface, which associates with the membrane lipid of the bilayer, and a hydrophilic core through which small ions and water can pass. The ionic environment of the extracellular fluid then communicates with that inside the cell, so that once this complex is inserted into the membrane, the cell cannot maintain its osmotic and chemical equilibrium. Water enters the cell because of the high internal oncotic pressure, and the cell swells and bursts. The assembly of C5b-C8 appears to form a small membrane channel that is increasingly enlarged and stabilized by the binding of multiple molecules of C9. One lesion penetrating the erythrocyte membrane is sufficient to destroy the cell. Cells with more complex metabolic machinery can internalize and destroy complement lesions that form on the cell surface, thereby providing some protection against complement attack.

CONTROL MECHANISMS

The complement system has evolved to aid in the host defense process by directly damaging invading organisms and by producing tissue inflammation. Maintaining tight regulatory control of this system is of critical importance to prevent complement-mediated destruction of the individual's own tissues. When complement is involved in causing disease, it usually is functioning normally but is misdirected, ie, damaging to the host tis-

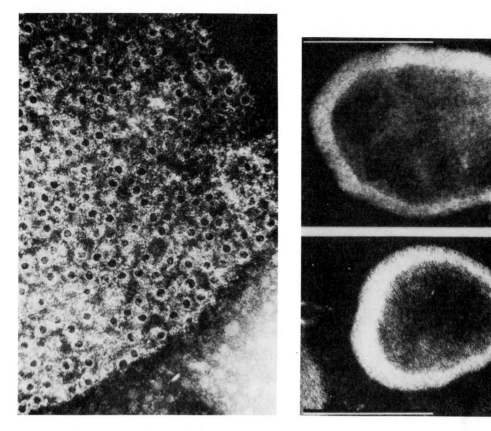

Figure 14-3. Lysis of cells by C5b-9, the MAC. **Left:** Surface of cells lysed by antibody and complement. Note the surface lesions. (Micrograph courtesy of R Dourmashkin.) **Right:** Two views of the purified lesions allowed to attach to lipid micelles. The hollow cylinder formed by the C5b-9 has allowed the electron-dense dye to enter the lipid droplet. (Photograph courtesy of S Bhakdi.)

sues. Many control proteins have evolved to defend against this attack.

The C1 Inhibitor

The first of these, C1 inhibitor (C1INH), recognizes activated $\overline{\text{C1r}}$ and $\overline{\text{C1s}}$ and destroys their activity. This glycoprotein (MW 105,000) not only inhibits $\overline{\text{C1r}}$ and $\overline{\text{C1s}}$, but also acts as an inhibitor of activated Hageman factor (see below) and all of the enzyme systems activated by Hageman factor fragments. Thus, C1INH regulates enzymes formed during activation of the kinin-generating system, the clotting system, and the fibrinolytic system. In each of these systems C1INH binds physically to the active site of the enzyme to destroy its activity and thereby is consumed. Interestingly, during this process the C1 is dissociated, with the C1INH binding to each of the C1r and C1s enzymatic sites and freeing C1q of its subunits. Since C1INH is consumed when acting as an inhibitor, 2 genes are necessary to provide the

relatively high plasma concentration of the protein gene product required for effective inhibitor activity. A relative deficiency occurs in patients with hereditary angioedema, who have a defect in one of the 2 genes responsible for formation of C1INH. These patients have one-half to one-third the normal level of C1INH and have frequent attacks of angioedema—painless swelling of deep cutaneous tissues—whose cause is still uncertain. It may arise from activation of the kinin-generating system or from activation of the complement system, with generation of peptides that cause vascular leakage.

C4-binding Protein, Factor I, & Factor H

C4-binding protein (C4BP) and a second protein, factor I, are responsible for regulation of C4b. C4BP binds to C4b and facilitates cleavage by the proteolytic enzyme factor I. On target surfaces, C4BP is not required for C4b cleavage by factor I, but its presence may accelerate the cleavage process.

Factor I also is responsible for the cleavage of C3b (Fig 14–4). In this case the required cofactor is termed factor H. Factor H acts as an obligate cofactor in the fluid phase and as an accelerator of C3 cleavage on cell surfaces (see Fig 14–4). In the presence of factors H and I, the C3b or C3(H₂O) α-chain is cleaved at 2 sites to form a partially degraded molecule, iC3b. This molecule, although inactive in continuing the complement cascade, is active in phagocytosis and will be discussed further below. Under the appropriate conditions, as discussed below, factor I can cleave iC3b further to form a molecule termed C3dg, which also interacts with specific receptors that recognize this C3 degradation peptide.

Vitronectin (S Protein)

Yet another control protein, S protein (also called vitronectin), interacts with the C5b67 complex as it forms in the fluid phase and interacts with its membrane-binding site to prevent the binding of C5b67 to biologic membranes. Following binding of S protein to fluid-phase C5b67, binding of C8 and C9 to the fluid-phase complex

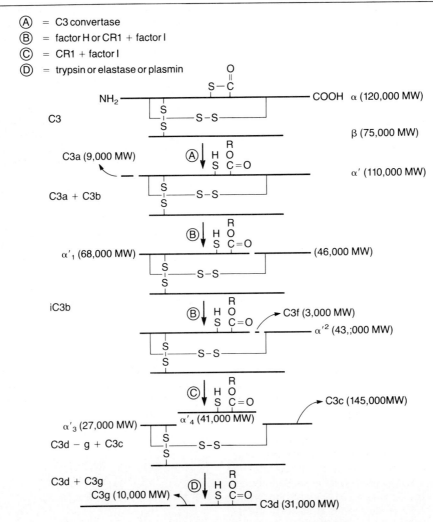

Figure 14–4. The C3 degradation pathway. The α and β chains of C3 are shown. Activation of C3 with the formation of C3a and C3b by the C3 convertases is shown (step A). C3b is degraded to iC3b by the action of factor H or CR1 plus factor I (step B). Two forms of iC3b have been described differing in loss of a 3-kDa fragment. In the presence of CR1 and factor I, C3c is released and C3dg remains target bound (step C). C3dg can be further degraded to C3d by proteolytic enzymes (step D). Specific cellular receptors exist for each of these fragments.

can proceed, but the complex does not insert into lipid membranes and does not lyse cells.

In the control of complement attack against host tissue, it would be beneficial if complement proteins such as C3b were rapidly degraded when bound to host cells but not degraded when bound to the surface of a microorganism. A process for accomplishing this goal has evolved. When deposited on a microorganism, C3b is often in a "protected site," which is protected from the action of the control proteins factors H and I. The C3b persists to activate the alternative pathway and destroy the organism. In contrast, on host cells C3b interacts with factors H and I and is degraded. The biochemical basis for this protection of C3b on an organism surface is not yet completely understood, but appears to relate to the presence of charged carbohydrates such as sialic acid on mammalian cells, facilitating the binding of factor H.

GENETIC CONSIDERATIONS

Most of the genes encoding proteins of the classic and alternative pathways have been cloned, and their amino acid sequences have been determined. Moreover, the activation peptides have been studied in some detail. Allotypic variants of many of the proteins have been found that show genetic polymorphisms, as demonstrated by differences in surface charge. Almost all of the variants of complement proteins show autosomal codominant inheritance at a single locus. The genes for C4, C2, and factor B are located within the major histocompatiblity locus on the short arm of chromosome 6 in humans and are termed class III histocompatibility genes. The significance of the intimate localization of histocompatibility genes and complement genes is unknown at present.

Interestingly, there are 2 C4 loci on each chromosome; thus, there are 4 C4 genes. The 2 loci code for proteins termed C4A and C4B, which differ in functional activity. Individuals with at least one null allele at one of the C4 loci are fairly common and are thought to be prone to the development of autoimmune disease. Genes for many of the regulatory proteins that interact with C4 and C3 are grouped as a supergene family on chromosome 1. This family is now known to encode factor H, C4-binding protein, decay-accelerating factor, CR1, and CR2. The gene products of this family have a 60-amino-acid domain made up of shorter repeating segments that repeat multiple times in the molecule. They presumably originate from a common gene precursor.

BIOLOGIC CONSEQUENCES OF COMPLEMENT ACTIVATION IN INFLAMMATION

In general, the larger fragments formed during complement component cleavage tend to continue the complement cascade, and the smaller fragments mediate features of inflammation. For example, the cleavage of C3 and C5 generates C3a and C5a fragments, which consist of the first 77 and 74 amino acids of the C3 and C5 α chains, respectively. Cleavage of C4 generates C4a, a MW 77,000 amino acid fragment from the α-chain of C4. All of these small activation peptides have anaphylatoxic activity; they cause smooth muscle contraction and degranulation of mast cells and basophils, with consequent release of histamine and other vasoactive substances that induce capillary leakage. C5a is the most potent of these anaphylatoxins.

C5a and C3a also have important immunoregulatory effects on T cell function, either stimulating (C5a) or inhibiting (C3a) aspects of cell-mediated immunity.

C5a has profound effects on phagocytic cells. It is strongly chemotactic for neutrophils and mononuclear phagocytes, inducing their migration along a concentration gradient toward the site of generation. It increases neutrophil adhesiveness and causes neutrophil aggregation. In addition, it dramatically stimulates neutrophil oxidative metabolism and the production of toxic oxygen species, and it triggers lysosomal enzyme release from a variety of phagocytic cells. Cellophane membranes used in renal dialysis machines and membrane oxygenators may activate the alternative pathway with C5a generation. This, in turn, may lead to neutrophil aggregation, embolization of the aggregates to the lungs, and pulmonary distress. It is suspected that C5a generation plays an important deleterious role in the development of adult respiratory distress syndrome.

The life span of these biologically potent peptides, C3a and C5a, is limited by a serum carboxypeptidase that cleaves off the terminal arginine from the peptides, in most cases markedly reducing their activity.

COMPLEMENT PROTEINS ASSOCIATED WITH CELL MEMBRANES

Receptors & Regulatory Molecules

On the surface of most cells are complement receptors, ie, interactive membrane proteins with important regulatory properties. Receptors for the C1q component of C1 have been identified on neutrophils and monocytes, the majority of B lymphocytes, and a small population of lymphocytes lacking both B and T cell markers. Binding via this receptor has been shown to activate cells for a variety of cellular functions, including phagocytosis and oxidative metabolism. C1q can also augment the cytotoxicity of human peripheral blood lymphocytes to antibody-sensitized chicken erythrocytes and supports antibody-independent cytolytic activity by certain lymphoblastoid cell lines. The C1q receptor does not interact with C1q in intact C1, but interacts once the C1 has been dissociated by the C1 inhibitor.

A. THE C3 RECEPTORS: The best-studied receptors are those that recognize C3 fragments (Table 14–2). Importantly, these receptors do not recognize native circulating C3 and are not blocked by the normal plasma protein. Receptors exist for C3b, iC3b, and C3dg. These receptors have a characteristic cellular distribution, with the C3b receptor (termed CR1) being prominent on erythrocytes, granulocytes, mononuclear phagocytes, and B lymphocytes in humans. In contrast, the C3bi receptor (CR3) is present only on phagocytic cells. The C3d receptor (CR2) is present on lymphoblastoid cells and B lymphocytes. These receptors bind the various C3 fragments as indicated. If the C3 is bound to an antigen or target particle, the antigen or target will bind via the C3

ligand to the surface of cells with the receptor. For phagocytic cells, binding of the target to the phagocyte surface can augment the ingestion process.

Thus, CR1 and CR3 are both important in the process of phagocytosis. However, they also serve several other functions. They both act as cofactors for the further degradation of C3 fragments by the serum enzyme factor I. In each case, C3 fragment bound to the receptor can be cleaved by factor I to the decay fragment C3dg. This fragment is not formed in the absence of complement receptors. CR3 plays a major role in cell adherence; phagocytes from CR3-deficient patients have marked abnormalities in adherence and ingestion. CR3 is one member of a family of proteins termed "integrens." Other members of the CR3 group of proteins are LFA1 and p150/95, the latter being a protein that binds C3b and C3dg and that has recently been identified as CR4. All members of the CR3 family are 2-chain proteins with the same β chain. Presumably, the β chain is important in membrane localization of the protein. Recently, a number of children with deficiency of all of the CR3 proteins have been identified. They present with a history of delayed separation of the umbilical cord at birth and frequent soft-tissue and cutaneous infections by a variety of organisms, especially staphylococci and *Pseudomonas aeruginosa*.

CR2 is a receptor for the C3d and C3dg frag-

Table 14–2. Cellular receptors for C3 fragments.

Designation	Complement Component Recognized	Protein Structure	Cells	Function
CR1	C4b/C3b, iC3b	1 chain (MW 165,000–240,000)	Erythrocytes, phagocytes, B lymphocytes, some glomerular podocytes, eosinophils, Langerhans cells	Aids target cell ingestion by phagocytes; acts as cofactor in the metabolism of C3b, allowing factor I to cleave C3b to C3dg.
CR3	iC3b	2 chains, α (MW 170,000) and β (MW 95,000)	Phagocytes	Aids in ingestion; important in adherence of cells to surface; acts as cofactor for further degradation of C3bi.
CR2	C3d, C3dg	1 chain (MW 140,000)	B lymphocytes, some T cells, epithelial cells, follicular dendritic cells, NK and ADCC effector lymphocytes	On B cells, has immunoregulatory properties; site of attachment of Epstein-Barr virus to lymphocytes and epithelial cells.
CR4	iC3b, C3dg	2 chains, α (MW 150,000) and β (MW 95,000)	Kupffer cells, other phagocytes	Not well studied; presumably aids in attachment and metabolism of C3 coated targets.
C3aR	C3a, C4a	?	Neutrophils, T cells, goblet cells, smooth muscle, mast cells, monocytes, eosinophils	Immunoregulation, anaphylatoxin (see text).
C3eR	C3e	?	Neutrophils	Causes release of PMN from marrow stores.

ments of C3. It is present on B lymphocytes and nasal epithelial cells. It appears to function on B lymphocytes to facilitate differentiation. Interestingly, it serves as the site for attachment and cellular penetration of the Epstein-Barr virus.

B. Regulatory Molecules: Several other cellular membrane proteins act not as receptors but rather to control untoward complement activation. **Decay-accelerating factor (DAF)** is a single-chain membrane protein (MW 70,000) that is a potent accelerator of C3 convertase decay, but, unlike CR1 and CR3, it has no factor I cofactor activity. Functionally, the protein acts to limit membrane damage if, by chance, complement is activated at the cell surface. C8-binding protein, also known as **homologous restriction factor (HRF),** acts to prevent successful completion and membrane insertion of the MAC. This membrane protein therefore acts to prevent cell lysis at yet another step in the complement cascade. It is called homologous restriction protein because it recognizes C8 and C9 of the same species far better than it recognizes late components of other species. Human homologous restriction protein on cells will prevent the action of human C8 and C9 on those cells far better than it will prevent the action of C8 and C9 from other species. Any potential advantage of this function is completely obscure.

Interestingly, DAF and HRF are bound to the cell surface by a **phosphoinositide glycosidic linkage** rather than by a transmembrane domain within the amino acid backbone of the protein. This phosphoinositide linkage is reported to give the protein far greater lateral mobility within the cell membrane, increasing its ability to intercept damage-causing complement complexes. In patients with paroxysmal nocturnal hemoglobinuria, phosphoinositide-linked proteins are incorrectly assembled or inserted into cellular membranes of hematologic cells, rendering these cells exquisitely sensitive to complement-mediated lysis.

Another protein, **membrane cofactor protein (MCP;** formerly glycoprotein 45–70), is present on most blood cells but not on erythrocytes. This protein, a product of the supergene C4b/C3b-binding family, acts as a cofactor to facilitate the cleavage of C3b and iC3b by factor I. It does not accelerate convertase decay or bind with sufficient affinity to act as a receptor.

THE KININ CASCADE

The kinin-generating system is a second important mediator-forming system in blood. Here there is one major final product, **bradykinin,** a nonapeptide with potent activity causing increased vascular permeability, vasodilatation, hypotension, pain, contraction of many types of smooth muscle, and activation of phospholipase A_2 with attendant activation of cellular arachidonic acid metabolism.

PROTEINS OF THE KININ CASCADE

There are 4 elements of the bradykinin-generating system: **Hageman factor, clotting factor XI, prekallikrein,** and **high-molecular-weight kininogen.** Factor XI circulates as a complex with high-molecular-weight kininogen in a molar ratio of 2:1. Prekallikrein also circulates in a complex with high-molecular weight kininogen in a molar ratio of 1:1. In contrast, Hageman factor circulates as an uncomplexed single-chain plasma protein.

STEPS IN KININ ACTIVATION

On interaction with a negatively charged surface such as is supplied experimentally by glass or naturally by many biologically active materials like the lipid A of gram-negative bacterial endotoxin, Hageman factor is cleaved and activated. The cleaved Hageman factor (HFa) has proteolytic activity and can cleave additional molecules of Hageman factor to generate more HFa. Cleavage of the single chain of Hageman factor (MW 80,000) yields heavy and light chains (MW 50,000 and 28,000, respectively) that remain linked by disulfide bonds. The active enzymatic site of Hageman factor resides in its light chain. Cleavage is also catalyzed by other proteolytic enzymes, particularly kallikrein. HFa can interact with the complex of factor XI and high-molecular weight kininogen to activate factor XI to factor XIa. This, in turn, can activate the intrinsic coagulation cascade. HFa can also interact with the high-molecular-weight kininogen–prekallikrein complex to cleave the single-chain prekallikrein into a 2-chain molecule (kallikrein), with the chains associated via a disulfide linkage. The cleaved molecule now has proteolytic enzymatic activity associated with the lower-molecular-weight chain. To facilitate these cleavages of both factor XI and prekallikrein, high-molecular-weight kininogen complexes are bound to the surface, presumably near the Hageman factor.

AMPLIFICATION & REGULATION OF KININ GENERATION

Active kallikrein is capable of further cleaving HFa, with further degradation of the heavy chain

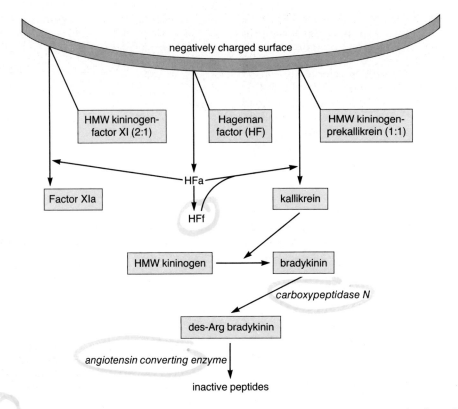

Figure 14-5. The kinin-generating pathway. Emphasized is the fact that complexes of high-molecular-weight (HMW) kininogen with both factor XI and prekallikrein associate on a surface with Hageman factor. The Hageman factor activates and in turn is responsible for the activation of factor XI and prekallikrein. Active kallikrein cleaves high-molecular-weight kininogen to release bradykinin.

but not the light chain. The resulting molecule, HFf, remains capable of activating the high-molecular-weight kininogen–prekallikrein complex, but it does not remain surface-bound and does not interact efficiently with the high molecular weight kininogen–factor XI complex. Prekallikrein is also a single-chain glycoprotein that is converted to an active form by cleavage within a disulfide bridge, resulting in a 2-chain molecule with the chains linked by disulfide bonds. The enzymatic site resides in the light chain, and the surface-binding site is on the heavy chain. Active kallikrein can cleave high molecular weight kininogen at several sites to release bradykinin from the kininogen. Bradykinin has a short half-life, interacting with carboxypeptidase N, which removes the C-terminal arginine to form the molecule termed des-Arg bradykinin. Des-Arg bradykinin no longer has the smooth muscle-contracting activity of bradykinin and cannot induce capillary plasma leakage when injected into skin, but it retains some of its vascular effects. Des-Arg bradykinin is, in turn, cleaved by angiotensin-converting en-

zyme to form low molecular weight peptides with consequent loss of biologic activity.

PLASMA INHIBITORS OF KININ GENERATION

The inhibitors of this mediator-generating system include C1 inhibitor, α_2-macroglobulin, and α_1-antitrypsin. C1 inhibitor and α_2-macroglobulin are the principal inhibitors of active kallikrein, with C1 inhibitor contributing most to inhibitory activity. C1 inhibitor and α_1-antitrypsin are the 2 major inhibitors of factor XIa, and C1 inhibitor is the principal inhibitor of active Hageman factor.

LOW-MOLECULAR-WEIGHT KININOGEN & TISSUE KALLIKREINS

A low molecular weight kininogen also exists in plasma. This protein has an identical heavy chain to that of high molecular weight kininogen. Low molecular weight kininogen can act as a source of bradykinin, but it is not easily cleaved by kallikrein. However, there are tissue kallikreins—low molecular weight kallikreins found in multiple tissues—that can cleave low molecular weight kininogen to lysylbradykinin (bradykinin with an additional linked lysine). Presumably, lysylbradykinin undergoes the same degradation pathway as does bradykinin.

FUNCTIONS OF KININS IN DISEASE

The physiologic role of the kinin-generating system is uncertain, and in only a few cases do we understand its role in disease. Free bradykinin and lysylbradykinin have been found in nasal secretions during rhinitis and viral nasal inflammation, and it is reasonable to believe that both blood and tissue kallikreins contribute to its presence. It is believed that kinins, via their ability to cause smooth muscle contraction and capillary leakage, contribute to asthma, but this is by no means proven at this time. Kinin generation has been found following antigen challenge of human lung fragments passively sensitized with specific IgE antibody, but the exact pathways involved in its generation are still uncertain. It has also been suggested that release of tissue kallikreins and activation of the kinin system is responsible for the severe pain of pancreatitis. The kinin-generating system has been reported to be involved in edema formation in hereditary angioedema, because kinins are present in fluid from suction-induced blisters over angioedema areas and because levels of circulating prekallikrein fall during attacks of this disease. Nevertheless, the kinin-forming system has not yet been conclusively proved to be responsible for the attacks of edema in hereditary angioedema.

REFERENCES

General

Borsos T: *The Molecular Basis of Complement Action.* Appleton-Century-Crofts, 1970.

Frank MM, Fries LF: Complement. Pages 679–702 in: *Fundamental Immunology,* 2nd ed. Paul WE (editor). Raven Press, 1989.

Harrison RA, Lachmann PJ: Complement technology. Chapter 39 in: *Handbook of Experimental Immunology,* 4th ed. Vol. 1. Weir DM (editor). Blackwell, 1986.

Classic Pathway

Cooper NR: The classical complement pathway: activation and regulation of the first complement component. Page 151 in: *Advances in Immunology.* Academic Press, 1985.

Kerr MA: The second component of human complement. *Methods Enzymol* 1981;**80**:54.

Tack BF: The β-Cys-τ-Glu thioester bond in human C3, C4, and α_2-macroglobulin. *Springer Semin Immunopathol* 1983;**6**:259.

Ziccardi RJ: The first component of human complement (C1): Activation and control. *Springer Semin Immunopathol* 1983;**6**:213.

Alternative Pathway

Pangburn MK, Muller-Eberhard HJ: The alternative pathway of complement. *Springer Semin Immunopathol* 1984;**7**:163.

Membrane Attack Complex

Mayer MM et al: Membrane damage by complement. *Crit Rev Immunol* 1981;**2**:133.

Muller-Eberhard HJ: The membrane attack complex of complement. *Annu Rev Immunol* 1986;**4**:503.

Control Mechanisms

Bock SC et al: Human C1 inhibitor: primary structure, with DNA cloning, and chromosomal localization. *Biochemistry* 1986;**25**:4292.

Frank MM, Gelfand JA, Atkinson JP: Hereditary angioedema: The clinical syndrome and its management. *Ann Intern Med* 1976;**84**:580.

Genetic Considerations

Alper CA, Rosen FS: Genetics of the complement system. Page 141 in: *Advances in Human Genetics.* Vol. 7. Harris H, Hirschhorn K (editors). Plenum, 1976.

Campbell RD et al: Structure, organization and regulation of the complement genes. *Annu Rev Immunol* 1988;**6**:161.

Biologic Effects

Goldstein IM: Complement: Biologically active products. Page 55 in: *Inflammation: Basic Principles and Clinical Correlates.* Gallin JE, Goldstein IM, Snyderman R (editors). Raven Press, 1988.

Hugli TE: Biochemistry and biology of anaphylatoxins. *Complement* 1986;**3**:111.

Hugli TE: Structure and function of the anaphylatoxins. *Springer Semin Immunopathol* 1984;**7**:193.

Reid KBM et al: Complement system proteins which interact with C3b or C4b. *Immunol Today* 1986;**7**:230.

Schapira M et al: Biochemistry and pathophysiology of human C1-inhibitor: Current issues. *Complement* 1986;**2**:111.

Cell Membrane Receptors & Regulatory Molecules

Berger M, Gaither TA, Frank MM: Complement receptors. *Clin Immunol Rev* 1983;**1**:471.

Pangburn MK, Schreiber RD, Muller-Eberhard HJ: Deficiency of an erythrocyte membrane protein with complement regulatory activity in paroxysmal nocturnal hemoglobinuria. *Proc Natl Acad Sci USA* 1983;**80:**5430.

Ross GD, Medof ME: Membrane complement receptors specific for bound fragments of C3. *Adv Immunol* 1985;**37:**217.

Schifferli JA, Ng YC, Peters DK: The role of complement and its receptor in the elimination of immune complexes. *N Engl J Med* 1986;**315:**488.

Zalman LS et al: Deficiency of the homologous restriction factor in paroxysmal nocturnal hemoglobinuria. *J Exp Med* 1987;**165:**572.

Kinins

Colman RW: Contact systems in infectious disease. *Rev Infect Dis* 1989;**4(suppl):**689.

Proud D, Kaplan AP: Kinin formation: Mechanisms and role in inflammatory disorders. *Annu Rev Immunol* 1988;**6:**49.

The Mucosal Immune System

Warren Strober, MD, and Stephen P. James, MD

15

The mucosal immune system is composed of the lymphoid tissues that are associated with the mucosal surfaces of the gastrointestinal, respiratory, and urogenital tracts. It has evolved under the influence of the complex and distinctive antigenic array present in mucosal areas and may be distinguished from the systemic (internal) immune system by a number of features. These include (1) a mucosa-related immunoglobulin, IgA; (2) a complement of T cells with mucosa-specific regulatory properties or effector capabilities; and (3) a mucosa-oriented cell traffic system for cells initially induced in the mucosal follicles to migrate to the diffuse mucosal lymphoid tissues underlying the epithelium. This last feature leads to the partial segregation of mucosal cells from systemic cells; thus, the mucosal immune system is a somewhat separate immunologic entity.

FUNCTIONS

The primary function of the mucosal immune system is to provide for host defense at mucosal surfaces. In this role it operates in concert with several nonimmunologic protective factors, including (1) a resident bacterial flora that inhibits the growth of potential pathogens; (2) mucosal motor activity (peristalsis and ciliary function) that maintains the flow of mucosal constituents, reducing the interaction of potential pathogens with epithelial cells; (3) substances such as gastric acid and intestinal bile salts that create a mucosal microenvironment unfavorable to the growth of pathogens; (4) mucus secretions (glycocalyx) that form a barrier between potential pathogens and the epithelial surfaces; and, finally, (5) substances such as lactoferrin, lactoperoxidase, and lysozyme that have inhibitory effects on one or another specific microorganism. Optimal host defense at the mucosal surface depends on both intact mucosal immune responses and nonimmunologic protective functions. Thus, antibiotic therapy that eliminates normal flora may result in infection, despite the existence of an intact immune system; mucosal infections are common in congenital and acquired immunodeficiency states even in the presence of normal nonimmunologic protective factors.

A second but equally important function of the mucosal immune system is to prevent the entry of mucosal antigens and thus protect the systemic immune system from inappropriate antigenic exposure. This occurs both at the mucosal surface, by preventing the entry of potentially antigenic materials, and in the circulation, by providing for the clearance of mucosal antigens via a hepatic clearance system. In addition, the mucosal immune system contains regulatory T cells that down regulate systemic immune responses to antigens which breach the mucosal barrier. Abnormalities of this aspect of mucosal immune function may be important in the development of autoimmunity.

ANATOMY

The mucosal immune system is a quantitatively important part of the immune system. The human gastrointestinal tract contains as much lymphoid tissue as the spleen does. The system can be morphologically and functionally subdivided into 2 major parts: (1) organized tissues consisting of the mucosal follicles (also called gut-associated lymphoid tissues [GALT] and bronchus-associated lymphoid tissues [BALT]) and (2) a diffuse lymphoid tissue consisting of the widely distributed cells located in the mucosal lamina propria (see Fig 15–1 and Chapter 2). The former (or organized) tissues are "afferent" lymphoid areas, where antigens enter the system and induce immune responses, and the latter or diffuse tissues are "efferent" lymphoid areas, where antigens interact with differentiated cells and cause the secretion of antibodies by B cells or induce cytotoxic reactions by T cells. As mentioned above, the 2 parts of the mucosal immune system are linked by a mucosal "homing" mechanism, so that sensi-

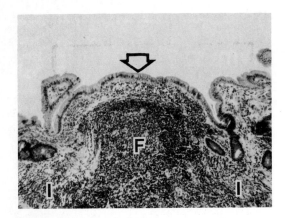

Figure 15-1. Histologic section of a human Peyer's patch lymphoid nodule from the terminal ileum. Antigens are taken up from the lumen through the follicle epithelium (arrow) for processing in the dome. The follicle (F) and its germinal center are composed largely of B cells. The interfollicular areas (I), composed of T cells, contain both high endothelial venules from which T lymphocytes enter follicles and lymphatics through which lymphocytes leave Peyer's patches. Magnification × 72. (Courtesy of Robert L Owen.)

tized cells from the lymphoid follicles travel to the diffuse lymphoid areas, where they can best interact with their inciting antigens. Finally, both the organized and the diffuse mucosal lymphoid areas are highly antigen-dependent; their numbers are remarkably reduced in germ-free states and expanded under conditions of increased antigenic stimulation.

Mucosal Lymphoid Aggregates

Mucosal lymphoid aggregates are morphologically different from those of the systemic lymphoid system. They receive antigen via the epithelium rather than through the lymphatic or blood circulation. More particularly, antigen enters through specialized epithelial cells called M cells (membranous cells) in the epithelium overlying the lymphoid aggregates (Fig 15-2).

A. M cells: M cells are flattened epithelial cells characterized by poorly developed brush borders, a thin glycocalyx, and a cytoplasm rich in pinocytotic vesicles, but they are virtually devoid of the proteolytic machinery found in absorptive epithelial cells. Antigen transport by M cells involves (1) initial binding to the M cell surface via as yet undefined binding sites, (2) uptake into pinocytotic vesicles, (3) vesicular transport across the cell body, and, finally, (4) release of material in an undegraded form into the subepithelial area.

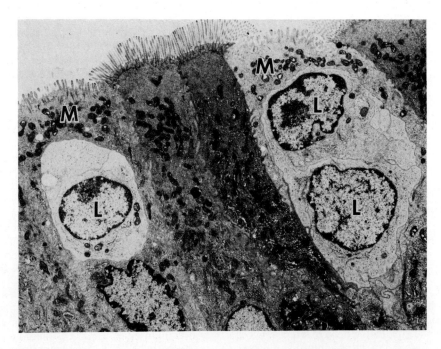

Figure 15-2. Transmission electron micrograph of the epithelium of a rat Peyer's patch lymphoid follicle. M cells (M) have short, irregularly shaped microvilli and surround intraepithelial lymphoid cells (L). Magnification × 6300. (Courtesy of Robert L Owen, MD).

Such transport is applicable to widely disparate substances including particulates (viruses, bacteria, and protozoa) and soluble proteins. However, neither binding nor uptake is totally indiscriminate. For instance, there is some evidence that the transport of bacteria by M cells is inhibited by specific antibodies, which may interact with bacterial determinants necessary for binding to M cells. This fact may explain the lack of uptake of resident microorganisms into M cells. Furthermore, some organisms that bind to M cells are taken up, whereas others are not. The ability to be taken up by M cells may have an impact on the virulence of an organism. For example, viral binding to and uptake by M cells may be an obligate means of entry of the organism and therefore a positive virulence factor, whereas uptake leading to antibody formation and immune elimination of the organism has a negative impact on virulence.

B. Dome Cells: The area just below the epithelium of the lymphoid aggregate (the so-called dome area) is rich in cells bearing class II major histocompatibility complex (MHC) antigens (macrophages, dendritic cells, and B cells) and therefore is rich in cells capable of antigen presentation following exposure to antigens in vitro or via oral antigen feeding in vivo. For this reason, any lack of response following oral antigen administration is not due to a lack of antigen-presenting cells in mucosal lymphoid aggregates (see the discussion of oral unresponsiveness below). M cells do not bear class II MHC antigens and are therefore probably not involved in antigen presentation; on the other hand, absorptive epithelial cells, particularly in the presence of inflammation, do express class II MHC antigens and have been shown to have antigen-presenting function in vitro.

The dome areas also contain many T cells. Although most of these cells bear CD4, a number bear neither CD4 nor CD8. This latter population may correspond to the cells recently identified as contrasuppressor cells (see the discussion of IgA regulation below).

C. Follicles: Below the dome area is the follicular zone, which contains the germinal centers. B cells predominate in this region, although scattered T cells are also present. As in other germinal centers, the B cells are highly differentiated and bear surface IgD; however, unlike other germinal-center B cells, a large fraction (up to 40%) bear surface IgA. Thus, the lymphoid aggregates of the mucosal immune system form the site of IgA B cell development, but the mucosal follicle is conspicuous for the absence of the terminally differentiated IgA B cells (IgA plasma cells), presumably because such cells leave the follicle before differentiating into plasma cells. The interfollicular areas between and around the follicles are also rich in T cells; most of the small population of

CD8 T cells in mucosal lymphoid aggregates are found in these areas.

Diffuse Mucosal Lymphoid Tissue

The diffuse lymphoid tissues of the mucosal immune system consist of cell populations present in 2 separate compartments: the **intraepithelial lymphocyte (IEL) compartment** and the **lamina propria lymphocyte (LPL) compartment.**

A. Intraepithelial Lymphocytes: The IEL are, as the name implies, a population of cells lying above the basement membrane, among the epithelial cells. Although this population is numerically smaller than the lamina propria cell population, it is nonetheless considerable, there being 6–40 IEL/100 epithelial cells under normal conditions and a larger number in various inflammatory states. The IEL population is phenotypically heterogeneous, consisting for the most part of CD3 and CD2 T cells that are also predominantly of the CD8 phenotype. Recently it has been shown that proliferation of human IEL can be induced by stimulation of these cells via the CD2 receptor but not the T cell receptor. The reason for such activation requirements is as yet unknown.

Studies with mice suggest that IEL have specialized immune effector functions, including natural killer (NK) cell activity, specific cell cytotoxicity, secretion of gamma interferon (IFN-γ) with an increase in epithelial cell expression of class II MHC antigens, and expression of γ/δ T cell receptors.

B. Lamina Propria Lymphocytes: The lymphocyte population beneath the epithelial layer in the lamina propria, the LPL, is distinguished from the IEL population in being about equally divided between B cells and T cells. The B cell population is dominated by IgA B cells (and plasma cells), but IgM, IgG, and IgE B cells (and plasma cells) are also present (in descending order of frequency). In IgA deficiency, IgM rather than IgA cells are the predominant cells in the gastrointestinal mucosa and the number of IgG B cells is not increased; on the other hand, in various inflammatory diseases of the mucosa (eg, ulcerative colitis), the population of B cells producing each of the isotypes, particularly those producing IgG, is increased. In both normal and diseased mucosal tissue, the B cell population is composed of cells that display spontaneous immunoglobulin secretion in vitro.

The mucosal T cell population is composed of both CD4 and CD8 cells, with the former being twice as numerous as the latter, just as in peripheral blood. Recent evidence suggests that these cells have undergone prior activation. This is supported by the findings that lamina propria T cells contain IL-2 receptor (IL-2R) mRNA, have increased class II MHC and IL-2R expression, and have high expression of mRNA for IL-2 and IFN-γ. Activated CD4 T cells act as helper cells in vitro; it is not surprising that the CD4 lamina propria T cells provide more help and less suppression than do the corresponding CD4 cells in other tissues. These findings and recent data that CD4 lamina propria T cells respond to specific antigens by secreting "helper" lymphokines rather than by proliferating have led to the concept that lamina propria T cells are a class of memory T cells.

Lamina Propria Macrophages

Cells with typical macrophage morphology are found in the diffuse mucosal areas throughout the mucosal immune system. In these areas they tend to be concentrated in the more superficial parts of the mucosa just below the epithelium. They may derive from the mucosal lymphoid aggregates (as do mucosal lymphocytes), because cells with monocyte morphology are found in the intestinal lymphatics that drain the intestinal tissue. A high proportion of lamina propria macrophages bear class II MHC and other surface markers associated with phagocytic cell activity, which suggests that they are in a more highly activated state than are the corresponding cells in other lymphoid areas. These cells probably are important in nonspecific host defense. In addition, they may produce cytokines (IL-1, IL-6) necessary for local B cell differentiation and other immune processes.

Lamina Propria NK & Lymphokine-Activated Killer (LAK) Cells

Cells bearing NK cell markers (CD16, CD56) are sparse in the lamina propria, and NK activity is difficult to demonstrate in LPL populations unless procedures to enrich for NK cells are used. On the other hand, definite, albeit low (as compared with the level in spleen or peripheral blood cells) NK activity is seen in primate and rodent LPL populations, which suggests that the lack of NK activity in human lamina propria is due in part to the fact that human habitats and habits are not conducive to stimulation of mucosal NK cells, even though the potential for such stimulation does exist. In contrast to cells having NK function, cells with lymphokine-activated killer (LAK) function are easily demonstrated among the LPL. LAK cells are either CD8 T cells or NK cells that manifest antigen-nonspecific cytotoxicity when exposed to IL-2. Because the lamina propria lacks cells with NK markers, the LAK activity in this population is likely to be mediated by T cells or other undefined cells. Finally, the LPL population contains CD8 T cells that can be activated by allogeneic cells, anti-CD3 antibody, and mitogens to manifest cytolytic or suppressor function; these

cells probably originate from precursor cells induced in the mucosal aggregates, although some might arise locally. Cytotoxicity is mediated by CD57-negative cells in the lamina propria but by CD57-positive cells in blood, showing that mucosal cytolytic effector cell populations may sometimes be phenotypically different from corresponding populations in the systemic immune system.

Lamina Propria Mast Cells

The mucosal areas are rich in mast cell precursors, which rapidly differentiate into mature mast cells when they are appropriately stimulated. Through their release of mediators, mast cells constitute an important mechanism by which inflammatory cells rapidly enter mucosal tissues and participate in local host defense.

In humans, mast cells in mucosal tissue have relatively small amounts of histamine and tryptic protease, whereas those in connective tissue contain relatively large amounts of histamine and possess both tryptic and chymotryptic proteases. Differential mast cell development in these 2 tissues may depend on the types of cells and cytokines present in their local environments. In this regard, mast cell precursors differentiate into mucosal mast cells under the influence of lymphokines secreted by T cells such as IL-3, whereas connective-tissue mast cells appear to require these factors as well as a factor(s) produced by fibroblasts. This may account for the rapid appearance of mast cells in mucosal tissues infected with nematode parasites, since presumably the parasites can stimulate mucosal T cells to secrete lymphokines that cause differentiation of mast cell precursors into mucosal mast cells. Thus, the significance of the mucosal mast cell type to the mucosal immune system (and to the body as a whole) may lie in its unique capacity to rapidly expand in number under the influence of a T cell–derived signal.

IMMUNOGLOBULIN A

Structure & Function

The central role of IgA in the mucosal immune response is one of the distinguishing features of the mucosal immune system. This is based on the fact that IgA has a number of properties that allow it to function more efficiently than other immunoglobulins in the mucosal environment.

The biochemical structure, genetics, and synthesis of IgA are discussed in Chapter 9. The features of this immunoglobulin that relate to its function in mucosal immunity are discussed here.

IgA is quantitatively the most important of the immunoglobulins, having a synthetic rate exceeding that of all other immunoglobulins combined when secretory as well as circulating IgA is taken into account. In humans it is encoded by 2 genes that lie in the immunoglobulin region of the genome downstream of each of two blocks of γ and ϵ heavy-chain genes. The first IgA gene encodes IgA1, the predominant circulating IgA (ca 80% of the total), as well as a major component of the IgA in mucosal secretions. The second IgA gene encodes IgA2, the IgA that is particularly abundant in the secretions, especially those of the distal gastrointestinal tract (ca 60% of the total). IgA1 differs from IgA2 in being susceptible to cleavage in its hinge region by proteases secreted by a number of different bacteria. Such cleavage can lead to markedly reduced functional activity; however, given the fact that IgA2 is also present in the part of the mucosa where IgA protease-producing bacteria reside, such proteases probably have little effect on the host defense function of the IgA system as a whole. Another difference between IgA1 and IgA2 is that the latter occurs in 2 allotypic forms, IgA2(m1) and IgA2(m2), which, in turn, are distinguished from one another by the fact that IgA2(m1) lacks interchain (H-L) disulfide bonds.

IgA manifests 3 structural features that relate specifically to its role as the mucosal immunoglobulin (Fig 15–3).

A. IgG Polymerization: The IgA heavy chain, in common with the IgM heavy chain, has an extra cysteine residue–containing C-terminal domain. This domain permits IgA to interact with a bivalent (or multivalent) molecule, also produced by B cells, known as J (joining) chain to form IgA dimers and trimers. IgA polymerization is important to IgA function because polymerized IgA (pIgA) has an increased capacity to bind to and agglutinate antigens.

B. Secretory Component: Only dimerized IgA can react with secretory component (SC), a protein (MW 95,000) produced by epithelial cells. SC acts as a transport receptor for IgA and becomes part of the secreted IgA molecule (see discussion below). It renders the IgA molecule less susceptible to proteolytic digestion and more mucophilic, thus enhancing the ability of the IgA molecule to interact with potential pathogens and to prevent their attachment to the epithelial surface. In addition, the IgA hinge region contains a glycosylated, proline-rich region that is generally more resistant to proteolysis by mammalian proteases than is IgG. On this basis, IgA has greater survivability in the gastrointestinal lumen than IgG or other immunoglobulins have. Such survivability, as already mentioned, is enhanced by the presence of secretory component.

C. Fc Region Properties: The Fc domain of IgA is characterized by certain unique properties,

both positive and negative. Unlike the IgM or IgG Fc region, the IgA Fc region does not react with components of either the classic or alternative complement pathway, except possibly when the IgA is highly polymerized or is in the form of an immune complex; even in the latter instance, it does not bind C3b and therefore does not recruit inflammatory cells and mediators. In addition, although IgA facilitates phagocytosis and other phagocytic cell functions in the presence of specific antigen, it actually down-regulates phagocytosis in the absence of the antigen.

These facts suggest that free IgA (ie, IgA not associated with antigen) has anti-inflammatory effects. This, of course, is a highly useful property in an area of the body that is replete with materials that can induce excessive inflammatory responses.

IgA has certain pro-inflammatory features as well. Its Fc region binds to lactoferrin and lactoperoxidase and thereby enhances the function of these nonspecific host defense elements. There is also evidence that IgA can interact via its Fc region with Fc receptors to mediate antibody-dependent cellular cytotoxicity reactions (ADCC).

Transport

As noted above, the capacity of dimeric IgA to bind to SC enhances it effectiveness as a mucosal immunoglobulin. More importantly, however, SC is the key factor in an IgA transport system in allowing the mucosal immune system to focus IgA at mucosal sites (Fig 15-4). The sequence of events occurring during IgA transport involves first the binding of polymeric IgA to SC (via a covalent interaction) on the basolateral surface of the epithelial cell (or hepatocyte, as noted below), followed by endocytosis of IgA into vesicles, movement of IgA-containing vesicles to the apical surface of the cell, and, finally, release of IgA-SC complexes into the mucosal lumen. This final step requires cleavage of the SC receptor molecule so that the receptor for IgA becomes part of the secreted IgA molecule. Cellular synthesis and translocation of SC is independent of the presence of IgA and usually exceeds the amount necessary for transport, leading to the secretion of free (unbound) SC.

IgA transport mediated by SC occurs in the epithelium of the digestive tract, the salivary glands, the bronchial mucosa, and the lactating mammary glands. It also occurs in the uterine epithelium, where it is regulated by the effects of estrogen on SC synthesis by uterine epithelial cells. IgA transport mediated by SC also takes place in the liver, in which case it results in secretion of IgA into the bile. This involves the biliary epithelial cells but not hepatocytes, as in rodents, implying that SC-mediated transport is less important in humans

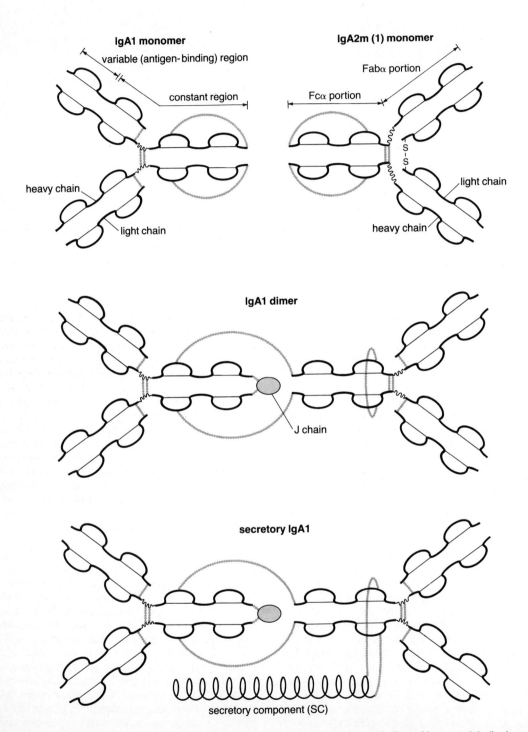

Figure 15-3. Diagrammatic representation of IgA structural forms. Hatched areas indicated immunoglobulin domains. Beads indicate disulfide bonds. In the actual IgA dimer and secretory IgA molecule, the J chain and secretory component molecules are intertwined with Cα heavy chains.

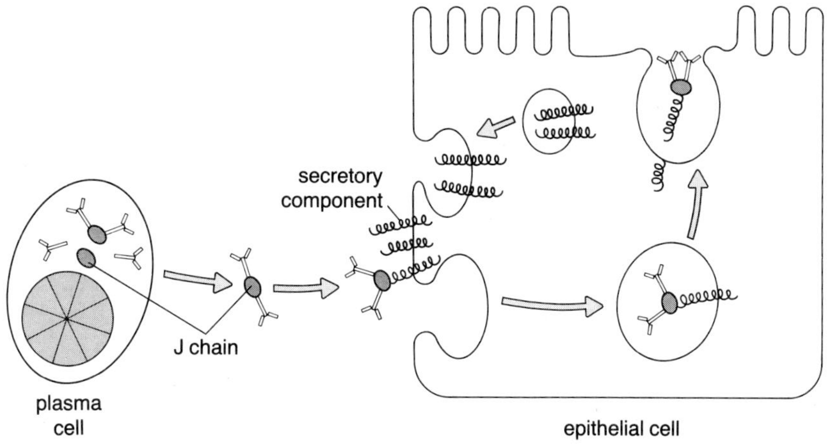

Figure 15-4. SC-mediated transport of IgA across the epithelial cell. Synthesis of SC (indicated as spirals) is independent of the transport process, and SC is released onto the luminal surface whether or not it is bound to IgA. Transport of IgA by this process does not result in its degradation.

than in certain other species. However, lessened SC-mediated transport in humans is compensated for by other hepatic uptake mechanisms. In this regard, IgA1 can be internalized by hepatic cells via asialoglycoprotein receptors as well as by Fc receptors.

Hepatic uptake of IgA may be one mechanism by which IgA secreted into the circulation is redirected back to the mucosa in species with well-developed SC-mediated hepatic transport capabilities, possibly to clear the circulation of potentially damaging antigenic material that has penetrated the mucosal barrier and become bound to circulating IgA. This mechanism has, in fact, obtained limited support from experiments in animals, but further study is necessary to establish its validity in humans.

Immune Exclusion

The ability of IgA to undergo SC-mediated transport or other clearance mechanisms facilitates the process of immune exclusion, whereby the mucosal immune system prevents the entry of antigenic molecules that could potentially evoke harmful immune responses. First, IgA molecules delivered into the secretions by SC-mediated transport can bind to antigens at the mucosal surface and thus lead to their entrapment in the mucus layer and their degradation by proteases before they become bound to and taken up by epithelial cells. That IgA antibody is best suited to this function is shown by the fact that individuals with selective IgA deficiency (ie, those who have low IgA levels and normal IgM and IgG levels) show increased absorption of macromolecules and high levels of circulating immune complexes

following ingestion of antigens. This may be the cause of the increase in autoimmunity associated with IgA deficiency. Second, there is good evidence in animals and some evidence in humans that injected antigens become bound to circulating IgA and are then cleared in the liver via SC-mediated transport. Thus, the mucosal immune system either prevents the entry of potentially harmful antigens to the circulation via the mucosa or facilitates their removal from the circulation. This has the effect of limiting the immune response to the antigens present in the mucosal area to the regulated response occurring in the mucosal immune system itself, as discussed below.

Secretory versus Circulating IgA

In recent years in vivo and in vitro studies of IgA synthesis and catabolism have allowed insights into the source of IgA present in various body compartments. The results of these studies show that in humans most circulating IgA is produced in the bone marrow and is in the form of IgA1 monomers, whereas secretory IgA is produced mainly at mucosal sites (either as IgA1 or IgA2 dimers or polymers). Polymeric IgA (whether IgA1 or IgA2) is more rapidly catabolized than monomeric IgA because polymeric IgA is subject to additional clearance mechanisms such as SC-mediated transport and asialoglycoprotein receptor-mediated uptake. In rats and rabbits, polymeric IgA accounts for about half of the circulating IgA, although most IgA delivered into the circulation is polymeric IgA. This is explained by the fact that in these species SC-mediated transport in the liver is a quantitatively important process and thus polymeric IgA is more rapidly cleared than monomeric IgA. The importance of hepatic clearance of polymeric IgA in rats and rabbits is underscored by the observation that in these species (but not in humans) biliary obstruction leads to increased IgA levels.

The separate origin of mucosal and circulating IgA in humans has led Conley and Delacroix to suggest that the IgA system in humans is bipartite, ie, is composed of 2 relatively independent synthetic centers that are separately regulated. An alternative view more in keeping with the concept that the bone marrow is not an inductive site for IgA B cells is that the IgA1 B cells that produce IgA in the marrow originate in the mucosa and secondarily colonize the marrow to form a separate (but subordinate) locus of IgA-producing B cells. In any case, the monomeric IgA1 arising from the bone marrow in humans may provide a selective advantage in that such IgA may be better suited than other forms of IgA to mediate the clearance of mucosal antigens from the circulation (as discussed above). This is because a monomeric IgA1 molecule may form smaller, more nonpathogenic complexes with circulating antigens than polymeric IgA, yet retain the capacity to undergo removal via interaction with appropriate receptors in the liver.

PRODUCTION OF OTHER IMMUNOGLOBULINS IN THE MUCOSA

Immunoglobulins other than IgA also play a role in the mucosal immune system. Mucosal synthesis of IgM, which can be transported across the epithelial cell via the SC-mediated mechanism, is measurable and physiologically significant. Its capacity to act as a mucosal immunoglobulin is underscored by the fact that it usually replaces IgA adequately to produce mucosal immunity in individuals with selective IgA deficiency. Mucosal synthesis of IgG, on the other hand, is quite low in most mucosal areas, and IgG cannot be transported across the epithelium. Nevertheless, it does have a mucosal role. It is synthesized in substantial amounts in the distal pulmonary tract and is an important antibody class in pulmonary secretions, which it probably enters by passive diffusion. IgE is also synthesized in mucosal tissues, particularly during parasitic infection or during certain pathologic (allergic) states. However, there is no preferential localization of IgE B cells in the mucosa and the number of B cells synthesizing IgE is small, as it is in other tissues. Recent studies with rats suggest that the mucosa may be an important site for IgE B cells during neonatal development.

REGULATION OF IgA SYNTHESIS AT MUCOSAL SITES

Several factors are involved in the preferential synthesis of IgA in mucosal follicles rather than in other lymphoid areas. Cells derived from mucosal lymphoid aggregates (Peyer's patches), but not those from the spleen, have the capacity to induce secretory IgM (sIgM)-positive B cells to undergo isotype switching to sIgA-positive B cells in vitro. Cells bringing about the isotype switching were identified as T cells, but it remains possible that other cells, including mucosal macrophages and stromal cells, also play a role (Fig 15–5). Although it is presumed that the switch cells produce an

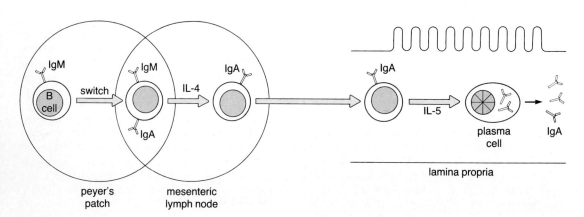

Figure 15–5. Regulation of the IgA response. This involves switching events on the mucosal follicle (Peyer's patch) and then a series of post-switch regulatory events in the mesenteric lymph node and lamina propria. The latter events are known to involve IL-4 and IL-5.

IgA-specific switch cytokine or lymphokine, such a material has yet to be identified. It is known, however, that neither IL-4 nor IL-5 can perform this function in the IgA system, unless perhaps they act in conjunction with other factors.

A second mechanism that accounts for the predominance of IgA B cells in the mucosal lymphoid aggregates involves the fact that B cells in mucosal areas come under the influence of post-isotype switch IgA-specific signals, ie, signals that favor terminal differentiation of IgA B Cells (Fig 15–5). A class of T cells that bear Fc receptors specific for IgA (FcαR) and that enhance post-switch differentiation of sIgA-bearing B cells have been identified. It is thought that such cells act through the release of IgA-binding factors which act on sIgA-positive B cells. There is evidence that certain T cells secrete IL-5, which, along with other lymphokines such as IL-6, may have preferential effects on IgA B cell differentiation. Either of these types of T cells having effects on IgA B cell differentiation may be more abundant in mucosal areas than elsewhere and may therefore act in concert with switch cells to lead to preferential IgA B cell maturation in the mucosal follicles.

Other types of IgA class-specific regulatory cells have been reported. One such cell is the "contrasuppressor" T cell obtained from Peyer's patches. These cells appear to counteract the effects of suppressor T cells on IgA responses to a greater extent than they counteract the effects of suppressor T cells on IgG or IgM responses. There is also a suppressor T cell that bears IgA-specific Fc receptors and that down-regulates IgA responses in a class-specific fashion. Cells of this type are induced in mice and humans bearing IgA plasmacytomas or myelomas, and in mice they mediate suppression of responses elicited by oral antigen administration. Thus, T cells bearing IgA-Fc receptors can act as both IgA-specific helper and suppressor cells and are, in this sense, analogous to cells having both positive and negative regulatory effects on IgE responses.

ORAL UNRESPONSIVENESS

The mucosal immune system responds negatively to the vast number of antigens from foods and normal bacterial flora in the mucosal environment. This unresponsiveness prevents the system from being overwhelmed by the antigens.

Oral unresponsiveness is more complete for antigens on the surface of erythrocytes, those associated with bacteria and viruses, and most protein antigens than it is for thymus-independent antigens and complex particulate antigens (including live viruses). This may explain why the mucosal system mounts immune responses to potential pathogens while remaining generally unresponsive to food antigens. Oral unresponsiveness is both B cell (antibody) and T cell mediated, but not necessarily to the same degree in all cases.

Adoptive transfer experiments with animals show that one cellular mechanism underlying oral unresponsiveness is the strong tendency for antigenic stimulation via mucosal follicles to induce **antigen-specific** suppressor T cells in Peyer's patches. However, it is not clear why suppressor circuits are initiated more readily in the mucosal system than elsewhere. The presence of **antigen-nonspecific** suppressor cells may be a second mechanism of oral unresponsiveness. Evidence for this comes from the observation that in animals that are genetically unresponsive to lipopolysaccharide (LPS; a B cell mitogen), oral responses to certain antigens are increased, suppressor T cell responses following oral challenge are reduced, and the phenomenon of oral unresponsiveness does not occur. Although the mechanism is unknown, it is significant that in the "normal" LPS-rich (B cell mitogen-rich) environment of the mucosa, antigen-nonspecific regulatory cells play an important role in down-regulating responses to specific antigens. A third possible mechanism is clonal inhibition (or clonal anergy) resulting from direct effects of antigens on B or T cells in mucosal follicles. Peyer's patches in sheep are sites of massive cell turnover and death; these cells may be undergoing negative clonal selection, just as they do in the thymus.

Abnormalities of oral unresponsiveness may relate to certain immunologic diseases. First, oral unresponsiveness appears to be decreased in several autoimmune mouse strains, which suggests that inappropriate reactivity to one or another antigen in the mucosal system may be a factor in the development of autoimmunity. This possibility gains credence from recent evidence that autoantibodies are structurally related to antibodies against simple antigenic determinants commonly present in the mucosal environment. Second, oral unresponsiveness is reduced in young children, resulting in hypersensitivity to certain oral antigens such as milk proteins. Third, genetically determined defects associated with oral unresponsiveness may form the basis of gluten-sensitive enteropathy or the inflammatory bowel diseases (see Chapter 40).

MUCOSAL HOMING

A characteristic feature of the mucosal immune system is the homing capability of cells developing in the mucosal follicles (Fig 15–6). As mentioned

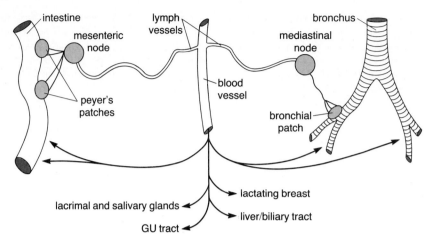

Figure 15-6. Cell traffic in the mucosal immune system. Cells originating in the mucosal follicles localize in subepithelial areas of many mucosal tissues. The ability to do so is governed by specific receptor-ligand interactions involving receptors on lymphoid cells and ligands on endothelial cells.

above, this mechanism acts to limit and focus the mucosal immune response to mucosal tissues. Studies of mucosal cell traffic show that B lymphoblasts arising in mesenteric or bronchial lymph nodes selectively localize to mucosal areas and that the majority (70–90%) of the localizing B cells are IgA B cells. T lymphoblasts from mesenteric node and thoracic duct lymph also localize to mucosal sites, both to the lamina propria and to the IEL compartment; however, compared with B cells, a smaller proportion of T cells arising in the mucosal follicles have this property. Small resting (or memory) B cells and T cells arising in the mucosal follicles also recirculate in the mucosal immune system.

Mucosal homing is not an antigen-trapping mechanism. Mucosal lymphoblasts migrate to antigen-free intestinal grafts in extraintestinal sites. Antigen challenge to an isolated area of mucosa results in the appearance of antigen-reactive cells in equal numbers at both exposed and nonexposed areas of mucosa, indicating that cell migration is not directed by antigen. After cells have migrated into the lamina propria, however, antigen does cause them to become sessile (fixed in tissue) and to proliferate. In fact, antigen-specific responses are enhanced at intestinal sites that have been previously exposed to antigen and reduced elsewhere in the intestine.

There is a growing body of data supporting the idea that mucosal homing is initiated by interactions between specific homing receptors on Peyer's patch-derived lymphocytes and ligands for such receptors on endothelial cells (addressins). These interactions are followed by cellular penetration of the endothelium and the entry of cells

into mucosal tissue proper. Thus, the capacity of a Peyer's patch lymphocyte to home to the lamina propria can be explained by the selective induction of homing receptors on lymphocytes developing at this site.

BREAST MILK IMMUNOLOGY

The lactating breast is an important component of the mucosal traffic "loop" and ensures that mucosal immunoglobulins and cells are available to protect the neonate during a critical period of relative immunologic incompetence. The concentration of IgA in initial breast secretions (colostrum) is extremely high, averaging 50 mg/mL (versus 2.5 mg/mL in adult serum). However, it falls rapidly to serum levels after the first 4 days, in part owing to the dilutional effect of increased secretion volume. The IgA of breast milk originates from IgA B cells in breast tissue, which migrated there from gastrointestinal and respiratory mucosal follicles. Such migration is dependent on as yet unidentified changes in breast tissue brought about by the action of hormones. The locally synthesized IgA is then transported across the epithelium by an SC-mediated transport mechanism.

Human colostrum and milk are rich in antibodies to a variety of organisms. The beneficial effect of such antibodies may not be obvious in developed countries, but it is readily apparent in underdeveloped countries, where exposure to environmental pathogens is much greater. In addition to protecting the newborn from infection, breast milk antibodies may play a role in establishing the normal flora and in preventing the uptake of certain macromolecules. The latter effect may be relevant to the development of allergies, but this is not yet certain.

Breast milk secretion also contains a significant number of cells, and its ingestion results in the transfer of as many as 10^8 cells/d to the newborn. Most of the cells in breast milk are macrophages and granulocytes, but small numbers of B and T lymphocytes are also present. The macrophages are functionally active and contain ingested IgA; thus, they may be a vehicle for the delivery of IgA to critical areas. Although the T cells are present in small numbers, they are able to transfer specific immune reactivity; suggesting that these cells gain entry to the newborn circulation.

SUMMARY

The antigenic environment of the mucosa is a chaotic mix of virtually the entire antigenic universe, to which may be added potential mitogens that could further stimulate the mucosal system. In this situation it is essential that the relevant immune system be capable of discriminating between stimuli that have possible pathogenic import and those that are harmless and would merely engage the system in a fruitless and wasteful response. The mucosal immune system is shaped to fulfill this need. On the one hand, it has a highly focused response to stimuli, which produces antibodies that interact with and eliminate potential pathogens, without at the same time evoking undue inflammation. Such responses also help to prevent entry and to facilitate clearance of unwanted antigens. On the other hand, it also elaborates suppressor elements that interact with ubiquitous antigens and thus down regulate responses both in the mucosal areas and in systemic lymphoid tissues. In pursuing these somewhat opposing goals, the mucosal immune system fulfills an important and critical "gatekeeper" function of the immune system, which ensures the integrity of the internal milieu.

REFERENCES

General
Mestecky J, McGhee J: Immunoglobulin A (IgA): Molecular and cellular interactions involved in IgA biosynthesis and immune response. *Adv Immunol* 1987;**40**:153.
Strober W, Brown WR: The mucosal immune system, In: *Immunological Diseases,* 4th ed. Samter M (editor). Little, Brown, 1988.

Antigen-Presenting Cells
Ermak TH, Owen RL: Differential distribution of lymphocytes and accessory cells in mouse Peyer's patches. *Anat Rec* 1986;**215**:144.
Richman LK, Graeff AS, Strober W: Antigen presentation by macrophage-enriched cells from the mouse Peyer's patch. *Cell Immunol* 1981;**62**:110.

M Cells
Sneller MC, Strober W: M cells and host defense. *J Infect Dis* 1986;**154**:737.

Intraepithelial Lymphocytes
Ernst PB, Befus AD, Bienenstock J: Leukocytes in the intestinal epithelium: An unusual immunological compartment. *Immunol Today* 1985;**6**:50.

Mucosal Mast Cells
Befus AD et al: Mast cells from the human intestinal lamina propria. *J Immunol* 1987;**138**:2604.
Irani AA et al: Two types of human mast cells that have distinct neutral protease compositions. *Proc Natl Acad Sci USA* 1986;**83**:4464.

Lamina Propria Lymphocytes
Fiocchi C et al: Modulation of intestinal immune reactivity by interleukin 2: Phenotypic and functional analysis of lymphokine-activated killer cells from human intestinal mucosa. *Dig Dis Sci* 1988;**33**:1305.
James SP et al: Intestinal lymphocyte populations and mechanisms of cell mediated immunity. *Immunol Allergy Clin N Am* 1988;**8**:369.

IgA Structure & Transport
Conley ME, Delacroix DL: Intravascular and mucosal immunoglobulin A: Two separate but related systems of immune defense? *Ann Intern Med* 1987;**106**:892.
Kilian J, Mestecky J, Russel MW: Defense mechanisms involving Fc-dependent functions of immunoglobulin A and their subversion by bacterial immunoglobulin A proteases. *Microbiol Rev* 1988;**52**:296.
Underdown BJ, Schiff JM: Immunoglobulin A: Strategic defense initiative at the mucosal surface. *Annu Rev Immunol* 1986;**4**:389.
Walker WA: Antigen handling by the small intestine. *Clin Gastroenterol* 1986;**15**:1.

Regulation of IgA Synthesis
Harriman GR et al: The role of IL-5 in IgA B cell differentiation. *J Immunol* 1988;**140**:3033.
Kawanishi H, Saltzman LE, Strober W: Mechanisms regulating IgA class-specific immunoglobulin production in murine gut-associated lymphoid tissues. *J Exp Med* 1983;**157**:433.
Kiyono H et al: Isotype-specific immunoregulation. IgA-binding factors produced by Fcα receptorpositive T cell hybridomas regulate IgA responses. *J Exp Med* 1985;**161**:731.

Oral Unresponsiveness

Mowat AM: The regulation of immune responses to dietary protein antigens. *Immunol Today* 1987; **8:**93.

Mucosal Cell Homing

Bienenstock J et al: Regulation of lymphoblast traffic and localization in mucosal tissues, with emphasis on IgA. *Fed Proc* 1983;**42:**3213.

Jalkanen S et al: Human lymphocyte and lymphoma homing receptors. *Annu Rev Med* 1987;**38:**467.

Breast Milk

Ogra PL, Losonsky GA, Fishaut M. Colostrum-derived immunity and maternal-neonatal interaction. *Ann NY Acad Sci* 1983;**409:**82.

Physiologic & Environmental Influences on the Immune System

16

The immune system has developed a high intrinsic capacity for recognizing and dealing with foreign substances. This capacity is controlled by a series of internal processes of self-regulation. In the intact host, however, the immune system has anatomic and physiologic relationships with other systems of the body, and there is a potential for it to be adversely or beneficially affected by environmental influences.

In contrast to the current wealth of information about the immune system itself, there is relatively little information about the relationship between the immune system, other physiologic systems, and the environment. Available data are very incomplete, but research interest in many of these areas is gaining momentum. This chapter will cover a selected group of topics dealing with external and internal influences on the immune system. These include psychoneuroimmunology, aging, nutrition, environmental chemicals, and uremia.

PSYCHONEUROIMMUNOLOGY

Abba I. Terr, MD

For many years a few investigators have been studying the interrelationships among the immune system, the nervous system, the endocrine glands, and psychologic behavior. There is evidence from clinical observations and experimentation and from animal studies that the immune response and its various effector mechanisms are regulated and modulated in part by neuroendocrine influences, in addition to internal regulation by its own feedback inhibition, regulatory lymphocytes, and the anti-idiotype network. The nervous system/immune system interaction appears to be bidirectional, and it is influenced by and expressed in behavioral and emotional terms. There are some important similarities between central nervous system and immune system function. Both respond to environmental stimuli, the nervous system sensing physical signals and the immune system sensing chemical structures.

Much of the research in this area deals with the effect of stress on the immune response. In this context, stress is usually defined as the host response to an adverse environmental event or stimulus, called a stressor, and the effects are related to inability to cope with the stressor. Coping mechanisms are defined subjectively and include both internal psychologic mechanisms and external social support systems.

ANATOMIC CONNECTIONS BETWEEN THE NERVOUS AND IMMUNE SYSTEMS

Although a direct nervous system/endocrine anatomic connection between the hypothalamus and the pituitary has been well established for some time, a similar study of innervation of the immune system has been undertaken only recently. There are, in fact, nerve endings in the thymus, spleen, and lymph nodes, primarily sympathetic efferents. In both humans and animals, autonomic nervous system fibers to the thymus appear embryologically before immature T cells do. In the bone marrow, spleen, and lymph nodes, the nerve endings appear in locations rich in T cells but not B cells.

PHYSIOLOGIC INTERRELATIONSHIPS

The nervous and immune systems are comparable in a number of ways. Both are characterized by a diversity of cell types and by cell-to-cell transmission of information by soluble factors such as lymphokines (in the immune system) and neurotransmitters (in the nervous system). Both systems have the capacity for short-lived and long-lived memory. Opportunities for cross-communication are becoming increasingly evident. Lymphocytes and macrophages have receptors capable of responding to the neurotransmitters acetylcholine and norepinephrine, endorphins, enkephalins, and a number of endocrine hormones including adrenocorticotropic hormone (ACTH), corticosteroids, insulin, prolactin, growth hormone, estradiol, and testosterone. Lymphocytes, in turn, are capable of producing and secreting ACTH and endorphinlike compounds, which could act as an autocrine feedback regulator of lymphocyte functions.

Neurons in the brain, particularly in the hypothalamus, can recognize immunocyte products (including prostaglandins, interferons, and interleukins) and chemical mediators from inflammatory cell products (including histamine and serotonin).

ANIMAL EXPERIMENTS

Short-term animal experiments have been performed primarily with rodents and primates. The relevance of these results to humans is obviously tenuous because of small but significant differences in the immune responses and obviously enormous differences in psychologic makeup. Many animal experiments have involved the effect of acute stressors on antibody responses, antibody-induced effects such as anaphylaxis, mitogen responses, and quantitative changes in circulating immunoglobulins and lymphocytes. Stressors have included physical stimuli, such as electric shock, loud noise, and acceleration, and purely psychologic stressors, such as infant-mother separation, peer separation, restraints, and overcrowding. Results have been mixed. Although early experiments showed that antibody production was increased after low-voltage electric shock, more recent studies have generally shown an early inhibition of antibody production, mitogenic responses of lymphocytes, and reduced lymphocyte counts. Longer-term experiments generally show that these effects are transient; this suggests that adaptation occurs. Immunologic effects are most pronounced when the animal is stressed in an inescapable condition, possibly stimulating the phenomenon of poor coping in humans. Some reports suggest that stressed animals have an increased incidence of infections and enhanced growth of injected syngeneic tumor cells. Since the immunologic measurements of lymphocyte counts and lymphocyte responses are usually performed with circulating cells, the effect of stress is caused at least in part by stress-induced glucocorticoid lymphopenia. However, a slight but reproducible suppressive effect on the immune response occurs in adrenalectomized animals. The results on tumor growth may reflect changes in vascularity or hormone effects independent of any effect on the immune system itself.

There are several compelling reports of Pavlovian conditioning of the immune response. Rats given saccharin as a conditioned stimulus along with the immunosuppressant drug cyclophosphamide as an unconditioned stimulus (but used in this case to produce nausea) were later fortuitously discovered to be conditioned for immune suppression with saccharin alone. This observation led to a series of experiments in which both antibody-mediated immunity and cell-mediated immunity (CMI) were depressed by conditioning. In a reverse type of experiment, conditioning was also used successfully to significantly reduce the dose of cyclophosphamide required to control systemic lupus in mice. Mediators from immunologically sensitized mast cells have also been released in vivo by a conditioned stimulus of an odor in guinea pigs and an audiovisual stimulus in rats.

The presence of an immune response on the brain has been shown by the fact that norepinephrine synthesis in the hypothalamus (as well as in the spleen) is inhibited at the peak of an induced immune response to a foreign antigen. Follow-up experiments showed that the inhibition was related to soluble factors secreted by lymphocytes, but the nature of these factors has not yet been determined.

Hemispheric lateralization of the central nervous system control of immunity is shown by the effect of experimental lesions in the cerebral neocortex. Left-sided neocortical lesions in mice caused a reduction in the number of spleen cells, T cell-dependent responses, natural killer (NK) cells, lymphokines, and regulatory T cells, whereas right-sided lesions produced the opposite effect. B cells and macrophages were not affected.

Finally, an interesting series of experiments reveals that immune responses were altered when surgical lesions were induced in the brain. Lesions in the anterior hypothalamus of mice inhibited immune responses, whereas lesions in the amygdala or hippocampus enhanced them, possibly via neural influences on spleen suppressor cell activity. In other studies, an induced immune response in mice produced changes in the electrical activity of brain neurons, an effect that was probably mediated by lymphokines.

A variety of endocrine hormones administered to different animals cause differing effect on immune responses. In general, glucocorticoids, androgens, estrogen, and progesterone inhibit antibody production, whereas growth hormone, thyroxine, and insulin enhance it. The effect of autonomic neurotransmitters is likewise a dual one, with parasympathetic agonists increasing and sympathetic agonists decreasing antibody production and cytotoxicity.

STUDIES IN HUMANS

Anecdotal reports based on clinical observations have long suggested that psychologic factors, particularly stressful life events, influence diseases related to the immune system. Clinicians and patients alike have long suspected that symptoms of infections and allergies are worsened by stressful events. Graves' disease is reported to appear after separation or loss of a close family member. A number of retrospective studies on bereavement suggest that it is associated with a susceptibility to diabetes, ulcerative colitis, rheumatoid arthritis, systemic lupus erythematosus (SLE), and cancer. However, spousal bereavement has also been associated with occurrence of schizophrenia, coronary artery disease, sudden accidents, and death.

The designs of clinical studies have usually taken one of 2 forms: cross-sectional analysis of immune responses in a susceptible population and prospective case-control studies.

Several investigators have used spousal bereavement to study immunologic changes secondary to a stressful life event in otherwise normal individuals. A prospective study of husbands of women with advanced breast cancer found that lymphocyte responses to mitogens diminished during the first 2 months following the wife's death, although total lymphocyte and lymphocyte subset counts, delayed-type hypersensitivity (DTH), and circulating levels of cortisol, prolactin, growth hormone, and thyroid hormone remained normal. In some studies, there are reports of an increase in the severity of respiratory infections accompanying these functional lymphocyte changes, but this information is based on patient reports rather than objective evidence. In general, possible confounding factors of weight loss, changes in diet, sleep alteration, lack of exercise, and use of drugs were not monitored.

The stress produced in first-year dental students as a result of their academic examinations produced a significant drop in salivary IgA secretion. In these studies it was noted that the basal secretory levels and response to stress correlated with the personality traits of each student. Those with an inherent need for personal relationships tended to have higher levels of secretory IgA. In another report, the stress of examinations caused a decrease in circulating CD4 cells and NK cell activity in medical students; this effect was most marked in students who expressed loneliness. Other studies have shown that although anxiety and depression may inhibit some manifestations of the immune response, subjects who coped well with stress showed an increase in NK cell activity. The significance of such observations for host defense is unclear. Although experiments using Pavlovian conditioning have not been done with human subjects, there are a number of anecdotal reports of suppression of immediate and delayed skin tests to allergens induced by hypnosis or meditation.

THE IMMUNOLOGY OF PSYCHIATRIC ILLNESS

In recent years an emphasis in psychiatry research has shifted to a search for a biologic, rather than a psychologic, cause for many psychiatric diseases, especially for the major depressive disorders. Depressive disease, also called affective disorder, has a 1–2% prevalence in the general population, is characterized by dysphoria, and may be accompanied by somatic symptoms. It may manifest as simple unipolar depression or as alternating manic-depressive bipolar disease. Immunologic studies are confounded by the fact that increased release of corticosteroids from the pituitary is a feature of major depressive disorder as well as a response to a wide range of stresses that may produce temporary depression in normal individuals. Case-control studies on depression have shown variable effects on circulating lymphocytes. On balance, counts of circulating lymphocytes and their subsets are not consistently changed, although mitogenic responses are often reported to be diminished. Controlling for the effects of diet and activity makes studies on this group of patients difficult. The investigators usually discontinue administration of antidepressant medications prior to obtaining blood samples for study, but a possible effect of drug withdrawal has not been carefully investigated.

Patients with schizophrenia also show variable and inconsistent changes in circulating lymphocyte concentrations. Mitogen responses were normal in patients with agarophobia and panic attacks. One interesting report showed evidence of a possible human leukocyte anitgen (HLA) linkage in a family study of depression, regardless of whether the disease was unipolar or bipolar. The association suggested that an HLA-associated gene may be involved in the susceptibility to the disease, which probably requires other factors for clinical expression.

NEUROPSYCHIATRIC STUDIES IN IMMUNOLOGIC DISEASES

This area has received much less research attention. An organic psychosis can occur in some forms of autoimmune disease, such as SLE, but the relevance of this to psychiatric illness in general is obscure. Recent clinical trials of recombinant lymphokines have revealed, in some cases, side effects including psychiatric symptoms. For example, interferon therapy characteristically produces a picture of depression with fatigue, drowsiness, disorientation, lethargy, withdrawal, and electroencephalogram (EEG) abnormalities.

A recent provocative report that certain immune diseases—autoimmune thyroiditis, celiac disease, regional ileitis, ulcerative colitis, childhood atopic allergy, and myasthenia gravis—are significantly more common among those who are naturally left-handed is reminiscent of the animal studies showing hemispheric dominance in immune responses, but these results should be considered preliminary.

SUMMARY

Clinical and experimental psychoneuroimmunology studies to date confirm the long-standing belief that the immune system does not function completely autonomously. The findings suggest many exciting research opportunities, but few if any conclusions can yet be drawn about the interrelationships of psychiatric and immunologic factors that can be applied to the diagnosis and treatment of specific diseases.

AGING & NUTRITIONAL EFFECTS ON IMMUNE FUNCTIONS IN HUMANS

Devendra P. Dubey PhD,
& Edmond J. Yunis, MD

The elderly are more susceptible than younger adults to develop certain infectious diseases with increased severity, and they are at greater risk of developing cancer and autoimmune diseases. This suggests that immune deficiencies may be a feature of the aged population. Studies generally agree that there is a decline in immune functions in older individuals but disagree about which specific immune functions are impaired. The conflicting results may be due to methodologic differences, differences in the selection of subjects for study, and lack of an accepted definition of "old" and "young." The changes in immune function due to disease may further confound the determination of intrinsic age-related decline in the immune function.

This section describes the age-related changes in the thymus, T cell responses to mitogens and antigens, lymphokine production, antibody production, and NK cell function. The T cell response to PHA, CMI, and T cell–dependent antibody production significantly decline, whereas T cell–independent antibody production is not significantly affected in healthy aged individuals.

AGING

The Thymus & Aging

The thymus plays a central role in T cell maturation and proliferation. One of the better-known phenomena associated with aging is the involution of the thymus. Morphologic studies reveal that although the weight and volume of the thymus may show large variations among individuals, they increase until 6 months of age and thereafter remain constant, although the morphology of the thymus changes significantly.

Structurally, the thymus can be divided into 4 major regions: epithelial cortex, cortex, corticomedullary region, and medulla. The outer region of the cortex contains many macrophages and large blastlike lymphocytes. The inner cortex and medulla contain medium-sized and smaller lymphocytes as well as Hassall's corpuscles. In addition to lymphoid cells, the thymus contains nonlymphoid cells: cortical and medullary epithelial cells, interdigitating reticulum cells, macrophages, and mast cells. Blood vessels are found in the cortex and medullary region and characteristically possess epithelial cells in the adventitia, which serves as a blood-thymus barrier. Hematopoietic stem cells from bone marrow travel through the bloodstream and enter the thymus through the epithelial cell lining of the cortex (Fig 16-1). Prothymocytes (or pre-T cells) differentiate within the microenvironment of the thymus. In the thymus 4 peptide hormones, thymulin, thymosin a, thymosin β, and thymopoietin, are synthesized. These hormones are involved in the proliferation and differentiation of T cells. In addition, direct contact with the thymic epithelium, which expresses HLA antigens, is required for the generation of functional T cells and their education to recognize antigens of the major histocompatibility complex (MHC) region. The thymus is believed to be linked with the central nervous system, the endocrine system, and the immune system and thus to participate in the regulation of immune function by a complex network of interactions. The most significant change in the

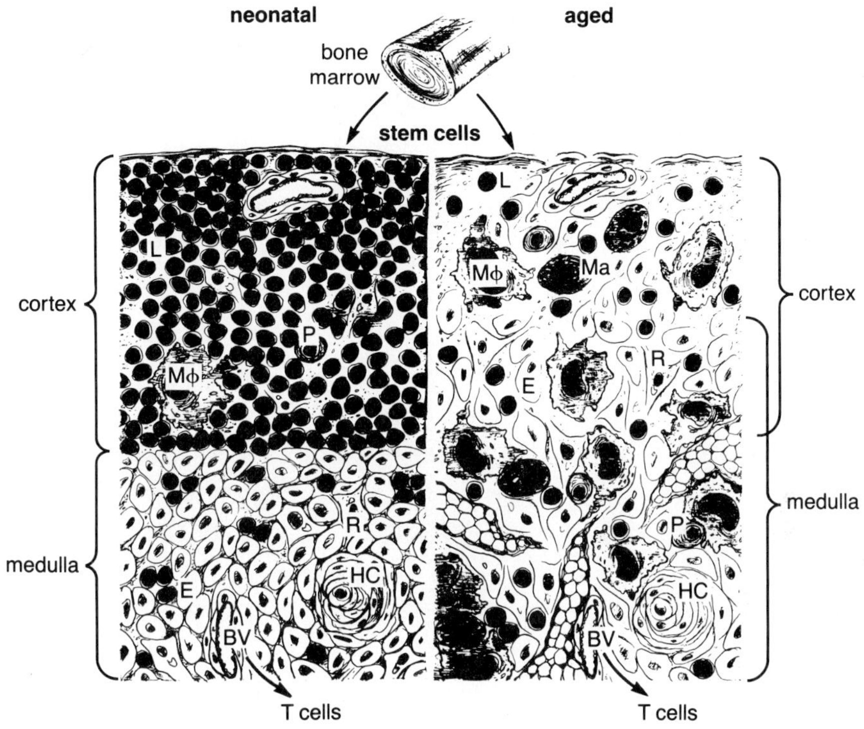

Figure 16-1. Schematic representation of age-related changes in the human thymus. The cortex is heavily populated with lymphocytes (L) in neonatal thymus, and the medulla contains Hassall's corpuscles (HC) and fewer lymphocytes. The aged thymus is involuted and atrophied and contains fat cells. The cortex has fewer lymphocytes, infiltrated with macrophages (Mφ) and mast cells (mα). The medulla is relatively unaffected. The stem cells that migrate to the thymus encounter the epithelial cells (E), which express class I and II antigens on their surface. Class I antigen is weakly expressed on the thymocytes in the cortical region and strongly expressed on thymocytes in the medullary region. It differentiates into mature T-cells with CD4 and CD8 antigen expression

thymus during aging is a decrease in the mass of the organ, in the number of lymphocytes, and in thymic hormone production (Fig 16-2).

T & B Lymphocyte Changes & Aging

The total number of lymphocytes and the number of T and B cells in the peripheral blood do not change with age. The relative proportions of CD4 and CD8 T cells are both slightly reduced with age. The reduction in CD4 cells is somewhat greater than in CD8 cells, resulting in lowered CD4/CD8 cell ratios. It is possible that although the changes are numerically small, they may be important to immune regulation. T lymphocyte proliferation is low in response to mitogens in the aged, without a corresponding reduction in the number of T cells.

The autologous mixed-lymphocyte reaction is considered an in vitro model with which to study T-T interaction in which both helper T (CD4) and suppressor/cytotoxic (CD8) cell functions are generated. The autologous mixed-lymphocyte response of lymphocytes from the aged is significantly lower than that of lymphocytes from the young, and could not be corrected by the addition of interleukin-2 (IL-2).

Other T cell functions defective in the elderly population are the ability to respond to or to stimulate allogeneic and autologous lymphocytes in mixed-lymphocyte reactions, reduced generation of cytotoxic T cells, and reduced capability to reject primary allografts and tumor cells. The level of interferon produced by lymphocytes from elderly donors exposed to herpes simplex virus is decreased.

The B cell responsiveness to pokeweed mitogen is dependent on T cell subsets. Lymphocytes from aged donors exhibit a lower frequency of pokeweed mitogen-induced plaque-forming cells in comparison with those from young subjects. This apparent decrease in B cell function could be due to an age-related decline in helper T cell function. This is supported by the observation that in the elderly population the proportion of CD45R, a

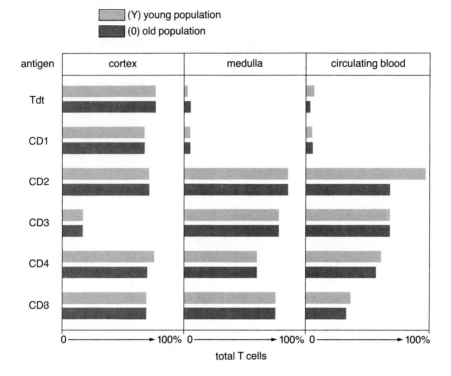

Figure 16-2. Age-dependent changes in the human thymocytes and peripheral blood lymphocytes. Immature thymocytes are found in the cortex. These cells express terminal deoxyribonucleotidyl transferase (Tdt). The expression of this enzyme is lost when thymocytes become mature. CD1 antigen is lost in the medullary region. The percentage of CD2- and Cd3-positive cells increases when the cells move from the cortex to the medulla. In the cortex CD4 is coexpressed with CD8. In the medulla, CD4 and CD8 antigens are expressed on different cells. A small percentage of cells in the medulla coexpress CD4 and CD8 antigens. With age there may be a slight decrease in the number of mature CD3 cells and an increase in the number of immature CD1 cells.

subset of CD4 T cells, is significantly lower than in younger age groups.

Activation of T cells plays a crucial role in the responsiveness of the host to a foreign antigen. Some of the early activation events are stimulation of phospholipase C and protein kinase C, mobilization of intracellular calcium, IL-2 production and its receptor expression, and activation of proto-oncogenes such as c-*myc* and c-*myb*. A defect in T cell responses to mitogen or antigens may reflect a defect in one or more steps of signal transduction. T cells of older people respond poorly to mitogen or antigen stimulation. Studies have not revealed any defect in the antigen-presenting capacity or other stimulatory characteristics of macrophages of older people. However, a defect in IL-2 production as well as expression of both high-affinity and low-affinity IL-2 receptors has been observed, and T cell proliferation cannot be restored by addition of exogenous IL-2. The binding of IL-2 receptor with the ligand (IL-2) and internalization of this complex are also impaired. A similar reduction in c-*myc*

gene expression in activated T cells has been reported. Definitive information on the other early steps in signal transduction, such as calcium mobilization and protein kinase C activation, is still lacking.

Humoral Immunity & Aging

An increased frequency of infections and autoimmune diseases is observed among the elderly. One of the most common causes of morbidity and mortality in this population is infections caused by certain bacteria such as *Streptococcus pneumoniae* and *Escherichia coli*. Polyclonal hyperimmunoglobulinemia and increased levels of autoantibodies are also common. The lack of a response to bacterial infection may be due to an age-related defect in antibody function. Although the total concentration of immunoglobulins remains unchanged with age, there is an increase in the level of IgA and IgG antibodies. Antibody responses to specific antigens such as flagellin, purified protein derivative (PPD), hepatitis B virus, and multivalent influenza virus vaccines are decreased. The subpopulation of CD8 T cells in the elderly population has been shown to decrease with age, suggesting that loss of regulatory suppressor T cell activity may explain the occurrence of autoantibodies in the elderly.

Recent studies show a decrease in the NK lytic activity but an increase or no change in the number of NK cells as defined by CD16 and CD57 (Leu 7) markers in healthy elderly individuals. However, others have observed a decrease in activity as well as in the number of NK cells in this age group.

SUMMARY

The functions of the immune system show some evidence of decline with age. Involution of the thymus is accompanied by reduced production of thymic hormones and an increase in the number of immature lymphocytes. The DTH response is reduced. Although the number of circulating T lymphocytes in peripheral blood does not show any significant decrease with age, a small decrease in the proportion of subsets of T cells responsible for immune regulation may lead to a reduced responsiveness to foreign antigens and increased autoimmunity. There is an age-dependent decline in in vitro T cell responses to mitogens such as PHA and concanavalin A. IL-2 and gamma interferon (IFN-γ) production by T cells is reduced. No change in the antigen-presenting capacity of macrophages has been observed. Data on NK cell activity of old individuals are controversial, and further study is needed. B cells do not show any significant decrease in number but have a reduced capacity to form hemolytic plaques by antibody secretion and are diminished in T cell–dependent antibody production. This reflects a possible defect in T cell subsets that regulate antibody production.

The importance of these changes is not yet clear. Many other factors, such as nutritional deficiency and stress, that may suppress immune function could induce immune deficiency and render older people vulnerable to life-threatening infections, autoimmunity, and cancers.

NUTRITION

Proteins, carbohydrates, lipids, vitamins, and minerals are essential for human maintenance and growth. Qualitative and quantitative changes in these nutrients may significantly affect the functions of the immune system. Cells of the immune system, when activated, are metabolically very active and synthesize and secrete molecules that are involved in cell-cell interaction. Thus, either a deficiency or an excess of specific nutrients can influence the synthesis of these molecules, thereby altering the regulation of immunity.

Malnutrition is a common cause of immune deficiency, with a particularly significant effect on CMI, phagocytosis, and the complement system. It may have long-term reversible or irreversible effects, depending on its severity and duration. Malnourishment of the mother can lead to nutritional deficiencies in utero that may affect the newborn's ability to respond to infections at birth. This in utero deficiency may involve both CMI and humoral immunity. In severe protein-calorie malnutrition, the humoral response and antibody production may return to a normal level after the subject is maintained on an adequate diet, but the deficiency in CMI may persist.

Protein-Calorie Malnutrition

Chronic nutritional deficiency may lead to different kinds of diseases such as kwashiorkor and marasmus. Kwashiorkor is an extreme case of protein-calorie malnutrition. Marasmus, a milder form of the disease, is a clinical manifestation of protein, fat, vitamin, or mineral deprivation during the early part of life. Patients with these diseases have a higher than normal incidence of bacterial and parasitic infections. Severe thymic atrophy is seen in malnourished children, especially in patients with kwashiorkor and to a lesser extent in those with marasmus. A severe case of kwashiorkor leads to acute thymic involution accompanied by loss of corticomedullary differentiation, a reduced number of thymocytes, and various degrees of depletion of lymph node germinal centers and paracortical cells in peripheral lymphoid tissues. The degree of thymic atrophy depends on the duration and severity of the nutritional deficiency. Lymphoid organs such as the thymus and lymph nodes become smaller, and there is lymphopenia, impaired response to PHA, low NK activity, and decreased cutaneous DTH reactions. These findings suggest that protein-caloric malnutrition affects CMI (Table 16–1). The effects of protein-calorie malnutrition on humoral immunity are less severe. B cell numbers and immunoglobulin levels are not affected significantly, but the antibody response may vary with the antigen and the form in which it is given. Although serum IgA levels are normal in protein-calorie-malnourished individuals, secretory IgA levels are low, suggesting that synthesis of secretory component by epithelial cells is impaired. In many cases, hypergammaglobulinemia of the IgM type is present. Patients with kwashiorkor characteristically have hypoproteinemia and hypoalbuminemia and yet

Table 16-1. Effects of protein deficiency on immune functions.

Cell-Mediated Immunity

Decreased cutaneous DTH, delayed skin homograft rejection, decreased thymic hormone activity.

Reduced circulating CD3 cells and CD4 subsets; increased relative proportion of TdT immature T cells.

Suppressed T cell responses to mitogens such as PHA and concanavalin A; reduced autologous mixed-lymphocyte reaction response.

Humoral Immunity

Normal level of serum antibody, reduced antibody response to T cell–dependent antigen (eg, sheep erythrocytes), secretion but normal T cell–independent antibody production.

Nonspecific Immune Functions

Normal antigen processing by macrophages; reduced phagocytosis.

Impaired PMN activity.

Table 16-2. Effects of vitamin deficiencies on immune functions.

Nutritional Status	Immune Effects
Vitamin A deficiency	Atrophy of thymus and spleen, decreased DTH decrease in circulating leukocytes and lymphocytes, reduced T and B cell responses to certain mitogens and antigens, reduced secretory IgA production; high infection rate; effect reversible after treatment with vitamin A.
Vitamin B_6 (pyridoxine) deficiency	Decreased DTH, prolonged survival of skin homografts; reduced T and B cell numbers, decreased antibody-forming cells, reduced phagocytic activity of neutrophils; impaired thymic epithelial cell functions. Mothers with B_6 deficiency have fetuses with much smaller thymus and spleen, and the newborns have reduced CMI.
Vitamin B_{12} deficiency	Decreased DTH, reduced T and B cell responses to mitogens and antigens, impaired phagocytic and bactericidal capacity of PMN; in humans, pernicious anemia with autoimmune phenomena.
Vitamin D deficiency	No consistent effects.
Vitamin E deficiency	Decreased DTH, decreased T and B cell responses to mitogens, decreased immunoglobulin production.
Folic acid deficiency	Decreased DTH, suppressed T cell responses to mitogens, reduced antibody production, no effect on PMN activity.
Vitamin C deficiency	No significant effect on T or B cell functions, temporary decrease in vitamin C in macrophages and PMN, reduced phagocytic capacity; the effect is reversible.

have relatively high levels of serum immunoglobulins.

Protein-calorie malnutrition also impairs macrophage functions and polymorphonuclear-neurophil (PMN) activity. Although cell numbers and phagocytosis may remain normal, the oxidative and glycolytic activity of these cells is significantly reduced. Since protein-calorie malnutrition may be accompanied by mineral, vitamin, fat, and carbohydrate deficiencies, it is important that the effects of deficiency or excess of these individual nutritional components on immune functions also be understood.

Vitamin Deficiency

Deficiencies in immune function due to protein-calorie deficiency may result from a lack of adequate vitamins. In vitro studies show that vitamins are involved in the synthesis of DNA and proteins as well as in the regulation of cell proliferation and maturation of immune cells. Table 16-2 describes the reported effects of vitamin deficiencies on immune function.

Trace Element Deficiency

Trace elements are essential for adequate nutrition. The deficiency or excess of copper, iron, zinc, manganese, or selenium in the diet generally suppresses immune function (Table 16-3), rendering the host vulnerable to infections and other disorders.

A. Iron: Lymphoid cells need iron for metabolic activities such as cell division, electron transport, and oxidation and reduction reactions. Iron is transported from extracellular fluids to the cell by the iron-binding protein transferrin. The iron-transferrin complex enters immune cells by binding with transferrin receptors and is transported inside the cells via endocytosis. The observation that patients with protein-calorie malnutrition invariably suffer from iron deficiency and a high frequency of infection suggests that an iron deficiency may impair the functioning of lymphoid cells.

B. Copper: A deficiency of copper is also associated with protein-calorie malnutrition and appears to occur more frequently with kwashiorkor than with marasmus. Menkes' kinky-hair syndrome is a fatal genetic disease, which is due to defective copper metabolism and reduced synthesis of ceruloplasmin. It results in an increase in

Table 16–3. Effects of trace element deficiency on immune functions.

Condition	Immune Status
Mn deficiency	Decreased CMI, reduced levels of serum immunoglobulin, reduced antibody-forming cells.
Fe deficiency	Decreased DTH reaction, reduced T cell mitogenic response, reduced lymphokine production by activated T cells; reduced antibody production, reduced phagocytosis by PMN.
Zn deficiency	Depressed DTH reactions, thymic atrophy, decrease in thymic hormone activity, decreased number of T cells and CD4 cells, reduced proliferation responses to PHA, increased number of CD8 cells; reduced NK cell activity, increased monocyte activity; decreased chemotaxis of monocytes and PMN.
Cu deficiency	Reduced function of monocytes.
Se deficiency	Decreased CMI, suppressed T cell response to mitogens and antigens, decreased phagocytosis by monocytes and macrophages.

the frequency of infection mainly as a result of defective functioning of the immune system.

C. Zinc: The discovery of nutritional zinc deficiency in the pathogenesis of several diseases such as sickle cell anemia, renal disorders, and the genetic disorder acrodermatitis enteropathica provided the impetus for a study of the mechanism of zinc-induced changes in cell metabolism and immunity. Zinc is an important cofactor for a large number of enzymes involved in DNA synthesis, such as DNA polymerase and thymidine kinases, which, in turn, regulate cellular functions. Zinc deficiency causes a profound im-

mune deficiency state in both humans and mice. Mice maintained on low-zinc diets during in utero development have an immune deficiency state, which was reversed when they were maintained on a diet supplemented with zinc.

D. Selenium: Selenium has profound effects on tumor development. Dietary supplementation of selenium, along with vitamin E, inhibits tumorigenesis and retards tumor growth in animals. A lack of selenium has been found to be associated with decreased CMI.

Fatty Acids

Fatty acids are the building blocks of several classes of lipids (neutral fatty acids, cholesterol esters, glycolipids), all of which make up to various degrees the structural components of the cell membranes. Various effects of deficiency have been associated with immunity (Table 16–4). The fluidity of these membranes is regulated to some extent by their cholesterol content, as is the maintenance of the structural and functional integrity of the cell.

Fatty acids are either unsaturated or saturated. The unsaturated fatty acid relevant to immune function is arachidonic acid. Prostaglandins, the product of arachidonic acid, play an important role in immunoregulation such as T cell proliferation and NK cell function. Lipids are precursors of vitamins A, E, K, and D as well as cholesterol. Biosynthesis of these vitamins and cholesterol is affected by the presence of exogenous lipids and cholesterol. In in vitro studies, high levels of cholesterol have been found to suppress immune function by inhibiting the cholesterol synthesis needed for the normal functioning of the immune cells. An excess in polyunsaturated fatty acids in the diet is highly immunosuppressive. One of the possible mechanisms of immunosuppression by fatty acids is that the polyunsaturated fatty acids influence membrane fluidity and hence the cell surface receptor distribution and function. Also, it has been suggested that since the polyunsat-

Table 16–4. Effects of fatty acid status on immune functions.

Fatty Acid Type	Effect when Deficient	Effect when in Excess
Polyunsaturated	Reduced humoral response for both T cell-dependent and T cell-independent antigens; decreased membrane fluidity.	Immunosuppression, delayed rejection of skin grafts, suppressed DTH, reduced lymphocyte response to mitogens and antigens, reduced chemotactic and phagocytic activity of neutrophils.
Saturated	Rarely encountered.	In vitro inhibition of lymphocyte response to some antigens and mitogens.
Cholesterol	Rarely encountered.	Inhibition of humoral and cutaneous hypersensitivity to antigens; reduced lymphocyte and macrophage function.

urated fatty acids linoleic acid and arachidonic acid are precursors of prostaglandins, the excess production of these immunoregulatory molecules may suppress T cell and NK cell function.

SUMMARY

Nutrition plays an important role in the maintenance of health. Both malnutrition and excess food intake enhance the incidence of infections and possibly cancers. Changes in CMI and humoral immunity are significantly modulated by nutrition. Nutritional deficiencies, such as protein-calorie deficiency, vitamin deficiency, trace-metal deficiency, and excess fatty acids, have profound effects on immune functions such as DTH, T cell responses to mitogens, antibody production, and NK activity. Some of these immune deficiencies are reversible with nutritional supplements.

THE EFFECT OF ENVIRONMENTAL CHEMICALS ON THE IMMUNE SYSTEM

Robert H. Waldman, MD

In recent years there has been concern about possible genetic, oncologic, and immunologic effects of industrial and agricultural chemicals. The chemicals suspected of having possible immunologic toxicity belong primarily to 2 major categories: halogenated hydrocarbons and heavy metals.

Human exposure can be occupational (eg, farmers exposed to pesticides, or workers who treat wood with pentachlorophenol), environmental (eg, contamination of well water with trichloroethylene), or accidental (eg, the explosion at Seveso, Italy, which contaminated the countryside with dioxins). Publicity regarding these exposures has led to considerable discussion by the general public and by the medical community about the magnitude of the effect of environmental chemicals on immunity.

This section reviews the state of knowledge about the effects of these chemicals on the human immune system, examines the magnitude of the problem as it relates to the immune system, and presents general principles for evaluating the medical and lay literature on this topic.

EVALUATION OF EXPOSED PERSONS

Because intentional exposure is not possible, evaluating the effects of potentially toxic chemicals on the human immune system is based on clinical observations and laboratory testing of persons accidentally exposed. Clinical observation is directed to finding evidence of increased susceptibility to infection in general and opportunistic infections in particular and of the specific cancers that occur in known varieties of immunodeficiency.

Opportunistic infections are discussed in detail in studies but they can be conveniently classified in 2 ways. One is by the type of organism: (1) disease caused by organisms that do not cause disease in normal hosts, eg, *Pneumocystis carinii;* (2) severe and generalized disease caused by organisms that normally cause mild, local disease, eg, *Candida albicans;* and (3) reactivation of disease that is normally quiescent eg, varicella-zoster infection. The second classification is by the type of immune abnormality. As examples, pyogenic bacteria are common pathogens in antibody deficiencies, whereas reactivation of tuberculosis occurs in depressed CMI. Cancers associated with immune deficiencies are restricted to certain types that are uncommon. There is no evidence for a generalized increase in common cancers (lung, breast, prostate) in immunosuppressed patients, but there is an increase in a few rare cancers, eg, Kaposi's sarcoma and extranodal B cell non-Hodgkin's lymphoma.

The second way to evaluate effects of potentially toxic chemicals on the immune system is by laboratory testing. Measurement of immunologic factors in the laboratory is undoubtedly helpful in evaluating patients who have opportunistic infections. A more dubious use of the laboratory is in the evaluation of healthy people, or patients with vague and subjective complaints. There are many limitations in laboratory testing. One must ensure that newer tests have been well standardized, especially for the ages of the people being tested; that the necessary conditions for handling the specimens are used; and that the laboratory carrying out the tests has had enough experience to be reliable. It should be remembered that the reference range is generally established to include 95% of normal individuals. Therefore, if 10 tests are performed (a white count and differential is a total of 7 tests) on a patient, there is a 50% chance of one or more "abnormalities." Also, it should be remembered that many drugs commonly taken by patients, eg, aspirin and oral contraceptives, as well as the common cold and other viral infections, may have clinically insignificant but measurable effects on immunologic laboratory testing. Pregnancy, stress, and aging also have measurable effects.

The high incidence of laboratory "abnormalities" means that to be significant with respect to an effect of chemicals on the human immune system, the changes should have some degree of consistency from patient to patient or from epidemiologic study to epidemiologic study. For example, if one patient has all normal tests except for an increased serum IgM level, another patient has high NK cell activity, another has a slightly low mitogen stimulation with pokeweed mitogen, etc, one must conclude that there is no pattern and therefore probably no effect of the chemical(s).

ANIMAL TESTING OF TOXIC CHEMICALS

The use of animal toxicity studies for evaluating the effects of chemicals on the human immune system has the same inherent limitations of all animal toxicity studies: (1) there are interspecies differences in sensitivities to agents; (2) the dosages used are usually much greater than those to which humans are exposed; (3) observed changes in short-term toxicity experiments may be transient and not clinically significant; and (4) the effects may be secondary; eg, the chemical may cause gastrointestinal effects, leading to undernutrition with secondary immunologic abnormalities.

Selection of animal species and strains for immunotoxicity experiments is usually based on traditional toxicology studies in which changes in the gross and microscopic pathology of visceral organs, weight, mortality, etc, are observed. The test chemical is given in a short-term, high-dose exposure, usually by ingestion or injection. Extrapolation of the results to long-term, low-dose exposure is entirely speculative.

Animal studies have shown effects on antibody production and T cell function of halogenated hydrocarbons, such as dioxins and dibenzofurans, and of polychlorinated biphenyls and pentachlorephenol. However, the effect of the last 2 is most probably due to contamination by small amounts of the first 2 classes of chemicals.

EPIDEMIOLOGIC STUDIES

There have been several epidemiologic studies of human exposure to potentially toxic chemicals, and these can conveniently be divided into those involving occupational exposure and those following accidents. Examples of occupational exposures include workers in the wood-treating industry (exposed to pentachlorophenol), those in the dry-cleaning industry (trichloroethylene and perchloroethylene), and those manufacturing transformers (polychlorinated biphenyls). Much atten-

tion has been given to the exposure of military personnel to dioxin (Agent Orange) during the Vietnam War. The level of exposure was chronic and generally low to moderate, ie, higher than the background exposure of the general public, but not as high as the exposure of those involved in accidents described below. This is evidenced by the rarity of chloracne, a hallmark of high levels of exposure to halogenated hydrocarbons.

There is no evidence in any group described above, or of any similar group, of clinically significant immunosuppression. No increase has been seen in opportunistic infections or immunologically related cancers, nor has any other abnormality been found that could be related to the immune system. Similarly, laboratory testing has revealed no significant or consistent abnormalities. One large, well-controlled study of Air Force personnel exposed to Agent Orange showed no laboratory abnormalities in immune factors in the exposed group compared with the control group, and yet the tests were sensitive enough to pick up significant differences between smokers and non-smokers.

There have been epidemiologic studies of populations exposed to accidental chemical spills. Examples of these are several industrial accidents leading to exposure of workers and, in the Seveso accident, inhabitants of the surrounding area to dioxins; the people of Times Beach, Missouri, who were exposed to dioxins; and rice oil ("Yusho") accidents in Japan and Taiwan, where polychlorinated biphenyls accidentally contaminated cooking oil. These accidents are usually, but not always, higher-dose exposures (the exposed persons in several instances developed chloracne) and are more acute. There were transient changes in some laboratory tests of immune functions in children who had suffered intense exposure after the Seveso accident, those exposed to the contaminated rice oil in Japan and Taiwan, and the inhabitants of Times Beach. In some, there were minor abnormalities in immunoglobulin levels, which later returned to normal. There have also been effects on some tests of CMI, such as depression of DTH skin test responses, which also returned toward normal. In addition, methodologic questions have been raised regarding some of these studies, particularly the data on skin test responses of the inhabitants of Times Beach.

SUMMARY

There is concern about potential toxicity to the immune system from environmental or occupational exposure to a variety of chemicals. The current methodology used to evaluate human immunotoxicity has many shortcomings, but clinical observations do not support a widespread fear that "toxic" chemicals in our work or general environments are harmful to our immune systems.

IMMUNOLOGIC EFFECTS OF UREMIA

Raymond G. Slavin, MD

A number of clinical features of uremia point to abnormalities in immune function; these include a high rate of infection and an increased incidence of cancers. Up to 60% of patients with chronic renal failure suffer from severe infection, and 40% of deaths are thought to be due to infection. Studies of animals with experimentally induced uremia and of uremic patients have shown that immune functions may be markedly altered. It should be emphasized that many of the studies showing these changes are not conclusive, and, indeed, results are often contradictory. One reason for these discrepancies, especially in human studies, is that many factors may contribute to the apparent immune competency of patients with end-stage renal disease. These include hemodialysis, drugs, blood transfusions, duration of failure, and physiologic and metabolic disturbances associated with uremia. All of these may alter immune function. In addition, the immune response in patients with uremia is dependent to some extent on the particular antigen tested.

Table 16–5 summarizes the immune function factors that are probably affected by uremia. The most striking immune abnormalities of uremia oc-

cur in cell-mediated reactions. The uniform lymphocytopenia that occurs in acute and chronic uremia and involves mainly T cells appears to be due to an alteration of lymphocyte trafficking, with circulating lymphocytes being redistributed to the bone marrow.

In general, intrinsic cell defects appear to be less important than serum-mediated ones in inhibiting CMI. Washed uremic lymphocytes or uremic lymphocytes incubated in normal serum respond normally to mitogens such as PHA. Addition of uremic serum to normal or uremic lymphocytes significantly suppresses cellular responses. Several factors in uremic serum have been shown to be responsible for this type of immunosuppression. An in vivo correlate can be seen in adoptive transfer experiments in guinea pigs. Animals that were sensitive to tuberculin and that were then made uremic lost their tuberculin skin reactivity, but lymph node cells from these sensitized, nonresponding uremic animals could transfer DTH to normal animals. In contrast, lymph node cells from normal sensitized guinea pigs could not transfer sensitivity to uremic animals. This suggests that immunologically competent lymphocytes are present in uremic guinea pigs but are rendered nonresponsive in the presence of the uremic state.

The response of spleen cells from chronically uremic rats to mitogens is significantly suppressed compared with that of spleen cells from control animals. The suppression appears to be mediated by a suppressor cell, probably a monocyte, that is also present in the peritoneum and lungs of uremic rats and in the peripheral blood of uremic humans. Sera from uremic rats induces increased suppressor activity of normal spleen cells.

The reduced response of uremic lymphoid cells to mitogens and antigens may be due, in part, to the inability of uremic cells to act as antigen-presenting cells. In uremic rats, the antigen-presenting ability of macrophages is significantly diminished.

In the area of humoral antibody, a decrease in immunoglobulin levels is seen in uremic humans, with the most profound changes being found in IgM levels. Antibody production varies with the antigen presented. In the experimental animal model of uremia in the rat, antibody production to bovine serum albumin is suppressed, whereas anti-sheep erythrocyte antibody is not affected.

A decrease in neutrophil chemotaxis has been reported to occur in humans with uremia. Sera of uremic patients contain a chemotactic-factor inhibitor that is specific for several chemoattractants. The inhibitor reacts directly and irreversibly with the chemoattractants and is heat-labile. It thus resembles the chemotactic factor inhibitor present in low titers in normal human sera.

Table 16–5. Immune function abnormalities in uremia.

Immune Function	Abnormalities
CMI	Lymphocytopenia Impaired delayed skin reactivity Decreased in vitro lymphocyte proliferation Prolonged homograft survival Impaired graft-versus-host reaction
Humoral antibody	Decrease in immunoglobulin levels Decrease in antibody production
Chemotaxis	Decrease in neutrophil chemotaxis

SUMMARY

The increased rate of infection and the high incidence of cancer associated with chronic renal failure point to possible abnormalities of immune function in this condition. Studies of experimentally induced uremia in animals and of humans with chronic renal failure indicate that a variety of defects occur in CMI, antibody production, and neutrophil chemotaxis, with the most significant changes being in cell-mediated reactions.

REFERENCES

Psychoneuroimmunology

Ader R (editor): *Psychoneuroimmunology.* Academic Press, Orlando, 1981.

Besedovsky HO, DelRey AE, Sorkin E: What do the immune system and the brain know about each other? *Immunol Today* 1983; **4**:342.

MacQueen G et al: Pavlovian conditioning of rat mucosal MAST cells to secrete rat mast cell protease II. *Science* 1989; **243**:83.

Riley V: Psychoneuroendocrine influences on immunocompetence and neoplasia. *Science* 1981; **212**:1109.

Schleifer SJ et al: Depression and immunity. *Arch Gen Psychiatry* 1985; **42**:129.

Aging

Crawford J, Cohen HJ: Relationship of cancer and aging. *Clin Geriatr Med* 1987; **3**:419.

Deguchi Y et al: Age-related changes of proliferative response, kinetics of expression of protooncogenes after the mitogenic stimulation and methylation level of the protooncogene in purified human lymphocyte subsets. *Mech Ageing Dev* 1988; **44**:153.

Ford PM: The immunology of aging. *Clin Rheum Dis* 1986; **12**:1.

Krishnaraj R, Blandford G: Age-associated alterations in human natural killer cells. I. Increased activity per conventional and kinetic analysis. *Clin Immunol Immunopathol* 1987; **45**:268.

Lighart GJ et al: Admission criteria for immunogerontological studies in man: The Senieur protocol. *Mech Ageing Dev* 1986; **28**:47.

Mackinodan T et al: Cellular, biochemical and molecular basis of T-cell senescence. *Arch Pathol Lab Med* 1987; **111**:910.

Miller RG: Age-associated decline in precursor frequency for different cell-mediated reactions with preservation of helper and cytotoxic effect per precursor cell. *J Immunol* 1984: **132**:63.

Nordin AA, Proust JJ: Signal transduction mechanisms in the immune system. Potential implications in immunosenescence. *Endocrinol Metab Clin* 1987; **16(4)**:919.

Saltzman RL, Peterson PK: Immunodeficiency of the elderly. *Rev Infect Dis* 1987; **9**:127.

Weksler ME: The senescence of the immune system. *Semin Immunol* 1986; **16**:53.

Nutrition

Beisel WR: Simple nutrients and immunity. *Am J Clin Nutr* 1982; **35**:417.

Chandra RK: Malnutrition. Pages 187–203 in: *Immunodeficiency Disorders.* Chandra RK (editor). Churchill Livingstone, 1982.

Chandra RK: Nutrition and immunity. *Trop Geogr Med* 1988;**40**:546.

Chandra RK: *Trace Elements, Immune Response and Infections.* Wiley, 1983.

Good RA, Lorenz E: Nutrition, immunity, aging and cancer. *Nutr Rev* 1988;**46**:62.

Gross RL, Newberne PM: Role of nutrition in immunologic function. *Physiol Rev* 1980; **60**:188.

Laouri D, Kleinknecht C: The role of nutritional factors in the course of experimental renal failure. *Am J Kidney Dis* 1985;**5**:147.

Lipschitz DA: Nutrition, aging and the immunohematopoietic system. *Clin Geriatr Med* 1987;**3**:319.

Walford RL et al: Dietary restriction and aging: historical phases, mechanisms and current directions. *J Nutr* 1987; **117**:1650.

Environmental Chemicals

Dean JH, Murray MJ, Ward EC: Toxic modification of the immune system. In: *Cassarett and Doull's Toxicology: The Basic Sciences of Poisons*, 3rd ed. Doull J, Klaassen CD, Amdur MO (editors). Macmillan, in press.

Hoffman RE et al: Health effects of long-term exposure to 2,3,7,8-tetrachlorodibenzo-p-dioxin. *JAMA* 1986;**255**:2031.

Klemmer HW et al: Clinical findings in workers exposed to pentachlorophenol. *Arch Environ Contam Toxicol* 1980; **9**:715.

Masuda Y, Yoshimura H: Polychlorinated biphenyls and dibenzofurans in patients with Yusho and their toxicologic significance: A review. *Am J Ind Med* 1984;**5**:31.

Reggiani G: Localized contamination with TCDD—Seveso, Missouri and other areas. Page 303 in: *Halogenated Biphenyls, Terphenyls, Naphtholenes, Dibenzodioxins, and Related Products.* Kimbrough R (editor). Elsevier/North Holland, 1980.

Reggiani G: Medical problems raised by the TCDD contamination in Seveso, Italy. *Arch Toxicol* 1978;**40**:161.

Uremia

Mezzano S et al: Analysis of humoral and cellular factors that contribute to impaired immune responsiveness in experimental uremia. *Nephron* 1984; **36**:15.

Johnston MFM, Slavin RG: Mechanisms of inhibition of adoptive transfer of tuberculin sensitivity in acute uremia. *J Lab Clin Med* 1976;**87**:457.

Hayry P et al. Is uremia immunosuppressive in renal transplantation? *Transplantation* 1982;**34**;168.

Alevy YG, Slavin RG, Hutcheson PA: Immune response in experimentally induced uremia. I. Suppression of mitogen responses by adherent cells in chronic uremia. *Clin Immunol Immunopathol* 1981;**19**:8.

17 Reproductive Immunology

Daniel V. Landers, MD, Richard A. Bronson, MD, Charles S. Pavia, PhD, & Daniel P. Stites, MD

The last few decades have seen a rapid expansion in our knowledge of the immunology of the reproductive process. Advancing research in molecular biology and monoclonal antibody technology has helped to outline the complex nature of the immunologic events that surround fertilization, implantation, and intrauterine tolerance, growth, and development of the embryo. Immune responses to self antigens on sperm or alloantegins in females are associated with alterations in fertility. Over the years, investigators from around the world have begun to unravel the mystery of the fetal-maternal allograft. Although our understanding is far from complete, we have accumulated a tremendous amount of information about the immunologic events surrounding reproduction. Numerous alterations in the maternal immune response have been identified that evolve from the very beginning of gestation. A great deal has been uncovered regarding the success of the fetus as an allograft at both the maternal-fetal-placental interface and the more distant sites of fetal-maternal cell contact. Research efforts continue to further our understanding of the immune mechanisms of sperm penetration, sperm antibodies, and immune mechanisms involved in the maintenance of early pregnancy. These investigative efforts have led to new insights into contraceptive therapy, primary infertility, recurrent spontaneous pregnancy loss, and management of patients with allotransplants or tumors.

REPRODUCTIVE IMMUNOLOGY IN THE FEMALE

The exact mechanisms involved in the apparent success of the fetus as an allograft are only partially understood. Several hypotheses have been proposed, each of which is supported by substantial scientific investigation. The mechanisms that link the various hypotheses and the many signals and unknown factors that initiate and regulate the system as a whole remain unclear. The basic hypothesis remains that there exist both physical and humoral barriers to immune rejection of the fetus. This rather simplistic view has remained substantially unchallenged; however, our understanding at the molecular level has progressed. It is clear that for the fetus to avoid immune recognition and attack by the maternal immune system, the maternal immune response must be blunted, the fetal antigen stimulus must be suppressed, or, as is most likely, both must occur. In normal human allograft rejection, T lymphocytes play a major role in recognition and cytolysis of foreign antigen-bearing cells. This role is primarily undertaken by cytotoxic T lymphocytes (CTL). The fetal allograft must be protected against these effector cells. This may occur by a variety of mechanisms, which are discussed below.

REGULATION OF MATERNAL RECOGNITION OF THE FETAL ALLOGRAFT

The unique structure of the placenta provides an interface of maternal blood for exchange of gases and nutrients by the fetus. The hemochorial nature of the placenta provides direct exposure of the syncytiotrophoblast layer of the chorionic villi to maternal circulating lymphocytes. While the syncytiotrophoblasts come into direct contact with maternal T cells, including CTL, no apparent recognition or cytolytic events are evident. Numerous studies have shown that syncytiotrophoblast membranes do not express class I human leukocyte antigens (HLA antigens). This lack of antigenic expression may account for the lack of cytolytic response; however, many unexplained phenomena still exist. There are additional interfaces between maternal and trophoblastic tissue. Syncytiotrophoblasts are shed into the intervillous spaces and transported intravascularly to distant maternal sites, including the lungs, without causing an inflammatory or immune response at these sites. Furthermore, cytotrophoblasts are known to migrate to the uterine spiral arteries following implantation, and they eventually replace maternal endothelium at that site. Thus, maternal lymphocytes interface with histocompatibility antigens on endovascular trophoblast without stimulating a significant immune response. Other theoretic mechanisms of fetal protection exist; eg, that fetal antigens may be only weakly expressed, but the normal production of maternal antibodies to fetal erythrocytes, immunoglobulins, trophoblasts, and HLA contradict this hypothesis.

Two classes of trophoblast antigens have been identified. These unique antigens include trophoblastic antigen 1 (TA1) and the trophoblast-lymphocyte cross-reactive (TLX) antigens. TA1 may be involved in the immune protection afforded the fetus during pregnancy. Their levels in the blood of pregnant women increase as pregnancy progresses. These antigens have inhibitory effects on mixed-lymphocyte reactions without affecting nonspecific lymphocyte responses to mitogens. TLX antisera cross-react with unstimulated peripheral blood lymphocytes, placenta endothelium, and villous fibroblasts. These antigens are allogeneic and species-specific. Together, TA1 and the TLX antigens may function in normal pregnancy by inducing maternal production of antibodies that block the immune response to TA1. Thus, absence of TLX antigen recognition due to sharing of maternal-paternal TLX antigen profiles may not allow anti-TA1 activity and may lead to subsequent fetal rejection.

THE UTERUS AS A SITE FOR IMMUNE REACTIVITY

Although the uterus was once considered an immunologically privileged site, much experimental evidence indicates that both afferent and efferent limbs of the immune response are operative in this reproductive organ. When placed into the nonpregnant uterus, allografts are promptly rejected and cause hypertrophy of the draining para-aortic lymph nodes. A secondary response occurs when there is a local challenge with tissue of the same antigenic specificity. In addition, local alloimmunization in the uterine environment has a dramatic effect on subsequent reproductive capabilities. Increased numbers of embryos develop in pregnant animals whose uterine horns have been presensitized against paternal histocompatibility antigens and have already expressed the local "recall flare," a delayed hypersensitivity reaction. The immunologic basis for this unexpected result is

unknown, although it suggests that maternal immune reactivity has a beneficial effect and may play a vital role in maternal-fetal coexistence.

Following sexual intercourse, allogeneic spermatozoa are not ordinarily recognized as foreign and are therefore not rejected in the immunocompetent maternal host. This may be related to the presence of nonspecific immunosuppressive factors in semen. A high-molecular-weight component present in human seminal plasma has a strong suppressive effect on mitogen, antigen, and allogeneic cell activation of human lymphocytes, whereas other substances in semen interfere with the microbicidal activity of antibody, complement, and granulocytes.

The events of implantation of the fertilized egg and ensuing invasion of uterine tissue by the trophoblast evoke an inflammatory reaction resulting in the formation of a highly specialized gestational tissue called the decidua. Besides possessing endocrinologic activity, decidual tissue may act as a selective barrier by preventing released fetal or trophoblastic antigens from reaching the neighboring afferent lymphatic vessels and by preventing access of sensitized maternal lymphocytes to the conceptus. The decidua may also release immunosuppressive factors and express natural killer (NK) activity very early during its development. The well-known fact that ectopic pregnancy can elicit decidual reactions in extrauterine sites suggests that this locally evoked reaction at the site of implantation and the later development of the placenta play key roles in maintaining the integrity of the fetus.

ALLOANTIGENICITY OF THE FETOPLACENTAL UNIT & AN IMMUNOLOGIC ROLE FOR THE PLACENTA

The placenta is a unique and complex organ. Its biologic existence is brief. Its structural elements are heterogeneous, and its functionally active cell types include the trophoblastic, lymphocytic, and erythroid series. Like the fetus, the placenta consists of tissue derived from 2 different parental genotypes. It produces protein and steroid hormones that regulate the physiologic activities of pregnancy. Concurrently, it acts as the fetal lung, kidneys, intestine, and liver. It is becoming evident that an immunologic role for this organ may be of paramount importance for the successful maintenance of mammalian pregnancy.

Both the maternal and paternal components of fetal transplantation antigens are expressed on cellular elements within the placenta. However, from an immunologic standpoint, the key question is whether transplantation antigens can be demonstrated on trophoblast membranes. These membranes are the interface in direct apposition to the maternal circulation in the human hemochorial placenta. As such, they present a direct challenge for both the afferent and efferent limbs of the immune response and could serve as the site of immune attack by immunologically competent maternal lymphocytes.

Whether or not transplantation antigens are expressed on trophoblasts has become a matter of intense controversy. The answer seems to be dependent upon the ontogenetic and phylogenetic expression of these antigens at various stages of gestation. It has been reported that placental antigens may be masked by histocompatibility or specific trophoblast antibodies, fibrinoid, fibrinomucoid, or immune complexes. Class I (HLA-A, -B, -C) antigens can be detected on early human placental cytotrophoblast, although it has been difficult to demonstrate any HLA antigens on other human trophoblast tissue, including the syncytiotrophoblast of the mature chorionic villus. Although class I MHC antigens are expressed on murine trophoblasts, it is not yet known whether transplantation antigens are present in an immunogenic form on mammalian trophoblast cells, an important key to our understanding of the many aspects of the immunologic interaction between mother and fetus. The demonstration that maternal lymphocytes are capable of killing cultured human trophoblast cells from their own placenta is evidence that trophoblast cells do display transplantation antigens. Extrauterine placental allografts are usually rejected by allogeneic recipients and provoke a state of alloimmunity—while transplants of trophoblast from early gestational tissue proceed to grow and develop unimpeded without eliciting a detectable rejection.

A variety of hormonal and immunologic events occurring during pregnancy could modulate maternal transplantation immunity against paternal antigens expressed on the placenta and trophoblast. Circulating alpha-fetoprotein, placental-ovarian steroids, protein hormones, and antibody have widely different concentrations in pregnancy serum than at their sites of production. These factors have been proposed as naturally occurring immunosuppressive factors. Although there is no firm evidence that these circulating factors adequately explain the cell regulatory events that occur in the maternal immune system, and the concentrations of gestational steroid and protein hormones in maternal serum never achieve a level that will suppress immunity in vivo, these substances, taken together, could exert a potent immunosuppressive effect at the fetal-maternal interface, where they are made and maintained at high levels throughout most stages of pregnancy. Interestingly, the trophoblast produces most of the major pregnancy-associated hormones that have been implicated as immunomodulators, which is consistent with evidence that trophoblastic cells themselves or soluble extracts or eluates of placental tissue inhibit various expressions of cell-mediated immunity.

Other immunologic properties have been ascribed to cells derived from the placenta. Trophoblastic tissue serves as an anatomic barrier between fetal and maternal tissues and thereby serves as the first line of defense against maternal antifetal alloimmunity. Maternal lymphocytes sensitized to fetal antigens could be excluded specifically, as are certain antibodies, or nonspecifically, by a generalized barrier to cellular traffic. During early gestation, the trophoblast actively invades and proliferates within the maternal decidua. Studies with mice show that different stages of the trophoblast are highly phagocytic and lymphoid cells from murine placentas mediate graft-versus-host (GVH) reactions, respond to mitogenic lectins, and synthesize antibodies. There is also some evidence that the placenta produces the antiviral agent interferon and the macrophage-derived immune factor interleukin-1. The expression of immunelike function by both trophoblastic elements and lymphoid stem cells may be one of several processes enabling the fetoplacental unit to protect itself from injury. This is accomplished by preventing harmful infectious agents and certain maternal antigens and antibodies from reaching the embryo and by limiting the passage of cells from mother to fetus. These defense mechanisms could be especially important during the early stages of in utero development, when the fetus is quite vulnerable since it has not yet acquired complete immune competence.

FETAL-MATERNAL EXCHANGE OF HUMORAL & CELLULAR COMPONENTS

The human placenta is hemochorial, which means that there is direct apposition between the maternal circulation and the syncytiotrophoblast that lines the chorionic villi of the placenta. Although fetus and mother are grossly separated, cells as well as soluble substances can pass through the placenta during gestation, particularly at the time of placental separation (Fig 17–1).

That such transplacental traffic results in allosensitization to transplantation antigens has been extrapolated from observations rather than proved by rigorously documented experiments. Syncytial trophoblast (more than 200,000 cells per day) is continuously released from the placenta and has been shown to circulate in human mater-

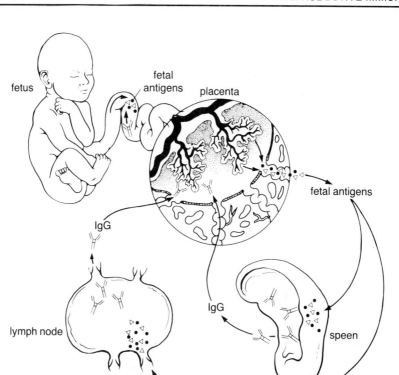

Figure 17-1. Maternal-fetal-placental complex. The anatomic features of the fetal-maternal relationship during pregnancy are depicted, with the placenta acting as a selective filter of leaking fetal or trophoblastic antigens that may sensitize maternal immune effector mechanisms. The passage of maternal immunity to the fetus is likewise regulated by the intervening layer of trophoblastic cells (where fetal and maternal tissues are in intimate proximity).

nal blood from the 18th week of gestation. Various blood elements that undoubtedly contain transplantation antigens can pass bidirectionally. This establishes adequate conditions for sensitization of the mother by fetal (paternal) transplantation antigens. Under experimental circumstances—or clinically after intrauterine blood transfusion—immunocompetent cells that gain entrance to the fetus can rarely cause GVH disease and runting. The placenta, then, provides only a partial barrier to transport of soluble or cellular elements and certainly should not be viewed as an absolute impediment to their traffic.

In addition, whereas under normal physiologic conditions the trophoblast seems to be invulnerable to immune attack, it is quite probable that some maternal reactivity to this tissue does arise, primarily to protect the pregnant host from extensive and otherwise unchecked growth and invasion of the trophoblast, as occurs in choriocarcinoma.

In the early stages of fetal development in primates, immune protection of the fetus is provided by maternally derived antibodies acquired exclusively by placental transmission. In other species,

immunoglobulins are transferred via the yolk sac or via intestinal absorption of colostrum during suckling. During gestation, only antibodies belonging to the IgG class are readily transferred from mother to fetus, and this process is most probably facilitated by the interaction of immunoglobulin molecules with Fc receptors present on the surface of trophoblastic membranes and other extraembryonic membrane components. With intrauterine infection, the fetus is capable of synthesizing IgM and IgA. The presence of high levels of these immuoglobulins in cord serum at birth is presumptive evidence of such infection.

The neonate is exposed to an environment that presents much greater risk of infection than was the case in the uterine shelter. Unless in utero infection has occurred, the newborn is usually not capable of mounting a quick and effective reaction against pathogenic organisms. Maternally acquired antibody provides initial protection against infection. The presence of maternal immunoglobulins in sufficiently high titer should protect against the initial invasion of certain pathogens that would otherwise multiply and disseminate without hindrance.

IMMUNOLOGIC CONSEQUENCES OF TRANSPLACENTALLY PASSED SUBSTANCES

Under certain circumstances, transferred maternal antibody is not beneficial to the fetus. This is most evident in hemolytic disease of the newborn mediated by either ABO or Rh blood group fetal-maternal incompatibilities. Situations involving ABO incompatibilities arise more frequently than does Rh hemolytic disease, but they usually take a milder course, with cases requiring transfusion being extremely rare. The disorder occurs primarily in blood group O mothers bearing fetuses of type A or B and is believed to be the result of the transfer of IgG anti-A or anti-B antibodies from mother to fetus. Although blood group A and group B women have antibody to type B and type A erythrocytes, respectively, these naturally occurring isoagglutinins are usually of the IgM class and therefore do not readily cross the placenta and cannot harm the fetus.

The more serious condition that can adversely affect fetal development results from Rh isoimmunization, which resembles the pathophysiology of ABO incompatibility yet manifests important immunologic differences. Rh antigens are expressed on blood cells only, whereas antigenic specificities related to A and B blood group determinants are widely distributed in nature and in the human body. During a pregnancy in which an Rh-negative mother is bearing an Rh-positive fetus, sensitization may occur if fetal erythrocytes cross into the maternal circulation via the placenta or when there is transplacental hemorrhage following the birth of the child or after an abortion. Alternatively, the mother could already be primed as a result of receiving an earlier transfusion of Rh-positive blood. Less than 1 mL of fetal blood can elicit a response. Maternal antibodies pass through the placenta, gain access to the fetal bloodstream, and cause the destruction of erythrocytes. Rh disease occurs rarely during the first pregnancy, with the vast majority of Rh-negative mothers becoming sensitized with increasing parity. The deleterious effects of isoimmunization can be prevented conveniently by administering Rh_0 (D) immune globulin to the mother immediately after delivery of her first Rh-positive child or following an abortion. The major suggested explanation for the action of anti-Rh immunoglobulins is that fetal erythrocytes present in the maternal circulation as a result of fetal detachment are destroyed and rapidly cleared, so that they are not available long enough to sensitize the mother effectively. Treatment must be administered after subsequent Rh-incompatible pregnancies, since there is no apparent development of tolerance following prophylactic therapy.

In certain situations, simultaneous ABO and Rh incompatibilities between mother and fetus may prevent the more destructive effects of Rh isoimmunization. The naturally occurring anti-A or anti-B antibodies in a group O, Rh-negative mother will effectively destroy Rh-positive erythrocytes crossing the placenta if the fetus is also of either group A or B blood type. The rapid removal of these cells by the already primed maternal immune system would make sensitization against Rh factor highly unlikely.

MATERNAL IMMUNE RESPONSE DURING PREGNANCY

Pregnancy has long been associated with a depression in cellular immunity, but the reason for this is far from clear. The human T lymphocyte is one of the major cellular components of the host defense response to foreign antigens, whether that antigen is an allograft, a virally infected cell, or any other foreign HLA antigen-bearing cell. The number and function of T cells change during pregnancy. Total lymphocyte counts fall during gestation; the maximal decrease occurs at 25–28 weeks of pregnancy. Most studies also show that T cell numbers are decreased. CD4 cells decrease and CD8 cells increase toward the end of pregnancy, resulting in a decrease in the CD4/CD8 cell ratio. Studies of NK cells during gestation show that although the number of these cells decreases, their level of activity is probably unchanged. In vitro tests of T cell function, using mitogens and mixed-lymphocyte reactions, show a decrease in proliferative response during pregnancy. T cell function in pregnancy has barely begun to be characterized.

Changes in humoral immunity also occur during gestation. The serum immunoglobulin concentrations increase, but alterations of specific immunoglobulin subclasses have not been well characterized.

MATERNAL-FETAL ANTIMICROBIAL IMMUNITY

Pregnant women seem to be at an increased risk of acquiring certain infectious diseases, particularly those controlled primarily by cell-mediated immunity (CMI). The pregnancy-related alteration in the immune response to infection includes changes in T lymphocyte subpopulations, polymorphonuclear leukocyte function, peripheral blood lymphocyte responses, serum immunoglobulin concentrations, immunosuppressive serum factors, and maternal immunologic recognition mechanisms. Although it has been assumed that these alterations relate in some way to maternal tolerance of the fetal allograft, it is not clear how they relate to pregnancy-specific alterations in susceptibility to infection.

A number of infectious agents are thought to behave differently in pregnant women, owing primarily to altered host defenses. These include some viral agents such as poliomyelitis virus, hepatitis A virus, influenza A virus, Epstein-Barr virus, variola virus, and cytomegalovirus; bacterial agents such as *Neisseria gonorrhoeae* and *Streptococcus pneumoniae;* parasites such as *Plasmodium* species; and fungi such as *Coccidioides immitis.*

The humoral immune alteration associated with pregnancy may play a role in this increased susceptibility. These changes involve a decrease in serum IgG concentration with advancing gestation. Some decrease in the levels of IgM and IgM-bearing lymphocytes has also been reported in the first trimester, but these levels do not continue to decrease with advancing gestation. The significance of these changes, however, is unclear, and they do not necessarily represent impaired humoral immunity. In fact, antibody production in response to infection during pregnancy is probably unaltered.

A variety of cellular immune functions are depressed during pregnancy as described above, including T cell numbers and functions; NK cell numbers and activity; and neutrophil, monocyte, and macrophage numbers. Among the agents thought to participate in this depression of CMI are steroid hormones produced in pregnancy, such as progesterone, estrogens, cortisol, alpha-fetoprotein, and uromodulin. Despite these alterations, there is little direct evidence to suggest significant alteration in the cellular component of the immune system during pregnancy. Furthermore, except for some notable exceptions such as rubella, cytomegalovirus infection, syphilis, and toxoplasmosis, the human fetus usually remains relatively unaffected by maternal infectious diseases.

IMMUNITY IN RECURRENT SPONTANEOUS ABORTION

Maternal immune recognition of the fetus is thought to play an important role in fetal acceptance. It is well known that an increased incidence of HLA antigen sharing between mates is associated with repeated spontaneous abortion when compared with normal fertile controls. In fact, the development of "hybrid vigor" may be related in part to polymorphism of HLA disparity between parents. The proposed theory is that an allogeneic incompatibility is necessary at an HLA or a closely linked locus for maternal recognition

and development of fetal acceptance. If such a recognition is lacking, cell-mediated allograft rejection or antibody response to foreign fetal antigen may lead to fetal loss. Numerous studies have found an association between repeated spontaneous abortion and HLA-sharing between mates. Furthermore maternal recognition of the allogeneic paternal TA1 or TLX antigen may lead to a blocking antibody that prevents a response to TA1. If mates share TLX antigen profiles prohibiting the maternal recognition of paternal TLX antigen, anti-TA1 activity may lead to rejection of the fetus. This hypothesis has yet to be confirmed.

Many centers now perform maternal immunization with paternal or donor lymphocytes in patients with 3 or more primary spontaneous abortions. The success rate in reducing abortion has been reported to be as high as 50–89%. The presumed mechanism of success is that the woman produces antipaternal alloantibodies, which play a role in protecting the fetus from immune-mediated rejection. There remains a great deal of difficulty in sorting out which patients indeed have immune-mediated recurrent losses and theoretically will benefit from this approach and which patients have another cause for their losses.

REPRODUCTIVE IMMUNOLOGY IN THE MALE

Since males are not exposed to histoincompatible gametes during reproduction, immune alterations involving the male reproductive system are necessarily autoimmune. Experimentally, auto- or alloimmunization to spermatozoa can in fact result in relative infertility in either the female or the male. Naturally occurring autoimmune reactions to sperm are uncommon but have become increasingly recognized as a consequence of vasectomy and in infertile couples. Recent findings suggest that potentially harmful immune responses associated with spermatozoa as antigens are inhibited by naturally occurring local and systemic immunoregulatory mechanisms.

NATURAL IMMUNITY TO SPERMATOZOA

Sera obtained from normal, fertile animals of many species, including rabbits, mice, and humans, have been found to contain antibodies that react with sperm of their own species and, to a lesser degree, with sperm of other species. In the rabbit, these naturally occurring antibodies enter the uterine secretions, probably as transudates from serum. Sperm recovered from the reproductive tract of female rabbits have immunoglobulins on the head region detectable by immunofluorescence. Interestingly, vigorously moving sperm recovered from the uterus did not fluoresce, whereas immotile sperm and those that showed evidence of senescence—as judged by alteration in the appearance of the acrosome—were bound by immunoglobulins. It has been proposed that binding of this naturally occurring antibody to spermatozoa may play a role in their clearance from the female reproductive tract, perhaps abrogating the immune response in the female to sperm-associated antigens, and in maintaining a state of tolerance.

The mechanism by which antibody binding to spermatozoa occurs appears to be through Fc receptors that have been demonstrated on alcohol-fixed sperm of both rabbits and pigs but were not present on the surface of living sperm of those species. While binding of intact immunoglobulins of the IgG class was noted, Fab fragments obtained from digests of purified rabbit IgG failed to bind to sperm.

It has recently been demonstrated that an IgG preparation from serum of unimmunized rabbits mediates complement-dependent sperm immobilization. This finding suggests that a naturally occurring antibody directed against a specific sperm-associated antigen is also present within the sera of some normal fertile bucks. Cytotoxic sperm-reactive antibodies have been found in the sera of nonimmunized inbred mice. Normal serum lysed spermatozoa of all strains tested, in the presence of complement. A 3-layer indirect immunofluorescence technique using normal mouse serum, rhodamine-conjugated goat antimouse serum, and rabbit antigoat antiserum also gave a distinct surface membrane fluorescence over the whole head, principal piece, and end piece of the sperm tail from any strain when tested using living spermatozoa in suspension. Absorption of normal serum with mouse spermatozoa removed both immunofluorescent and cytotoxic activity. The cytotoxic titer of sperm-reactive antibody in normal mouse serum was low—in the range of 1:8.

Naturally occurring antisperm antibodies have been detected by indirect immunofluorescence in 90% of sera of children of both sexes before puberty. The incidence declines thereafter to about 60% and persists throughout life. These naturally occurring antibodies were readily absorbed by sperm and testicular extracts but not by other human tissues. The constant staining pattern with several hundred serum samples also suggested they were unlikely to be alloantibodies. They were directed against neither blood group antigens nor sperm-coating antigens, since the antibodies were not absorbed by seminal plasma. Of special importance, these sperm-reactive naturally occurring antibodies did *not* stain the surface of viable sperm in suspension but rather were directed against intracellular antigens. Sera possessing antiacrosomal antibodies, when absorbed with lyophilized *Staphylococcus aureus, Escherichia coli, Pseudomonas aeruginosa, Klebsiella pneumoniae,* and *Candida albicans,* no longer reacted with sperm by indirect immunofluorescence. In contrast, reactivity against other regions of the sperm surface was not absorbed by microorganisms.

The sera of children, female blood donors, pregnant women, and women from infertile couples have also been screened for naturally occurring sperm-reactive antibodies. Analysis of the immunofluorescent staining patterns and titers of these antibodies revealed that while 68% of children's sera were positive, only one of 84 samples tested was titered to 1:16 dilution. Similarly, for female blood donors, while 79% were positive, only 3 of 80 sera were positive at 1:16 or greater. Conversely, in women with unexplained infertility, 15 of 29 sera tested showed at least one sperm-reactive antibody at a titer 1:16 or greater. Interestingly, while 9 sera from infertile women with an immunofluorescence titer of at least 1:64 were tested by means of a microscopic sperm agglutination test, none were positive. The antibody-antigen system detected by immunofluorescence is different from that detected by sperm agglutination, again suggesting that naturally occurring sperm-reactive antibodies are not directed against antigens on the sperm surface.

The sera of 2115 male partners of infertile couples have been studied by a sperm agglutination test in a gel. Three percent were found to have sperm agglutinins with titers of 1:32 or greater. This low incidence of agglutinating antibodies contrasts markedly with the high incidence of antibodies reactive with sperm subsurface antigens.

Against this background of naturally occurring sperm-reactive antibodies, there has been much confusion over the role of antisperm antibodies in impaired human reproduction. The subsurface nature of Fc receptors, the mediation of immunoglobulin binding to sperm of many species via the Fc portion of the immunoglobulin molecule, and the absence of immunoglobulin binding to living human spermatozoa have not been fully appreciated. It is now clear that sera of normal fertile men and women do not contain antibodies directed against antigenic determinants of the sperm surface and that their presence is a reflection of an aberrant immune response that may lead—depending upon isotype, antibody specificity, and titer—to altered sperm function.

ETIOLOGY OF AUTOIMMUNITY TO SPERMATOZOA

Sperm Antigens

The expression of antigens on sperm is central to the consideration of their immunogenicity in the reproductive tract, much the same as is the presence of antigens on placental trophoblast. Sperm antigens could theoretically elicit either auto- or alloimmunity, and either type could result in partial or complete infertility. Alternatively, these antigens could be nonimmunogenic in the normal environment of the reproductive tract.

Autoimmune diseases of the testis may be prevented by sequestration of autoantigens on germ cells by the presence of a blood-testis barrier. However, not all such antigens appear to be sequestered, since they can be detected in seminiferous tubules, where they are accessible to circulating antibodies and T cells. Active systemic or local immunoregulatory mechanisms must then be operative. Such mechanisms might include (1) activity of suppressor cells, (2) nonspecific suppression in the testis, (3) failure of antigen presentation in the testis, or (4) lymphocyte trafficking bypassing the testis.

The specific antigens to which antisperm antibodies are directed have yet to be defined. Newer techniques in immunoaffinity chromatography are making their identification in the near future likely. Evidence exists that antisperm antibodies in some women may be directed against antigens adsorbed to the sperm surface from seminal plasma at the time of ejaculation. Whether seminal plasma components may also be autoantigenic is unknown.

That these sperm antigens are tissue-specific antigens rather than alloantigens is indicated by an inability to detect HLA expression on mature human spermatozoa and the finding that antisperm antibodies detected in serum of men with autoimmunity to sperm also react similarly with spermatozoa from a panel of normal fertile men. Following exposure to serum possessing sperm-reactive antibodies, unfixed frozen sections of human stomach, thyroid, ovary, and adrenal have failed to show evidence of IgG binding by immunofluorescence. The vast majority of sera from men with autoimmunity to sperm also are free of antithyroid and antinuclear antibodies as well as rheumatoid factor.

To determine whether sperm-immobilizing antibodies in women are directed against peptide or carbohydrate portions of sperm antigens, ejaculated sperm have been treated with periodic acid which denatures carbohydrates. In some instances this reduces the subsequent ability of antibodies to immobilize these sperm, which suggests a role for carbohydrate antigens. Protein antigens are also involved as targets for these antibodies, emphasizing the complex nature of the target molecules for immobilizing antibodies to sperm.

The only sperm-specific antigen well characterized at present is LDH-X, an isoenzyme of LDH restricted mainly to sperm. ABO blood group antigens are expressed on sperm only in secretors, and this important fact suggests that they are absorbed from seminal plasma. Whether these antigens are expressed in the absence of such absorption is clinically moot, as no evidence for antibodies to ABO antigens in infertility has been found. However, anti-blood group antibodies in sera of women may react with adsorbed blood group substances on sperm surfaces from secretory males giving false-positive antigen-antibody tests. The presence of Rh antigens and the haploid expression of the genes determining these blood group antigens remains controversial.

Histocompatibility antigens may be intrinsically expressed on sperm and not absorbed from seminal plasma. Ia antigens in the mouse are clearly detectable on sperm from epididymis and ductus deferentes, the regions of the male reproductive tract where seminal plasma has not yet been formed. Whether both parental haplotypes are expressed in sperm remains unresolved. The presence of HLA antigens on sperm is controversial. Recently, studies with monoclonal antibodies directed at framework determinants of HLA-A, -B, -C, and -D antigens and employing very sensitive radioimmunoassays and immunofluorescence assays failed to find any HLA antigens in epididymal or ejaculated sperm.

There is fragmentary evidence for weak expression of both class I and II HLA antigens of sperm as well as the presence of mRNA for class II HLA antigens. Evidence for the presence of HLA-D antigens, the probable human analogs of murine Ia antigens, has been derived primarily from the ability of sperm to stimulate lymphocytes in allogeneic mixed sperm lymphocyte cultures. Conclusions from these experiments have been criticized by some because the sperm stimulator cell population was contaminated with small numbers of other cells from the reproductive tract, especially leukocytes known to express HLA-D antigens. Serologic methods for HLA antigens that do not employ monoclonal reagents may harbor non-HLA antibodies, thereby giving false-positive results. A definitive resolution to this very important issue of HLA expression on sperm awaits further studies with these specific reagents.

H-Y antigen, which is encoded as a male-specific antigen by a gene on the Y chromosome and is central to primary sex differentiation, appears to be expressed on sperm. If sperm expressed exclusively either Y- or X-determined antigens, sex determination by antibodies directed at either X- or Y-bearing sperm would theoretically be possible. However, most investigators have not been able to show haploid expression of genes determining H-Y or H-X antigens on sperm. Thus, the possibility of exploiting haploid gene expression for sex determination appears remote.

Unresolved questions in the important area of sperm antigens include (1) whether transplantation antigens are expressed in a haploid or diploid mode, (2) the identity of a sperm-specific antigen, and (3) the definition of antigens that give rise to antibodies which cause infertility in males or females.

Sperm Antibodies

A high incidence of sperm-reactive antibodies has been detected in the sera of homosexual men. Oral sex or deposition of sperm within the rectum during intercourse may result in immunization to sperm antigens. The distribution of immunoglobulin isotypes of sperm-reactive antibodies in the sera of these homosexual men is quite different from that seen in heterosexual men from infertile couples. While tail-directed antibody of the IgG class, and, to a lesser extent, IgA, predominate in the latter group, head-directed IgMs are found more frequently in the sera of homosexuals. The nature of the antigens to which these antibodies are directed is unknown.

It has been suggested that genital tract infections may lead to the development of autoimmunity to sperm. However, such individuals may constitute only a small proportion of the total population of men in whom sperm-reactive antibodies are detected. In a study of 324 consecutive ejaculates submitted for semen analysis and sperm antibody studies, 46 were found to possess autoantibodies to sperm. The incidence of pyospermia (greater than 1 million PMN per milliliter), as judged by acridine orange staining and fluorescence microscopy, was comparable in the 2 groups at 10.8% and 15.2% of those antibody-negative versus antibody-positive. Four of 46 ejaculates of autoimmune men were found to have more than 5 million PMN per milliliter, versus 9 of 278 ejaculates that were antibody-negative. Although this observation does not preclude a prior acute infection, it suggests that chronic genital tract infection is an unlikely cause of autoimmunity to sperm. Most men studied also denied knowledge or symptoms of acute prostatitis or epididymitis.

Role of Seminal Plasma Lymphocytes

A large number of lymphocytes, ranging from 42,000 to 29 million, have been identified in the semen of normal heterosexual men. Recently, by using monoclonal T cell probes and immunoperoxidase staining, a population of intraepithelial CD8-positive suppressor T lymphocytes has been identified within the human epididymis. It has been postulated that these cells might play a role in preventing the development of autoimmunity to spermatozoa by acting locally to limit B cell differentiation and production of specific antibody against sperm-associated antigens. Alternatively, these T cells might suppress antigen processing and presentation by macrophages.

METHODS OF DETECTING SPERM-REACTIVE ANTIBODIES

Many techniques have been described over the years for detection of sperm-reactive antibodies in serum and other body fluids. It has become increasingly apparent that there are 2 sources of immunoglobulins within the male genital tract. These include those present as transudates from serum and those locally secreted. Therefore, circulating sperm-reactive antibodies may not be representative of those antisperm antibodies present in semen. Infertile couples were tested for the presence of antisperm antibodies, either when impaired sperm cervical mucus-penetrating ability was noted on postcoital testing despite normal semen analysis or in the face of idiopathic infertility. During a 5-year period, 1825 semen specimens were submitted to the Laboratory of Human Reproduction at North Shore University Hospital, Manhasset, NY. Sperm were washed free of seminal fluid by low-speed centrifugation and tested directly by immunobead binding for the presence of surface-bound immunoglobulins. Humoral antisperm antibodies were detected by incubation of known antibody-free spermatozoa (husband or donor) in dilute patient serum (1:4), following which sperm were washed free of serum and tested by immunobead binding. Autoantibodies were detected on the sperm surfaces in 13% of ejaculates. In 846 men, matched serum and semen specimens were studied, and humoral antibodies could be compared with those present within the genital tract. Twenty percent of men were found to have sperm-reactive antibodies in their blood without any detected on spermatozoa.

Although humoral antibodies may enter the seminal plasma as transudates, total immunoglobulin levels in semen are about 90% of those seen in serum. Male infertility has previously been noted in association with high titers of circulating anti-sperm antibodies. Indeed, in cases where sperm-reactive antibodies were present in blood but not detected within the ejaculate, serum immunobead-binding levels were low. Bearing in mind that immune phenomena wax and wane and that these men with low-grade autoimmunity to sperm require further surveillance, it would seem that the absence of antisperm antibodies in the ejaculate means that they do not provide an immune basis for infertility.

Conversely, 15% of men were found to have antibodies present on the sperm surface, but no antibodies were detected in serum. These antibodies are primarily of the IgA class, although IgGs may also be detected. The predominance of IgA antibodies in semen—and their absence in serum—suggests local production within the genital tract. Whether these autoantibodies originate in the accessory gland secretions (and are encountered by sperm at the time of ejaculation) or within the epididymis is unknown.

In combination, one-third of serologic tests performed to detect antisperm antibodies provided misleading information that could lead to an error in clinical management. These results emphasize the need to study the ejaculate directly rather than solely using serologic tests in the diagnosis of immune-mediated male infertility.

DETECTION OF SPERM-ASSOCIATED IMMUNOGLOBULINS

Several methods are now clinically available to determine whether spermatozoa themselves are immunoglobulin-bound. These include the mixed agglutination reaction, a direct antiglobulin assay using ^{125}I-radiolabeled heterologous antibody, direct enzyme-linked immunosorbent assay (ELISA), and immunobead binding. Although each of these tests allows one to determine, in a semiquantitative way, the extent of autoimmunity to sperm, immunobead binding in particular provides a measure of the proportion of spermatozoa in the ejaculate antibody bound by each of the 3 major immunoglobulin isotypes (IgG, IgA, and IgM). The precise amount of immunoglobulin associated with the individual spermatozoal surface, however, still cannot be determined by current methods.

DETECTION OF HUMORAL ANTIBODIES

Sperm Immobilization Tests

Antibodies absolutely dependent on complement to produce immobilization of sperm were initially described by Fjällbrant in 1965 and Isojima in 1968. In these assays, donor sperm from the male to be tested—or from a normal control—

are washed and incubated with serial dilutions of heat-inactivated test serum or other secretions. These can be derived from the male to be tested or from female partners. A source of complement (usually fresh guinea pig serum) is added. A time end point for immobilization (Fjällbrant) of 90% sperm—or a percentage of motile sperm at a standard time (Isojima)—is compared microscopically with sperm incubated in control sera and complement alone. Complement-dependent immobilization, while highly specific in that false-positive reactions are uncommon, will not detect the presence of non-complement-fixing immunoglobulins. The degree of antibody present on the sperm surface also appears to play a role in the extent of complement-dependent immobilization. Results obtained from immobilization tests have a definite relationship to immunologic infertility. However, correlation of sperm-immobilizing antibodies with agglutinating antibodies is not perfect.

Since seminal plasma contains complement inhibitors, complement-dependent cytotoxicity tests cannot be applied to detection of autoantibodies to sperm in semen. Although sperm agglutination, antiglobulin tests, radiolabeled protein A, and ELISA have all been applied to the study of antisperm antibodies within the seminal plasma, they suffer from the fact that the majority of sperm-reactive antibodies present within the ejaculate may be cell-associated (sperm-bound) rather than cell-free. If antibody concentrations are limiting relative to the number of antigenic sites on the sperm surface, there may be no residual antibody within the seminal plasma despite its presence bound to spermatozoa. Those antibodies detected within seminal plasma may then not be reflective of immunoglobulins associated with sperm.

Sperm Agglutination Tests

Agglutination tests are a sensitive and specific means of detecting sperm antibodies. The 2 main procedures for sperm agglutination are the gelatin agglutination test of Kibrick and the microagglutination test read macroscopically. In the Franklin-Dukes method, no gelatin is used, and agglutination is read on slides or in a microtiter tray in the microscope. Agglutination may be primarily head-to-head or tail-to-tail, rarely head-to-tail. Tail-to-tail agglutination usually occurs in female sera and head-to-head in male sera. The antigens detected by this test are not fully characterized.

Failure to give careful attention to controls in sperm antibody tests has often led to misleading results, especially with relatively undiluted sera. Obviously, obtaining a standard source of viable human sperm presents difficulties. Known positive and negative control sera must be included.

Glossary of Terms Commonly Used in Immunology

Abrin: A potent toxin which is derived from the seeds of the jequirity plant and which agglutinates erythrocytes (a lectin).

Accessory cells: Lymphoid cells predominantly of the monocyte and macrophage lineage that cooperate with T and B lymphocytes in the formation of antibody and in other immune reactions.

Active immunity: Protection acquired by deliberate introduction of an antigen into a responsive host.

Activated lymphocytes: Lymphocytes that have been stimulated by specific antigen or nonspecific mitogen.

Activated macrophages: Mature macrophages in a metabolic state caused by various stimuli, especially phagocytosis or lymphokine activity.

Activation: A process in which the members of the complement sequence are altered enzymatically to become functionally active.

Adaptive Immunity: A series of host defenses characterized by extreme specificity and memory mediated by antibody or T cells.

Addressins: Ligands on mucosal endothelial cells for specific homing receptors on lymphocytes derived from Peyer's patches.

Adjuvant: A compound capable of potentiating an immune response.

Adoptive transfer: The transfer of immunity by immuno-competent cells from one animal to another.

Adrenergic receptors: Receptors for various adrenergic agents of either the α or the β class that are present on a variety of cells and from which the action of various adrenergic drugs can be predicted.

Agglutination: An antigen-antibody reaction in which a solid or particulate antigen forms a lattice with a soluble antibody. In reverse agglutination, the antibody is attached to a solid particle and is agglutinated by insoluble antigen.

Alexin (also **alexine**)**:** A term coined by Pfeiffer to denote a thermolabile and nonspecific factor that, in concert with sensitizer, causes bacteriolysis.

Allele: One of 2 genes controlling a particular characteristic present at a locus.

Allelic exclusion: The phenotypic expression of a single allelle in cells containing 2 different allelles for that genetic locus.

Allergens: Antigens that give rise to allergy.

Allergoids: Chemically modified allergens that give rise to antibody of the IgG but not IgE class, thereby reducing allergic symptoms.

Allergy (hypersensitivity): A disease or reaction caused by an immune response to one or more environmental antigens, resulting in tissue inflammation and organ dysfunction.

Allogeneic: Denotes the relationship that exists between genetically dissimilar members of the same species.

Allogeneic effect: A form of general immunopotentiation in which specific stimulation of T cells results in the release of factors active in the immune response.

Allograft (also **homograft**)**:** A tissue or organ graft between 2 genetically dissimilar members of the same species.

Allotype: The genetically determined antigenic difference in serum proteins, varying in different members of the same species.

α/β T cells: T cells in which α and β chains of the T cell receptor are rearranged and expressed on the surface. Most T cells are of this type.

Alpha-fetoprotein (AFP): An embryonic α-globulin with immunosuppressive properties that is structurally similar to albumin.

Alternative complement pathway (also **properdin pathway**)**:** The system of activation of the complement pathway through involvement of properdin factor D, properdin factor B, and C3b, finally activating C3 and then progressing as in the classic pathway.

Am marker: The allotypic determinant on the heavy chain of human IgA.

Amboceptor: A term coined by Ehrlich to denote a bacteriolytic substance in serum that acts together with complement or alexin, ie, antibody.

Anamnesis (also **immunologic memory**)**:** A heightened responsiveness to the second or subsequent administration of antigen to an immune animal.

Anaphylactoid reaction: Clinical response similar to anaphylaxis but not caused by an IgE mediated allergic reaction.

Anaphylatoxin: A substance produced by complement activation that results in increased vascular permeability through the release of pharmacologically active mediators from mast cells.

Anaphylatoxin inactivator: An α-globulin with a molecular weight of 300,000 that destroys the biologic activity of C3a and C5a.

Anaphylaxis: A reaction of immediate hypersensitivity present in nearly all vertebrates that results from sensitization of tissue-fixed mast cells by cytotropic antibodies following exposure to antigen.

Anergy: A state of diminished or absent cell-mediated immunity as shown by the inability to react to a battery of common skin test antigens.

Angiogenesis factor: Released by macrophages and causes neovascularization of surrounding tissues.

Antibody: A protein which is produced as a result of the introduction of an antigen and which has the ability to combine with the antigen that stimulated its production.

Antibody-combining site: The configuration present on an antibody molecule that links with a corresponding antigenic determinant.

Antibody-dependent cell-mediated cytotoxicity (ADCC): A form of lymphocyte-mediated cytotoxicity in which an effector cell kills an antibody-coated target cell, presumably by recognition of the Fc region of the cell-bound antibody through an Fc receptor present on the effector lymphocyte.

Antigen: A substance that reacts with antibodies or T cell receptors evoked by immunogens.

Antigen-presenting cell (APC): A cell that processes a protein antigen by fragmenting it into peptides that are presented on the cell surface in concert with class II major histocompatibility molecules for interaction with the appropriate T cell receptor. B cells, T cells, dendritic cells, and macrophages can perform this function.

Antigen processing: The series of events that occurs following antigen administration and antibody production.

Antigen-binding site: The part of an immunoglobulin that binds antigen.

Antigenic competition: The suppression of the immune response to 2 closely related antigens when they are injected simultaneously.

Antigenic determinant (see **Epitope**).

Antigenic modulation: The spatial alteration of the arrangement of antigenic sites present on a cell surface brought about by the presence of bound antibody.

Antigenic shift: Periodic changes over time in the surface antigens of certain viruses. These are caused by genetic mutations.

Antilymphocyte serum: Antibodies that are directed against lymphocytes and that usually cause immunosuppression.

Antitoxins: Protective antibodies that inactivate soluble toxin protein products of bacteria.

Armed macrophages: Macrophages capable of antigen-specific cytotoxicity as a result of cytophilic antibodies or arming factors from T cells.

Association constant (K value): The mathematical representation of the affinity of binding between antigen and antibody.

Atopy: A genetically determined state of hypersensitivity to common environmental allergens, mediated by IgE antibodies.

Attenuated: Rendered less virulent.

Autoantibody: Antibody to self antigens.

Autoantigens: Self antigens

Autocrine: Effects of hormones on the cell that actually produces them.

Autograft: A tissue graft between genetically identical members of the same species.

Autoimmunity: Immunity to self antigens (autoantigens):

Autoradiography: A technique for detecting radioactive isotopes in which a tissue section containing radioactivity is overlaid with x-ray or photographic film on which the emissions are recorded.

B cell (also **B lymphocyte**): Strictly, a bursa-derived cell in avian species and, by analogy, a bursa-equivalent derived cell in nonavian species. B cells are the precursors of plasma cells that produce antibody.

Bacteriolysin: An antibody or other substance capable of lysing bacteria.

Bacteriolysis: The disintegration of bacteria induced by antibody and complement in the absence of cells.

Beta lysin: A highly reactive heat-stable cationic protein that is bactericidal for gram-positive organisms.

Biosynthesis: The production of molecules by viable cells in culture.

Blast cell: A large lymphocyte or other immature cell containing a nucleus with loosely packed chromatin, a large nucleolus, and a large amount of cytoplasm with numerous polyribosomes.

Blast transformation: See **Lymphocyte activation.**

Blocking antibody: See **Blocking factors.**

Blocking factors: Substances that are present in the serum of tumor-bearing animals and are capable of blocking the ability of immune lymphocytes to kill tumor cells.

Bradykinin: A 9-amino-acid peptide that is split by the enzyme kallikrein from serum α_2-globulin precursor and that causes a slow, sustained contraction of the smooth muscles.

Bursa of Fabricius: The hindgut organ located in the cloaca of birds that controls the ontogeny of B lymphocytes.

Bursal equivalent: The hypothetical organ or organs analogous to the bursa of Fabricius in nonavian species.

C region (constant region): The carboxy-terminal portion of the H or L chain that is identical in immunoglobulin molecules of a given class and subclass apart from genetic polymorphisms.

C terminus: The carboxy-terminal end of a protein molecule.

Cachectin: A factor present in serum, which causes wasting and is identical to tumor necrosis factor alpha.

Capping: The movement of cell surface antigens toward one pole of a cell after the antigens are cross-linked by specific antibody.

Carcinoembryonic antigen (CEA): An antigen that is present on fetal endodermal tissue and is reexpressed on the surface of neoplastic cells, particularly in carcinoma of the colon.

Carrier An immunogenic substance that, when coupled to a hapten, renders the hapten immunogenic.

Cationic proteins: Antimicrobial substances present within granules of phagocytic cells.

Cell-mediated immunity: Immunity in which the participation of lymphocytes and macrophages is predominant.

Cell-mediated lymphocytolysis: An in vitro assay for cellular immunity in which a standard mixed-lymphocyte reaction is followed by destruction of target cells that are used to sensitize allogeneic cells during the mixed lymphocyte reaction.

Centimorgan: A unit of physical distance on a chromosome, equivalent to a 1% frequency of recombination between closely linked genes. Also called a map unit.

Central lymphoid organs: Lymphoid organs that are essential to the development of the immune response, ie, the thymus and the bursa of Fabricius.

Chase-Sulzberger phenomenon: See **Sulzberger-Chase phenomenon.**

Chemokinesis: Reaction by which chemical substances determine rate of cellular movement.

Chemotaxis: A process whereby phagocytic cells are attracted to the vicinity of invading pathogens.

Chromatography: A variety of techniques useful for the separation of proteins.

cis-Pairing: Association of two genes on the same chromosome encoding a protein.

Class I antigen: Histocompatibility antigen encoded in humans by A, B, and C loci and in mice by D and K loci.

Class II antigen: Histocompability antigen encoded in humans by DR, DP and DQ loci.

Class III antigens: C4 and factor B are complement components encoded within the MHC.

Classic complement pathway: A series of enzyme-substrate and protein-protein interactions that ultimately leads to biologically active complement enzymes. It proceeds sequentially C1, 423 567 89.

Clonal anergy: Theory that B cell tolerance is induced by antigen-B cell contact during obligatory paralyzable phase or tolerance-sensitive phase of B cell differentiation.

Clonal deletion: A concept related to Burnet's clonal selection theory, which suggests that tolerance to self antigens results from deletion of autoreactive lymphocyte clones in embryonic life.

Clonal selection theory: The theory of antibody synthesis proposed by Burnet that predicts that the individual carries a complement of clones of lymphoid cells which are capable of reacting with all possible antigenic determinants. During fetal life, clones reacted against self antigens are eliminated on contact with antigen.

Clone: A group of cells all of which are the progeny of a single cell.

Cluster of differentiation: One or more cell surface molecules, detectable by monoclonal antibodies, that define a particular cell line or state of cellular differentiation.

c-myc gene: Member of a candidate set of cancer-related genes or cellular oncogenes.

Coelomocyte: A wandering ameboid phagocyte found in all animal invertebrates containing a coelom.

Cohn fraction II: Primarily gamma globulin that is produced as the result of ethanol fractionation of serum according to the Cohn method.

Combinatorial joining: A process whereby one exon can combine alternatively with a variety of other gene segments, thereby multiplying the diversity of the gene products.

Complement: A system of serum proteins that is the primary humoral mediator of antigen-antibody reactions.

Complement fixation: A standard serologic assay used for the detection of an antigen-antibody reaction in which complement is fixed as a result of the formation of an immune complex. The subsequent failure of lysis of sensitized erythrocytes by complement that has been fixed indicates the degree of antigen-antibody reaction.

Complementarity: In genetics, the term indicates that more than one gene is required for the expression of a particular trait.

Concanavalin A (Con A): A lectin that is derived from the jack bean and stimulates the predominantly T lymphocytes.

Concomitant immunity: The ability of a tumor-bearing animal to reject a test inoculum of its tumor at a site different from the primary site of tumor growth.

Congenic (originally **congenic resistant**): Denotes a line of mice identical or nearly identical with other inbred strains except for the substitution at one histocompatibility locus of a foreign allele introduced by appropriate crosses with a second inbred strain.

Contact senstivity: A type of delayed hypersenstivity reaction in which sensitivity to simple chemical compounds is manifested by skin reactvity.

Contrasuppression: Effects of immunoregulatory circuit that inhibit suppressor influences in a feedback loop.

Copolymer: A polymer of at least 2 different chemical moieties, eg, a polypeptide with 2 different amino acids.

Coproantibody: An antibody present in the lumen of the gastrointestinal tract.

Crossmatching: A laboratory test using cells from a recipient and serum from a donor to detect antibodics directed at recipient's cells.

Cross-reacting antigen: A type of tumor antigen present on all tumors induced by the same or a similar carcinogen.

Cross-reaction: The reaction of an antibody with an antigen other than the one that induced its formation.

Cutaneous basophil hypersensitvity: An immunologically mediated inflammation in the skin with a prominent basophil infiltration occuring about 24 hours after injection of the sensitizing antigen.

Cyclo-oxygenase pathway: Enzymatic metabolism of cell membrane-derived arachidonic acid whereby prostaglandins are produced.

Cytokine: A factor such as a lymphokine or monokine produced by cells that affect other cells.

Cytotropic antibodies: Antibodies of the IgG and IgE classes that sensitize cells for subsequent anaphylaxis.

D gene region: Diversity region of genome encoding heavy chain sequences in the hypervariable region of immunoglobulin H chain.

Degranulation: A process whereby cytoplasmic granules of phagocytic cells fuse with phagosomes and discharge their contents into the phagolysosome thus formed.

Delayed hypersensitivity: A cell-mediated immune response producing a cellular infiltrate and edema that are maximal between 24 and 48 hours after antigen challenge.

Dendritic cells: Mononuclear cells that present antigens in lymphoid tissue but are distinct from the monocyte-macrophage lineage.

Determinant groups: Individual chemical structures present on macromolecular antigens that determine antigenic specificity.

Dextrans: Polysaccharides composed of a single sugar.

Diapedesis: The outward passage of cells through intact vessel walls.

Direct agglutination: The agglutination of erythrocytes, microorganisms, or other substances directly by serum antibody.

Direct immunofluorescence: The detection of antigens by fluorescently labeled antibody.

Disulfide bonds: Chemical S-S bonds between sulfhydryl-containing amino acids that bind together H and L chains as well as portions of H-H and L-L chains.

Domains (also **homology regions**): Segments of H or L chains that are folded 3-dimensionally and stabilized with disulfide bonds.

E rosette: A formation of a cluster (rosette) of cells consisting of sheep erythrocytes and human T lymphocytes.

EAC rosette: A cluster of *e*rythrocytes sensitized with *a*mboceptor (*a*ntibody) and *c*omplement around human B lymphocytes.

EAE (experimental allergic encephalomyelitis): An autoimmune disease in which an animal is immunized with homologous or heterologous extracts of whole brain, the basic protein of myelin, or certain polypeptide sequences within the basic protein, emulsified with Freund's complete adjuvant.

ECF-A (eosinophil chemotactic factor of anaphylaxis): An acidic peptide, molecular weight 500, that, when released, causes influx of eosinophils.

Effector cells: A term that usually denotes T cells capable of mediating cytotoxicity, suppression or helper function.

Electrophoresis: The separation of molecules in an electrical field.

Encapsulation: A quasi-immunologic phenomenon in which foreign material is walled off within the tissues of invertebrates.

Endocytosis: The process whereby material external to a cell is internalized within a particular cell. It consists of pinocytosis and phagocytosis.

Endogenous pyrogen (IL-1): Factor produced by macrophages and other cells. Causes fever by reducing prostaglandins in region of hypothalamus.

Endotoxins: Lipopolysaccharides that are derived from the cell walls of gram-negative microorganisms and have toxic and pyrogenic effects when injected in vivo.

Enhancement: Improved survival of tumor cells in animals that have been previously immunized to the antigens of a given tumor.

Epitope: The simplest form of an antigenic determinant present on a complex antigenic molecule, which combines with antibody or T cell receptor.

Equilibrium dialysis: A technique for measuring the strength or affinity with which antibody binds to antigen.

Equivalence: A ratio of antigen-antibody concentration where maximal precipitation occurs.

Euglobulin: A class of globulin proteins that are insoluble in water but soluble in salt solutions.

Eukaryote: A cell or organism possessing a true nucleus containing chromosomes bounded by a nuclear membrane.

Exon: The coding segment of a DNA strand.

Exotoxins: Diffusible toxins produced by certain gram-positive and gram-negative microorganisms.

F$_1$ generation: The first generation of offspring after a designated mating.

F$_2$ generation: The second generation of offspring after a designated mating.

Fab: An antigen-binding fragment produced by enzymatic digestion of an IgG molecule with papain.

F(ab)$'_2$: A fragment obtained by pepsin digestion of immunoglobulin molecules containing the 2 H and 2 L chains linked by disulfide bonds. It contains antigen-binding activity. An F(ab)$'_2$ fragment and Fc fragment make up an entire monomeric immunoglobulin molecule.

Fc fragment: A crystallizable fragment obtained by papain digestion of IgG molecules that consists of the C-terminal half of 2 H chains linked by disulfide bonds. It contains no antigen-binding capability but determines important biologic characteristics of the intact molecule.

Fc receptor: A receptor present on various subclasses of lymphocytes for the Fc fragment of immunoglobulins.

Felton phenomenon: Immunologic unresponsiveness or tolerance induced in mice by the injection of large quantities of pneumococcal polysaccharide.

Fetal antigen: A type of tumor-associated antigen that is normally present on embryonic but not adult tissues and that is reexpressed during the neoplastic process.

Fibronectin: A protein that has an important role in the structuring of connective tissue.

Fluorescence: The emission of light of one color while a substance is irradiated with a light of a different color.

Forbidden clone theory: The theory proposed to explain autoimmunity that postulates that lymphocytes capable of self sensitization and effector function are present in tolerant animals, since they were not eliminated during embryogenesis.

Freund's complete adjuvant: An oil-water emulsion that contains killed mycobacteria and enhances immune responses when mixed in an emulsion with antigen.

Freund's incomplete adjuvant: An emulsion that contains all of the elements of Freund's complete adjuvant with the exception of killed mycobacteria.

G cells: Gastrin-secreting cells in mucosa of the gastric antrum.

Gamma globulins: Serum proteins with gamma mobility in electrophoresis that make up the majority of immunoglobulins and antibodies.

Gammopathy: A paraprotein disorder involving abnormalities of immunoglobulins.

γ/δ T cells: T cells expressing γ and δ chains of the T cell receptor. The function of this minor T cell population is unknown.

Generalized anaphylaxis: A shocklike state that occurs within minutes following an appropriate antigen-antibody reaction resulting from the systemic release of vasoactive amines.

Genetic switch hypothesis: A hypothesis that postulates that there is a switch in the gene controlling heavy chain synthesis in plasma cells during the development of an immune response.

Genetic theory of antibody synthesis: A theory that predicts that information for synthesis of all types of antibody exists in the genome and that specific receptors are preformed on immunocompetent cells.

Germinal centers: A collection of metabolically active lymphoblasts, macrophages, and plasma cells that appears within the primary follicle of lymphoid tissues following antigenic stimulation.

Gm marker: An allotypic determinant on the heavy chain of human IgG.

Graft-versus-host (GVH) reaction: The clinical and pathologic sequelae of the reactions of immunocompetent cells in a graft against the cells of the histoincompatible and immunodeficient recipient.

Granuloma: An organized structure of mononuclear cells that is the hallmark of cell-mediated immunity.

Granulopoietin (colony-stimulating factor): A glycoprotein with a molecular weight of 45,000 derived from monocytes that controls the production of granulocytes by the bone marrow.

H chain: See **Heavy chain.**

H-2 locus: The major genetic histocompatibility region in the mouse.

Halogenation: A combination of a halogen molecule with a microbial cell wall that results in microbial damage.

Haplotype: The portion of the phenotype determined by closely linked genes of a single chromosome inherited from one parent.

Hapten: A substance that is not immunogenic but can react with an antibody of appropriate specificity.

Hassall's corpuscles (also **Leber's corpuscles** or **thymic corpuscles**): Whorls of thymic epithelial cells whose function is unknown.

Heavy chain (H chain): One pair of identical polypeptide chains making up an immunoglobulin molecule. The heavy chain contains approximately twice the number of amino acids and is twice the molecular weight of the light chain.

Heavy chain diseases: A heterogeneous group of paraprotein disorders characterized by the presence of monoclonal but incomplete heavy chains without light chains in serum or urine.

Helper T cells: A subtype of T lymphocytes that cooperate with B cells in antibody formation.

Hemagglutination inhibition: A technique for detecting small amounts of antigen in which the agglutination of antigen-coated erythrocytes or other particles by specific antibody is inhibited by homologous antigen.

Hematopoietic system: All tissues responsible for production of the cellular elements of peripheral blood. This term usually excludes strictly lymphocytopoietic tissue such as lymph nodes.

Hemolysin: An antibody or other substance capable of lysing erythrocytes.

Heterocytotropic antibody: An antibody that can passively sensitize tissues of species other than those in which the antibody is present.

Heterodimer: A 2-component molecule made up of different but closely joined segments, eg, T cell receptor α and β chains.

Heterologous antigen: An antigen that participates in a cross-reaction.

High dose (high zone) tolerance: Classic immunologic unresponsiveness produced by repeated injections of large amounts of antigen.

High endothelial venules: Specialized blood vessels present in lymphoid tissues with cuboidal endothelium, which allow passage of lymphocytes between cells into tissues.

Hinge region: The area of the H chains in the C region between the first and second C region domains. It is the site of enzymatic cleavage into $F(ab)'_2$ and Fc fragments.

Histamine: A bioactive amine of molecular weight 111 that cause smooth muscle contraction of human bronchioles and small blood vessels, increased permeability of capillaries, and increased secretion by nasal and bronchial mucous glands.

Histamine releasing factor: A lymphokine released from sensitized lymphocytes or antigenic stimulation that causes basophil histamine release.

Histocompatible: Sharing transplantation antigens.

HLA (human leukocyte antigen): The major histocompatibility genetic region in humans.

Homing receptors: Cell surface molecules that direct the cell to specific locations in other organs or tissues.

Homocytotropic antibody: An antibody that attaches to cells of animals of the same species.

Homologous antigen: An antigen that induces an antibody and reacts specifically with it.

Homopolymer: A molecule consisting of repeating units of a single amino acid.

Homozygous typing cells (HTC): Cells derived from an individual who is homozygous at the HLA-D locus used for the MLR typing of the D locus in humans.

Horror autotoxicus: A concept introduced by Ehrlich, proposing that an individual is protected against autoimmunity or immunization against self antigens even though these antigens are immunogenic in other animals.

Hot antigen suicide: A technique in which an antigen is labeled with a high-specific-acitivity radioisotope (^{131}I). It is used either in vivo or in vitro to inhibit specific lymphocyte function by attachment to an antigen-binding lymphocyte, subseqently killing it by radiolysis.

Humoral: Pertaining to molecules in solution in a body fluid, particularly antibody and complement.

Hybridoma: Transformed cell line grown in vivo or in vitro that is a somatic hybrid of 2 parent cell lines and contains genetic material from both.

Hydrophilic: A hydrophilic compound is soluble in water; a hydrophilic group binds water on the exterior surfaces of proteins and cell membranes.

Hydrophobic: A hydrophobic compound is insoluble in water; a hydrophobic group is pushed to the interior of proteins or membranes, away from water.

Hyperacute rejection: An accelerated form of graft rejection that is associated with circulating antibody in the serum of the recipient and which can react with donor cells.

Hypersensitivity: See **Allergy.**

Hypervariable regions: At least 4 regions of extreme variability which occur throughout the V region of H and L chains and which determine the antibody combining site of an antibody molecule.

Hyposensitization: See **Desensitization.**

I region: That portion of the major histocompatibility complex which contains genes that control immune responses.

Ia antigens (I region-associated antigens): Antigens that are controlled by Ir genes and are present on various tissues.

Idiotope: An epitope (antigenic determinant) on an idiotype.

Idiotype: A unique antigenic determinant present on homogeneous antibody or myeloma protein. The idiotype appears to represent the antigenicity of the antigen-binding site of an antibody and is therefore located in the V region.

IgA: The predominant immunoglobulin class present in secretions.

IgD: The predominant immunoglobulin class present on human B lymphocytes.

IgE: A reaginic antibody involved in immediate hypersensitivity reactions.

IgG: The predominant immunoglobulin class present in human serum.

IgM: A pentameric immunoglobulin comprising approximately 10% of normal human serum immunoglobulins, with a molecular weight of 900,000 and a sedimentation coefficient of 19S.

7S IgM: A monomeric IgM consisting of one monomer of 5 identical subunits.

Immediate hypersensitivity: An antibody-mediated immunologic sensitivity that manifests itself by tissue reactions occurring within minutes after the antigen combines with its appropriate antibody.

Immune adherence: An agglutination reaction between a cell bearing C423 and an indicator cell, usually a human erythrocyte, which has a receptor for C3b.

Immune complexes: Antigen-antibody complexes.

Immune elimination: The enhanced clearance of an injected antigen from the circulation as a result of immunity to that antigen brought about by enhanced phagocytosis of the reticuloendothelial system.

Immune exclusion: The normal prevention of entry of antigens across mucosal membranes by secretory IgA.

Immune response genes (Ir genes): Genes that control immune responses to specific antigens.

Immune suppression: A variety of therapeutic maneuvers to depress or eliminate the immune response.

Immune surveillance: A theory that holds that the immune system destroys tumor cells, which are constantly arising during the life of the individual.

Immunization: See **Sensitization.** Natural or artificial induction of an immune response, particularly when it renders the host protected from disease.

Immunobeads: Small plastic spheres coated with antibodies or antigens, which are used to indicate immune reactions by agglutinaton.

Immunocytoadherence: A technique for identifying immunoglobulin-bearing cells by formation of rosettes consisting of these cells and erythrocytes or other particles containing a homologous antigen.

Immunodominant: The part of an antigenic determinant that is dominant in binding with antibody.

Immunoelectrophoresis: A technique combining an initial electrophoretic separation of proteins followed by immunodiffusion with resultant precipitation arcs.

Immunofluorescence: A histo- or cytochemical technique for the detection and localization of antigens in which specific antibody is conjugated with fluorescent compounds, resulting in a sensitive tracer that can be detected by fluorometric measurements.

Immunogen: A substance that, when introduced into an animal, stimulates the immune response. The term immunogen may also denote a substance that is capable of stimulating an immune response, in contrast to a substance that can only combine with antibody, ie, an antigen.

Immunogenicity: The property of a substance making it capable of inducing a detectable immune response.

Immunoglobulin: A glycoprotein composed of H and L chains that functions as antibody. All antibodies are immunoglobuins, but it is not certain that all immunoglobulins have antibody function.

Immunoglobulin class: A subdivision of immunoglobulin molecules based on unique antigenic determinants in the Fc region of the H chains. In humans there are 5 classes of immunoglobulins designated IgG, IgA, IgM, IgD, and IgE.

Immunoglobulin class switch: The process in which a B cell precursor expressing IgM and IgG receptors differentiates into a B cell producing IgG, IgA, or IgE antibodies without change in specificity for the antigenic determinant.

Immunoglobulin subclass: A subdivision of the classes of immunoglobulins based on structural and antigenic differences in the H chains. For human IgG there are 4 subclasses: IgG1, IgG2, IgG3, IgG4.

Immunoglobulin supergene family: A structurally related group of genes that encode immunoglobulins, T cell receptors, β_2-microglobulin, and others.

Immunomodulation: A variety of methods for therapeutic manipulation of the immune response.

Immunopathic: Referring to damage to cells, tissues, or organs from immune responses.

Immunopotency: The capacity of a region of an antigen molecule to serve as an antigenic determinant and thereby induce the formation of specific antibody.

Immunotherapy: Either hyposensitization in allergic diseases or treatment with immunostimulants or immunosuppressive drugs or biologic products.

Indirect agglutination (also **passive agglutination**)**:** The agglutination of particles or erythrocytes to which antigens have been coupled chemically.

Indirect immunofluorescence (also **double antibody immunofluorescense**)**:** A technique whereby unlabeled antibody is incubated with substrate and then overlaid with fluorescently conjugated anti-immunoglobulin to form a sandwich.

Information theory of antibody synthesis: A theory that predicts that antigen dictates the specific structure of the antibody molecule.

Innate immunity: Various host defenses present from birth that do not depend on immunologic memory.

Inoculation: The introduction of an antigen or antiserum into an animal in order to confer immunity.

Integrins: A family of cell membrane-bound factors that promote cell adhesion.

Interferon: A heterogeneous group of low-molecular-weight proteins elaborated by infected host cells that protect noninfected cells from viral infection.

Interleukin: Chemically defined factor released from leukocytes or other cells, which has defined biologic effects.

Interleukin-1: Macrophage-derived factor (previously called LAF, or leukocyte-activating factor) that promotes short-term proliferation of T cells.

Interleukin-2: A lymphocyte-derived factor (previously called TCGF, or T cell growth factor) that promotes long-term proliferation of T cell lines in culture.

Interleukin-3: A T cell product that induces proliferation and differentiation in other lymphocytes and some hematopoietic cells.

Interleukin-4: (formerly **BCGF**)**:** A factor that is produced by helper T cells and stimulates the growth of T and B cells.

Interleukin-5: A factor that is produced by helper T cells and stimulates B cells and eosinophils.

Interleukin-6: A factor that is produced by fibroblasts and stimulates B cell immunoglobulin production.

Interleukin-7: A factor that is produced by stromal cells and causes early T and B cell lymphopoiesis.

Interleukin-8: A factor that is produced by macrophages and chemoattracts T cells and neutrophils.

Introns: Noncoding regions of DNA interspersed among the exons.

Inv marker: See **Km marker.**

Ir genes: See **Immune response genes.**

Isoagglutinin: An agglutinating antibody capable of agglutinating cells of other individuals of the same species in which it is found.

Isoantibody: An antibody that is capabable of reacting with an antigen derived from a member of the same species as that in which it is raised.

Isohemagglutinins: Antibodies to major erythrocyte antigens present in members of a given species and directed against antigenic determinants on erythrocytes from other members of the species.

Isotype: Antigenic characteristics of given class or subclass of immunoglobulin H and L chains.

Isotype switching: The process of changing synthesis of heavy-chain isotypes, eg, from μ to γ in B cells.

J chain: A glycopeptide chain that is normally found in polymeric immunoglobulins, particularly IgA and IgM.

Jarisch-Herxheimer reaction: A local or occasionally generalized inflammatory reaction that occurs following treatment of syphilis and other intracellular infections; it is presumably caused by the release of large amounts of antigenic material into the circulation.

Jones criteria: Signs and symptoms used to diagnose acute rheumatic fever.

Jones-Mote reaction: See **Cutaneous basophil hypersensitivity.**

K cell: A killer cell responsible for antibody-dependent cell-mediated cytotoxicity.

Kallikrein system: See **Kinin system.**

Kappa (κ) chains: One of 2 major types of light chains.

Kinin: A peptide that increases vascular permeability and is formed by the action of esterases on kallikreins, which than act as vasodilators.

Kinin system (also **kallikrein system**)**:** A humoral amplification system initiated by the activation of coagulation factor XII, eventually leading to the formation of kallikrein, which acts on a α-globulin substrate, kininogen, to form a bradykinin.

Km marker (also **Inv**)**:** An allotypic marker on the κ L chain of human immunoglobulins.

Koch phenomenon: A delayed hypersensitivity reaction by tuberculin in the skin of a guinea pig following infection with *Mycobacterium tuberculosis.*

Kupffer cells: Fixed mononuclear phagocytes of the reticuloendothelial system that are present within the sinusoids of the liver.

Kveim test: A delayed hypersensitivity test for sarcoidosis in which potent antigenic extracts of sarcoid tissue are injected intradermally and biopsied 6 weeks later in order to observe the presence of a granuloma, indicating a positive test.

L chain: See **Light chain.**

Lactoferrin: An iron-containing compound that exerts a slight antimicrobial action by binding iron necessary for microbial growth.

Lambda (λ) chain: One of 2 major types of light chains.

Langerhans cell: Bone marrow-derived macrophage with Ia cell surface antigens found in the epidermis.

Late-phase reaction: An inflammatory response that occurs about 6–8 hours after antigen exposure in IgE-mediated allergic diseases.

Latex fixation test: An agglutination reaction in which latex particles are used to passively adsorb soluble protein and polysaccharide antigens.

Lectin: A substance that is derived from a plant and has panagglutinating activity for erythrocytes. Lectins are commonly mitogens as well.

Leukocyte inhibitory factor (LIF): A lymphokine that inhibits the migration of polymorphonuclear leukocytes.

Leukotriene: A vasodilatory lipoxygenase metabolite of arachidonic acid.

Ligand: Any molecule that forms a complex with another molecule, such as an antigen used in a precipitin or radioimmunoassay.

Light chain (L chain): A polypeptide chain present in all immunoglobulin molecules. Two types exist in most species and are termed kappa (κ) and lambda (λ).

Lineage infidelity: Expression following neoplastic transformation of molecules on cells that are foreign to the lineage of the cell itself.

Linkage disequilibrium: An unexpected association of linked genes in a population.

Lipopolysaccharide (also **endotoxin**)**:** A compound derived from a variety of gram-negative enteric bacteria that have various biologic functions including mitogenic activity for B lymphocytes.

Lipoxygenase pathway: Enzymatic metabolism of cell membrane-derived arachidonic acid whereby leukotrienes are produced.

Local anaphylaxis: An immediate hypersensitivity reaction that occurs in a specific target organ such as the gastrointestinal tract, nasal mucosa, or skin.

Locus: The specific site of a gene on a chromosome.

Low dose (low zone) tolerance: A transient and incomplete state of tolerance induced with small subimmunogenic doses of soluble antigen.

Lymphocyte: A mononuclear cell 7–12 μm in diameter containing a nucleus with densely packed chromatin and a small rim of cytoplasm.

Lymphocyte activation (also **lymphocyte stimulation, lymphocyte transformation,** or **blastogenesis**)**:** An in vitro technique in which lymphocytes are stimulated to become metabolically active by antigen or mitogen.

Lymphocyte-defined (LD) antigens: A series of histocompatibility antigens that are present on the majority of mammalian cells and are detectable primarily by reactivity in the mixed lymphocyte reaction (MLR).

Lymphokines (also **mediators of cellular immunity**)**:** Soluble products of lymphocytes that are responsible for the multiple effects of a cellular immune reaction.

Lymphoreticular: Referring to lymphocyte and monocyte-macrophage system and stromal elements that support its growth.

Lymphotoxin (LT): A lymphokine that results in direct cytolysis following its release from stimulated lymphocytes.

Lysosomes: Granules that contain hydrolytic enzymes and are present in the cytoplasm of many cells.

Lysozyme (also **muramidase**)**:** The cationic low-molecular-weight enzyme present in tears, saliva, and nasal secretions that reduces the local concentration of susceptible bacteria by attacking the mucopeptides of their cell walls.

M cells: Membranous epithelial cells that overlie lymphoid tissues in the small intestine and allow limited passage of intraintestinal antigens.

M protein: Antigenic component of surface of streptococci. Cross-reacts with muscle antigens.

M protein: See **Myeloma protein.**

Macrophage chemotactic factor (MCF): A lymphokine that selectively attracts monocytes or macrophages to the area of its release.

Macrophage-activating factor (MAF): A lymphokine that will activate macrophages to become avid phagocytic cells.

Macrophages: Phagocytic mononuclear cells that derive from bone marrow monocytes and subserve accessory roles in cellular immunity.

Major basic protein: A toxic protein from the eosinophil membrane that produces tissue damage in allergic and inflammatory diseases.

Major histocompatibility complex (MHC): Genes located in close proximity that determine histocompatibility antigens of members of a species.

Mast cell: A tissue cell that has high-affinity receptors for IgE and generates inflammatory mediators in allergy.

Membrane attack complex: The terminal complement components that, when activated, cause lysis of target cells.

β₂-Microglobulin: A protein (MW 11,600) that is associated with the outer membrane of many cells, including lymphocytes, and that functions as a structural part of the histocompatibility antigens on cells.

Migration inhibitory factor (MIF): A lymphokine that is capable of inhibiting the migration of macrophages.

Mitogens (also **phytomitogens**)**:** Substances that cause DNA synthesis, blast transformation, and ultimately division of lymphocytes.

Mixed lymphocyte culture (mixed leukocyte culture) (MLC): An in vitro test for cellular immunity in which lymphocytes or leukocytes from genetically dissimilar individuals are mixed and mutually stimulate DNA synthesis.

Mixed lymphocyte reaction (MLR): See **Mixed lymphocyte culture.**

Molecular mimicry: Immunlogic cross-reactivity between determinants on an environmental antigen (such as a virus) and a self antigen, a notion that has been proposed to explain autoimmunity.

Monoclonal hypergammaglobulinemia: An increase in immunoglubulins produced by a single clone of cells containing one H chain class and one L chain type.

Monoclonal antibodies (Monoclonal immunoglobulin molecules): Identical copies of antibody that consist of one H chain class and one L chain type.

Monoclonal protein: A protein produced from the progeny of a single cell called a clone.

Monokine: Substance released from macrophage or monocyte that affects the function of another cell.

Monomer: The basic unit of an immunoglobulin molecule that is composed of 4 polypeptide chains: 2 H and 2 L.

Mononuclear phagocyte system: Mononuclear cells found primarily in the reticular connective tissue of lymphoid and other organs that are prominent in chronic inflammatory states.

Mucosal homing: The ability of immunologically competent cells that arise from mucosal follicles to traffic back to mucosal areas.

Mucosal immune system: The lymphoid tissues associated with the mucosal surfaces of the gastrointestinal, respiratory, and urogenital tracts, which produce a unique immunoglobulin (secretory IgA) and T cell immunity for these mucosal surfaces.

Multiple myeloma: A paraproteinemic disorder consisting typically of the presence of serum paraprotein, anemia, and lytic bone lesions.

Myeloma protein (M protein): Either an intact monoclonal immunoglobulin molecule or a portion of one produced by malignant plasma cells.

Myeloperoxidase: An enzyme that is present within granules of phagocytic cells and catalyzes peroxidation of a variety of microorganisms.

N terminus: The amino-terminal end of a protein molecule.

Natural antibody: Antibody present in the serum in the absence of apparent specific antigenic contact.

Neoantigens: Nonself antigens that arise spontaneously on cell surfaces, usually during neoplasia.

Network hypothesis: Jerne's theory of immunoregulation by a cascade of idiotype-anti-idiotype reactions involving T cell receptors and antibodies.

Neutralization: The process by which antibody or antibody in complement neutralizes the infectivity of microorganisms, particularly viruses.

NK cells (natural killer cells): Cytotoxic cells belonging to the cell class responsible for cellular cytotoxicity without prior sensitization.

Nonresponder: An animal unable to respond to an antigen, usually because of genetic factors.

Northern blotting: A method for detecting RNA fragments in an RNA mixture which are separated by gel electrophoresis, blotted, and probed with labeled DNA or RNA oligmers.

Nucleoside phosphorylase: An enzyme that catalyzes the conversion of inosine to hypoxanthine and is rarely deficient in patients with immunodeficiency disorders.

Nude mouse: A hairless mouse that congenitally lacks a thymus and has marked deficiency of thymus-derived lymphocytes.

Null cells: Cells lacking the specific identifying surface markers for either T or B lymphocytes.

NZB mouse: A genetically inbred strain of mice in which autoimmune disease resembling systemic lupus erythematosus develops spontaneously.

Oligoclonal bands: Immunoglobulins with restricted electrophoretic mobility in agarose gels found in cerebrospinal fluid of patients with multiple sclerosis and some other central nervous system diseases.

Oncofetal antigens: Antigens expressed during normal fetal development that reappear during cancer development, eg, carcinoembryonic antigen.

Oncogene: A gene of either viral or mammalian origin that causes transformation of cells in culture.

Oncogenesis: The process of producing neoplasia or malignancy.

Ontogeny: The developmental history of an individual organism within a group of animals.

Opportunistic infection: The ability of organisms of relatively low virulence to cause disease in the setting of altered immunity.

Opsonin: A substance capable of enhancing phagocytosis. Antibodies and complement are the 2 main opsonins.

Oral unresponsiveness: The process by which the mucosal immune system normally prevents immune responses to foods and intestinal bacteria while responding to potential pathogens.

Osteoclast activating factor (OAF): A lymphokine that promotes the resorption of bone.

Palindrome: In molecular biology, a self-complementary length of DNA which when read from the 5′ to the 3′ end displays an equivalent sequence whether read from the left or the right or forward or backward.

Paracrine: Effects of a hormone that are only local.

Paralysis: The pseudotolerant condition in which an ongoing immune response is masked by the presence of overwhelming amounts of antigen.

Paraproteinemia: A condition occurring in a heterogeneous group of diseases characterized by the presence in serum or urine of a monoclonal immunoglobulin.

Paratope: An antibody-combining site for epitope, the simplest form of an antigenic determinant.

Passive cutaneous anaphylaxis (PCA): An in vivo passive transfer test for recognizing cytotropic antibody responsible for immediate hypersensitivity reactions.

Passive immunity: Protection achieved by introduction of preformed antibody or immune cells into a nonimmune host.

Patching: The reorganization of a cell surface membrane component into discrete patches over the entire cell surface.

Peripheral lymphoid organs: Lymphoid organs not essential to the ontogeny of immune responses, ie, the spleen, lymph nodes, tonsils, and Peyer's patches.

Peritoneal exudate cells (PEC): Inflammatory cells present in the peritoneum of animals injected with an inflammatory agent.

Peyer's patches: Collections of lymphoid tissue in the submucosa of the small intestine that contain lymphocytes, plasma cells, germinal centers, and T cell-dependent areas.

Pfeiffer phenomenon: A demonstration showing that cholera vibrios introduced into the peritoneal cavity of an immune guinea pig lose their mobility and are lysed regardless of the presence of cells.

Phagocytes: Cells that are capable of ingesting particulate matter.

Phagocytosis: The engulfment of microorganisms or other particles by leukocytes.

Phagolysosome: A cellular organelle that is the product of the fusion of a phagosome and a lysosome.

Phagosome: A phagocytic vesicle bounded by inverted plasma membrane.

Phylogeny: The developmental and evolutionary history of a group of animals.

Phytohemagglutinin (PHA): A lectin that is derived from the red kidney bean *(Phaseolus vulgaris)* and that stimulates predominantly T lymphocytes.

Phytomitogens: Glycoproteins that are derived from plants and stimulate DNA synthesis and blast transformation in lymphocytes.

Pinocytosis: The ingestion of soluble materials by cells.

Plaque-forming cells: Antibody-producing cells capable of forming a hemolytic plaque in the presence of complement and antigenic erythrocytes.

Plasma cells: Fully differentiated antibody-synthesizing cells that are derived from B lymphocytes.

Plasmin: A fibrinolytic enzyme capable of proteolytically digesting C1.

Plasminogen activator: An enzyme secreted by macrophages that converts a plasma zymogen to active plasmin.

Platelet-activating factor: An inflammatory mediator that activates platelets and inflammatory cells and is considered to be important in the bronchial inflammation of asthma.

Pokeweed mitogen (PWM): A lectin that is derived from pokeweed *(Phytolacca americana)* and that stimulates both B and T lymphocytes.

Polyclonal hypergammaglobulinemia: An increase in γ-globulin of various classes containing different H and L chains.

Polyclonal mitogens: Mitogens that activate large subpopulations of lymphocytes.

Polyclonal proteins: A group of molecules derived from multiple clones of cells.

Polymerase chain reaction (PCR): A technique to amplify segments of genetic DNA or RNA of known composition with primers in sequential repeated steps.

Polymers: Immunoglobulins composed of more than a single basic monomeric unit; eg, an IgA dimer consists of 2 units.

Postcapillary venules: Specialized blood vessels lined with cuboid epithelium located in the paracortical region of lymph nodes through which lymphocytes traverse.

Prausnitz-Küstner reaction: The passive transfer by intradermal injection of serum containing IgE antibodies from an allergic subject to a nonallergic recipient.

Pre-B cells: Large immature lymphoid cells with diffuse cytoplasmic IgM that eventually develop into B cells.

Precipitation: A reaction between a soluble antigen and soluble antibody in which a complex lattice of interlocking aggregates forms.

Primary follicles: Tightly packed aggregates of lymphocytes found in the cortex of the lymph node or in the white pulp of the spleen after antigenic stimulation. Primary follicles develop into germinal centers.

Primed lymphocyte typing (PLT): A variation on the MLR in which cells are primed by allogeneic stimulation and reexposed to fresh stimulator cells. Used to type for HLA-D determinants.

Private antigen: A tumor or histocompatibility antigen restricted either to a specific chemically induced tumor or to the specific product of a given allele.

Prokaryote: An organism without a true nucleus which contains a single, linear chromosome.

Properdin system: A group of proteins involved in resistance to infection. The 2 main constituents consist of factor A and factor B. Properdin factor A is identical with C3, a β-globulin of MW 180,000. Properdin factor B is a β_2-globulin of MW 95,000. It is also called C3 proactivator, glycine-rich β-glycoprotein (GBG), or β_2-glycoprotein II. Properdin factor D is an α-globulin of MW 25,000 also called C3 proactivator convertase or glycine-rich β-glycoproteinase (GB-Gase).

Prostaglandins: A variety of naturally occurring aliphatic acids with various biologic activities, including increased vascular permeability, smooth muscle contraction, bronchial constriction, and alteration in the pain threshold.

Prothymocytes: Immature precursors of mature thymocytes that develop within the thymus gland.

Proto-oncogene: A viral oncogene present in normal mammalian DNA.

Prozone phenomenon: Suboptimal precipitation that occurs in the region of antibody excess during immunoprecipitation reactions.

Public antigen: Determinant common to several distinct or private antigens.

Pyogenic microorganisms: Microorganisms whose presence in tissues stimulates an outpouring of polymorphonuclear leukocytes.

Pyrogens: Substances that are released either endogenously from leukocytes or administered exogenously, usually from bacteria, and that produce fever in susceptible hosts.

Pyroglobulins: Monoclonal immunoglobulins that precipitate irreversibly when heated to 56 °C.

Quellung: The swelling of the capsules of pneumococci when the organisms are esposed to pneumococcal antibodies.

Radioimmunoassay: A variety of immunologic techniques in which a radioactive isotope is used to detect antigens or antibodies in some form of immunoassay.

Reagin: Synonymous with IgE antibody. Also denotes a complement-fixing antibody that reacts in the Wassermann reaction with cardiolipin.

Recombinant: An animal that has experienced a recombinational event during meiosis, consisting of crossover and recombination of parts of 2 chromosomes.

Recombinatorial germ line theory: Theory proposed by Dreyer and Bennett which states that variable-region and constant-region immunoglobulin genes are separated and rejoined at DNA levels.

Rejection response: An immune response with both humoral and cellular components directed against transplanted tissue.

Respiratory burst: The process by which neutrophils and monocytes kill certain microbial pathogens by conversion of oxygen to toxic oxygen products.

Reticuloendothelial system: See **Mononuclear phagocyte system**

Retrovirus: A virus that contains and utilizes reverse transcriptase, eg, human immunodeficiency virus or human T cell leukemia virus.

Rheumatoid factor (RF): An anti-immunoglobulin antibody directed against denatured IgG present in the serum of patients with rheumatoid arthritis and other rheumatoid diseases.

Ricin: A poisonous substance that derives from the seed of the castor oil plant and agglutinates erythrocytes (a lectin).

Rocket electrophoresis (Laurell technique): An electro-immunodiffusion technique in which antigen is electrophoresed into agar containing specific antibody and precipitates in a tapered rocket-shaped pattern. This technique is used for quantitation of antigens.

S region: The chromosomal region in the H-2 complex containing the gene for a serum β-globulin.

S value: Svedberg unit. Denotes the sedimentation coefficient of a protein, determined usually by analytic ultracentrifugation.

Schultz-Dale test: An in vitro assay for immediate hypersensitivity in which smooth muscle is passively sensitized by cytotropic antibody and contracts after the addition of an antigen.

Second set graft rejection: An immunologic rejection of a graft in a host that is immune to antigens contained in that graft.

Secretory IgA: A dimer of IgA molecules with a sedimentation coefficient of 11S, linked by J chain and secretory component.

Secretory immune system: A distinct immune system that is common to external secretions and consists predominantly of IgA.

Secretory Component (T piece): A molecule of MW 95,000 produced in epithelial cells and associated with secretory immunoglobulins, particularly IgA and IgM.

Sensitization: See **Immunization.** Natural or artificial induction of an immune response, particularly when it causes allergy in the host.

Sensitized: Synonymous with immunized.

Sensitizer: A term introduced by Pfeiffer to denote a specific thermostable factor capable of bacterial lysis when combined with alexin.

Sequential determinants: Determinants whose specificity is dictated by the sequence of subunits within the determinant rather than by the molecular structure of the antigen molecule.

Serologically defined (SD) antigens: Antigens that are present on membranes of nearly all mammalian cells and are controlled by genes present in the major histocompatibility complex. They can be easily detected with antibodies.

Serology: Literally, the study of serum. Refers to the determination of antibodies to infectious agents important in clinical medicine.

Serotonin (5-hydroxytryptamine): A catecholamine of MW 176 that is stored in murine mast cells and human platelets and has a pharmacologic role in anaphylaxis in most species except humans.

Serum sickness: An adverse immunologic response to a foreign antigen, usually a heterologous protein.

Shwartzman phenomenon: A nonimmunologic phenomenon that results in tissue damage both at the site of injection and at widespread sites following the second of 2 injections of endotoxin.

Side chain theory: A theory of antibody synthesis proposed by Ehrlich in 1896 suggesting that specific side chains that form antigen receptors are present on the surface membranes of antibody-producing cells.

Single radial diffusion (radioimmunodiffusion): A technique for quantitating antigens by immunodiffusion in which antigen is allowed to diffuse radially into agar containing antibody. The resultant precipitation ring reflects the concentration of the antigen.

Skin-reactive factor (SRF): A lymphokine that is responsible for vasodilation and increased vascular permeability.

Slow-reacting substances of anaphylaxis: A term used to describe the smooth muscle-constricting effect of several leukotrienes.

Slow virus: A virus that produces disease with a greatly delayed onset and protracted course.

Solid phase radioimmunoassay: A modification of radioimmunoassay in which antibody is adsorbed onto solid particles or tubes.

Southern blotting: A method for identifying DNA segments that have been digested with restriction endonucleases and electrophoresed in a gel according to size. The DNA segments are blotted onto nitrocellulose and reacted with complementary radiolabeled or enzyme-labeled probes.

Spherulin: A spherule-derived antigen from *Coccidioides immitis* used in delayed hypersenstivity skin testing for coccidioidomycosis.

Splits: Subtypes of human leukocyte antigens.

Sulzberger-Chase phenomenon: Abrogation of dermal contact sensitivity to various chemicals produced by prior oral feeding of the specific agent.

Suppressor T cells: A subset of T lymphocytes that suppress antibody synthesis by B cells or inhibit other cellular immune reactions by effector T cells.

Surface phagocytosis: The enhancement of phagocytosis by entrapment of organisms on surfaces such as leukocytes, fibrin clots, or other tissue surfaces.

Switch: Refers to change in synthesis between heavy chains within a single immunocyte from μ to γ—eg, during differentiation. V regions are not affected by H chain switch.

Syngeneic: Denotes the relationship that exists between genetically identical members of the same species.

T antigens: Tumor antigens, probably protein products of the viral genome present only on infected neoplastic cells.

T cell (T lymphocyte): A thymus-derived cell that participates in a variety of cell-mediated immune reactions.

T cell rosette: See **E rosette.**

T piece: See **Secretory piece.**

Theliolymphocytes: Small lymphocytes that are found in contiguity with intestinal epithelial cells and whose function is unknown.

Thymopoietin (originally **thymin**): A protein of MW 7000 which is derived originally from the thymus of animals with autoimmune thymitis and myasthenia gravis and which can impair neuromuscular transmission.

Thymosin: A thymic hormone protein of MW 12,000 that can restore T cell immunity in thymectomized animals.

Thymus: The central lymphoid organ that is present in the thorax and controls the ontogeny of T lymphocytes.

Thymus-dependent antigen: Antigen that depends on T cell interaction with B cells for antibody synthesis, eg, erythrocytes, serum proteins, and hapten-carrier complexes.

Thymus-independent antigen: Antigen that can induce an immune response without the apparent participation of T lymphocytes.

Tolerance: Traditionally denotes that condition in which responsive cell clones have been eliminated or inactivated by prior contact with antigen, with the result that no immune response occurs on administration of antigen.

Toxoids: Antigenic but nontoxic derivatives of toxins.

Transcription: The synthesis of RNA molecules from a DNA template.

Transfer factor: A dialyzable extract of immune lymphocytes that is capable of transferring cell-mediated immunity in humans and possibly in other animal species.

Transgenic: Referring to an organism that contains a foreign gene.

Translation: The process of formation of a peptide chain from individual amino acids to form a protein molecule.

***trans*-Pairing:** Association of two genes or opposite chromosomes encoding a protein.

Transplantation antigens: Antigens that are expressed on the surface of virtually all cells and induce rejection of tissues transplanted from one individual to a genetically disparate individual.

Trophoblast: Cell layer in placenta in contact with uterine lining. Produces various immunosuppressive substances, eg, hormones.

Tryptic peptides: Peptides produced as a result of tryptic digestion of a protein molecule.

Tumor-specific-antigens: Cell surface antigens that are expressed on malignant but not normal cells.

Ultracentrifugation: A high-speed centrifugation technique that can be used for the analytic identification of proteins of various sedimentation coefficients or as a preparative technique for separating proteins or different shapes and densities.

Ultrafiltration: The filtration of solutions or suspensions through membranes of extremely small graded pore sizes.

Uropods: Long pseudopods extending form lymphocyte cytoplasm covered by cellular plasma membrane.

V antigens: Virally induced antigens that are expressed on viruses and virus-infected cells.

V (variable) region: The amino-terminal portion of the H or L chain of an immunoglobulin molecule, containing considerable heterogeneity in the amino acid residues compared to the constant region.

V region subgroups: Subdivisions of V regions of kappa chains based on substantial homology in sequences of amino acids.

Vaccination: Immunization with antigens administered for the prevention of infectious diseases (term originally coined to denote immunization against vaccinia or cowpox virus).

Variolation: Inoculation with a virus of unmodified smallpox (variola).

Viropathic: Damage to host tissues that is produced directly by the presence of pathogenic viral infection.

Viscosity: The physical property of serum that is determined by the size, shape, and deformability of serum molecules. The hydrostatic state, molecular charge, and temperature sensitivity of proteins.

Wasting disease (also **runt disease**): A chronic, ultimately fatal illness associated with lymphoid atrophy in mice who are neonatally thymectomized.

Western blotting (also **Immunoblotting**): A technique to identify particular antigens in a mixture by separation on polyacrylamide gels, blotting onto nitrocellulose, and labeling with radiolabeled or enzyme-labeled antibodies as probes.

Xenogeneic: Denotes the relationship that exists between members of genetically different species.

Xenograft: A tissue or organ graft between members of 2 distinct or different species.

Zone electrophoresis: Electrophoresis performed on paper or cellulose acetate in which proteins are separated almost exclusively on the basis of charge.

Acronyms & Abbreviations Commonly Used in Immunology

ABA Azobenzenearsenate.
ACTH Adrenocorticotropic hormone.
ADCC Antibody-dependent cell-mediated cytotoxicity.
AEF Allogeneic effect.
AFC Antibody-forming cells.
AFP Alpha-fetoprotein.
AIDS Acquired immunodeficiency syndrome.
ALG Antilymphocyte globulin.
ALS Antilymphocyte serum.
Am Allotypic marker on IgA.
AMP Adenosine monophosphate.
ANA Antinuclear antibody.
APC Antigen-presenting cells.
ARC AIDS-related complex.
ATG Antithymocyte globulin.

B27 HLA antigen with strong disease association.
BAF B cell-activating factor.
BALT bronchus associated lymphoid tissue.
BCG Bacillus Calmette-Guérin.
BCDF B cell differentiation factors.
BCGF B cell growth factors.
Bf Properdin factor B.
BSA Bovine serum albumin.
BUDR, BUdR 5-Bromodeoxyuridine.

C Complement.
CALLA Common acute lymphocytic leukemia antigen.
cAMP Cyclic adenosine monophosphate.
CBH Cutaneous basophil hypersensitivity.
CD Cluster of differentiation.
CDC Centers for Disease Control.
CD3 Antigenic marker on T cell associated with T cell receptor.
CD4 An antigenic marker of helper/inducer T cells (also designated OKT 4, T4, Leu 3).

CD8 An antigenic marker of suppressor/cytotoxic T cells (also designated OKT 8, T8, Leu 2).
cDNA Complementary DNA.
CFA Colonization factor antigens (also Freund's complete adjuvant).
CFU Colony-forming unit.
CFU-C Colony-forming unit of cells grown in culture.
CFU-GEMM Colony forming unit of granulocytes, erythrocytes, monocytes and megaharyocytes.
CFU-GM Colony stimulating factor of granulocytes and macrophages.
CFU-S Colony-forming unit of cells grown in the spleen.
cGMP Cyclic guanosine monophosphate.
C$_H$ Constant domain of H chain.
CIg Cytoplasmic immunoglobulin.
C$_L$ Constant domain of L chain.
cM Centimorgan.
c-myc An oncogene.
CMI Cell-mediated immunity.
CML Cell-mediated lympholysis.
Con A Concanavalin A.
C3PA C3 proactivator.
CRI–CR6 Six distinct receptors for C3 fragments found on various cell types.
CREG Cross reactive group.
CRP C-reactive protein.
CSA Colony-stimulating activity.
CSF Colony-stimulating factor.
CTL Cytotoxic lymphocytes.
CTLL Cloned mouse cytotoxic T lymphocytic line.

DC Dendritic cells.
D$_H$ Diversity region of immunoglobulin heavy-chain gene.
DNCB 2,4-Dinitrochlorobenzene.
DNFB Dinitrofluorobenzene.

DNP Dinitrophenyl.
DP Human class II MHC allele (formerly called SB).
DQ Human class II MHC allele (formerly called DC, MB, and DS).
DR D-related HLA locus in humans.
DTH Delayed-type hypersensitivity.

EA Erythrocyte amboceptor (sensitized erythrocytes).
EAC Erythrocyte amboceptor complement.
ECF Eosinophil chemotactic factor.
ECF-A Eosinophil chemotactic factor of anaphylaxis.
ECP Eosinophil cationic protein.
EDTA Ethylenediaminetetraacetate.
EIA Enzyme immunoassay.
ELISA Enzyme-linked immunosorbent assay.
ENA Extractable nuclear antigen.
EP Endogenous pyrogen.
EPO Eosinophilic peroxidase.
ER Endoplasmic reticulum.

F$_1$ First generation.
F$_2$ Second generation.
FA Fluorescent antibody.
Fab Antigen-binding fragment.
FACS Fluorescent-activated cell sorter.
Fc Crystallizable fragment.
FCC Follicular center cell.
FCM Flow cytometry.
FCR Fractional catabolic rate.
FcϵR Fc receptor specific for IgE.
FcγR Fc receptor specific for IgG.
FcμR Fc receptor specific for IgM.
FeLV Feline leukemia virus.
FITC Fluorescein isothiocyanate.
FUDR Fluorodeoxyuridine.

GALT Gut-associated lymphoid tissue.
GBG Glycine-rich beta-glycoprotein.
G-CSF Granulocyte colony stimulating factor.
GEF Glycosylation-enhancing factor.
GFR Glomerular filtration rate.
GGG Glycine-rich gamma-glycoprotein.
GIF Glycosylation inhibition factor.
GLO Glyoxylase.
Gm Allotypic marker on human IgG.
GM-CSF Granulocyte-manophage colony stimulating factor.
GMP Guanosine monophosphate.
gp Glycoprotein.
gp70 Glycoprotein antigen (MW 70,000) on viral envelope of C type murine viruses.
GPA Guinea pig albumin.
GVH Graft-versus-host (disease).
GVHR Graft-versus-host reaction.

HAT Hypoxanthine, aminopterin, and thymidine.
HbF Fetal hemoglobin.
HDL High-density lipoproteins.
H&E Hematoxylin and eosin (stain).
HETE Hydroxyeicosatetraenoic acid.
HEV High endothelial venules.
HIV Human immunodeficiency virus.
HLA Human leukocyte antigen.
(H₂L₂)n General formula for immunoglobulin molecule.
HMW-NCF High-molecular-weight neutrophil chemotactic factor.
HPETE Hydroperoxyeicosatetraenoic acid.
HPLC High-performance liquid chromatography.
HRF Homologous restriction factor.
HPRT Hypoxanthine phosphoribosyl transferase.
HSA Human serum albumin.
HSF Histamine-sensitizing factor, also hepatocyte stimulating factor.
5-HT 5-Hydroxytryptamine (serotonin).
HTC Homozygous typing cells.
HTLV Human T cell leukemia virus.
HuFcR Human Fc receptor.

ICAM Intracellular adhesion molecule.

Id Idiotype.
IDU Idoxuridine.
IEF Isoelectric focusing.
IEL Intraepithelial lymphocyte.
IEP Immunoelectrophoresis.
IFA Indirect fluorescent antibody.
IFE Immunofixation electrophoresis.
IFN Interferon.
IL-1–IL-8 Interleukin 1–8.
Inv Allotypic marker on human kappa chain (κm).
Ir Immune response (genes).
ISG Immune serum globulin.

J segment Joining segment of DNA encoding immunoglobulins.
J_H Joining region of immunoglobulin-bearing chains.

K (cells) Killer (cells).
K562 Erythroleukemic cell line.
KAF Bovine conglutinin: conglutinin activating factor.
KLH Keyhole limpet hemocyanin.

LAF Leukocyte-activating factor (see IL-1).
LAK Lymphokine-activated killer (cells).
LAV Lymphadenopathy-associated virus.
LCMV Lymphocytic choriomeningitis virus.
LD Lymphocyte-defined.
LDCC Lectin-dependent cell-mediated cytotoxicity.
LDCF Lymphocyte-derived chemotactic factors.
LDH Lactate dehydrogenase.
LDL Low-density lipoproteins.
LFA Lymphocyte functional antigen(s).
LGL Large granular lymphocytes.
LIF Leukocyte inhibitory factor.
LMI Leukocyte migration inhibition.
LPL Lamina propria lymphocyte
LPS Lipopolysaccharide.
LT Leukotriene.
LT Lymphotoxin or lymphocytotoxin.
Lyb Lymphocyte antigens on murine B cells.
Lyt Lymphocyte antigens on murine T cells.
M-CSF Monocyte-macrophage colony stimulating factor.

MAC (Complement) membrane attack complex.
Mac-1 Macrophage-1 glycoprotein.
MAF Macrophage-activating (-arming) factor.
MALT Mucosa-associated lymphoid tissue.
MBP Major basic protein.
MCF Macrophage chemotactic factor.
MCP Membrane cofactor protein.
MDP Muramyl dipeptide.
MeBSA Methylated bovine serum albumin.
MER Methanol extraction residue (of phenol-treated BCG).
MF Mitogenic factor.
MHA Major histocompatibility antigen.
MHC Major histocompatibility complex.
MIF Migration inhibitory factor.
MLC Mixed lymphocyte (leukocyte) culture.
MLR Mixed lymphocyte (or leukocyte) response or reaction.
MMI Macrophage migration inhibition.
MPG Methyl green pyronin.
MPO Myeloperoxidase.
MTX Methotrexate.
MuLV Murine leukemia virus.
MW Molecular weight.

NCF Neutrophil chemotactic factor.
NF Nephritic factor.
NK Natural killer (cells).
NZB New Zealand black (mice).
NZW New Zealand white (mice or rabbits).

OAF Osteoclast activating factor.
OS Obese strain.

PAF Platelet-activating factor.
PAP Peroxidase antiperoxidase.
PAS p-Aminosalicylic acid; periodic acid-Schiff (reaction).
PCA Passive cutaneous anaphylaxis.
PCR Polymeric chain reaction.
PEC Peritoneal exudate cells.
PFC Plaque-forming cells.
PG Prostaglandin.
Pg5 Urinary pepsinogen.
PGE Prostaglandin E (PGE₁, PGE₂, PGe₂α).

PGM₃ Phosphoglucomutase 3.
PHA Phytohemagglutinin.
pIgA Polymeric IgA.
PLL Poly-L-lysine.
PMA Phorbol myristate acetate; a tumor promotor that stimulates monocytes and lymphocytes nonspecifically.
PMN Polymorphonuclear neutrophil.
PNA Peanut agglutinin.
PPD Purified protein derivative (tuberculin).
PVP Polyvinylpyrrolidone.
PWM Pokeweed mitogen.

R Roentgen unit of radiation.
RBC Red blood cell; red blood count.
RE Reticuloendothelial.
RES Reticuloendothelial system.
RFLP Restriction length fragment polymorphism
RIA Radioimmunoassay.
RIF Receptor-inducing factor.
RIST Radioimmunosorbent test.
RNP Ribonuclear protein.

S S value or sedimentation coefficient.
SAC Staphylococcal protein A of Cowan I strain.
SC Secretory component.
SCID Severe combined immunodeficiency disease.
SD Serologically defined.
sIg Surface immunoglobulin.
sIgA Secretory IgA.
SIRS Soluble immune response suppressor.
SMAF Specific macrophage arming factor.
SNagg Serum normal agglutinator.
SpA Staphylococcal protein A.
SRBC Sheep red blood cells.
SRS-A Slow-reacting substance of anaphylaxis.

TA Transplantation antigens.
TA1 Trophoblast antigen 1.
Tac T cell activation receptor.
TAF T cell-activating factor.
Tc Cytotoxic T cells.
TCGF T cell growth factor (see IL-2).
TCR T cell receptor.
TD Thymus-dependent.

TGF Transforming growth factor.
Th Helper T cells.
Thy Thymus-derived.
TI Thymus-independent.
TIL Tumor infiltrating lymphocyte.
TL Thymic lymphocyte (antigen) on prothymocytes.
TLI Total lymphoid irradiation.
TLX Trophoblast lymphocyte cross reactive antigen.
TMP Thymocyte mitogenic protein.
TNF Tumor neurons factor.
TNP Trinitrophenyl.
Tp Precursor T cells.
Ts Suppressor T cells.
TSA Tumor-specific antigen.
TX Thromboxane.

VEA Virus envelope antigen.
V_H Variable domain of heavy chain.
V_L Variable domain of light chain.

Z-DNA Methylated DNA coiled into a left-handed helix.

Index

Page numbers followed by *t* or *f* indicate tables or figures, respectively